The Clinical Neuropsychiatry of Stroke

This fully revised new edition covers the range of neuropsychiatric syndromes associated with stroke, including cognitive, emotional, and behavioral disorders such as depression, anxiety, and psychosis. Since the last edition there has been an explosion of published literature on this topic and the book provides a comprehensive, systematic, and cohesive review of this new material. There is growing recognition among a wide range of clinicians and allied healthcare staff that poststroke neuropsychiatric syndromes are both common and serious. Such complications can have a negative impact on recovery and even survival; however, there is now evidence suggesting that pre-emptive therapeutic intervention in high-risk patient groups can prevent the initial onset of the conditions. This opportunity for primary prevention marks a huge advance in the management of this patient population. This book should be read by all those involved in the care of stroke patients, including psychiatrists, neurologists, rehabilitation specialists, and nurses.

Robert Robinson is a Paul W. Penningroth Professor and Head, Department of Psychiatry; Roy J. and Lucille A., Carver College of Medicine, The University of Iowa, IA, USA.

The Clinical Neuropsychiatry of Stroke

Second Edition

Robert G. Robinson

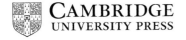

CAMBRIDGE
UNIVERSITY PRESS

CAMBRIDGE UNIVERSITY PRESS
Cambridge, New York, Melbourne, Madrid, Cape Town, Singapore, São Paulo

CAMBRIDGE UNIVERSITY PRESS
The Edinburgh Building, Cambridge CB2 2RU, UK
Published in the United States of America by Cambridge University Press, New York

www.cambridge.org
Information on this title: www.cambridge.org/9780521840071

First published 2006

Printed in the United Kingdom at the University Press, Cambridge

A catalogue record for this book is available from the British Library

Library of Congress Cataloguing in Publication data

ISBN-13 978-0-521-84007-1 hardback
ISBN-10 0-521-84007-4 hardback

Every effort has been made in preparing this book to provide accurate and
up-to-date information which is in accord with accepted standards and practice
at the time of publication. Although case histories are drawn from actual cases,
every effort has been made to disguise the identities of the individuals involved.
Nevertheless, the authors, editors and publishers can make no warranties that the
information contained herein is totally free from error, not least because clinical
standards are constantly changing through research and regulation. The authors,
editors and publishers therefore disclaim all liability for direct or consequential
damages resulting from the use of material contained in this book. Readers are
strongly advised to pay careful attention to information provided by the
manufacturer of any drugs or equipment that they plan to use.

Dedication

As with the first edition of this book, I want to dedicate it to all of my friends and colleagues whose hard work, dedication, intelligence and training made this work possible. The older I get, the longer is the list of colleagues who have worked with me on these studies and who deserve much of the credit for this new growth in our knowledge of poststroke neuropsychiatric disorders. I am particularly grateful to Dr. Thomas Price and the late Dr. Frank Benson who gave me the chance to begin these studies by sharing their enthusiasm, ideas and patients. Dr. Sergio Starkstein, Dr. Philip Morris, Dr. Rajesh Parikh and now Dr. Ricardo Jorge have been the backbone, guiding lights, and steam engine behind this work. Their dedication to research, their innovative ideas and their perseverance to see this work through to publication has brought us all to our current state of knowledge. My latest colleagues have written many of the new papers outlined in this book as part of their training as well as a reflection of their hard work, intelligence and commitment. Drs. Kishi, Kimura, Murata, Manes, Shimoda, Narurshima, Chemerinski and Takezawa have all contributed significantly to this work. To each and every one of you I express my eternal gratitude.

Contents

Preface

In the second edition of *The Clinical Neuropsychiatry of Stroke*, I have tried to include all of the recent findings concerning the neuropsychiatric syndromes associated with stroke published since 1998 when the original edition of this text was released. Integrating the substantial amount of literature which has been generated over the past 7 years has been a large task. The number of publications related to the single topic of poststroke depression has more than doubled in the 7 years before the first edition of this text (i.e., from 1990 to 1997), compared with the 7 years since the first edition (i.e., 1998 to 2004) (source: http://www.ncbi.nlm.nih.gov/). This reflects the growing worldwide interest in poststroke depression as well as the numerous other stroke related neuropsychiatric disorders and the growing recognition by clinicians that neuropsychiatric syndromes are both common and have a negative influence on patients' emotional state, physical recovery, cognitive recovery, and even survival following stroke. Thus, identifying effective interventions based on controlled treatment trials represents an essential task in the care of patients with stroke. The recent demonstration by Rasmussen *et al.* (2003) (see Chapter 23) that the negative physical consequences of poststroke depression may be significantly reduced by prophylactic treatment with antidepressants represents a major advance in the care of patients with stroke. I do not know of any psychiatric disorder in which the initial onset of the condition has been prevented by therapeutic intervention (i.e., primary prevention). In fact, with the exception of infectious disease, primary prevention in all fields of medicine has not progressed as quickly as we would have hoped. In psychiatry, secondary and tertiary prevention (i.e., early treatment before the full syndrome appears and prevention of recurrence) has been demonstrated in a variety of conditions but primary prevention has not been established for any psychiatric disorder. Primary prevention requires the identification of a very high risk population so that the risk of treating patients who would never have developed the disorder is out weighed by the benefit of preventing the disorder in the large number who would have developed it. Patients with stroke represent a high risk population for the development of several psychiatric disorders. This may lead to enhanced recovery, decreased suffering as well as decreased mortality and morbidity. Therefore, based on the significant advances in the field and the increased need for clinicians in all specialty areas to be aware of the importance of neuropsychiatric disorders in patients with stroke, a second edition seemed appropriate. Hopefully, the field will continue to advance and further therapeutic successes will establish even more effective methods of treating stroke victims in the future.

REFERENCE

Rasmussen, A., Lunde, M., Poulsen, D. L., *et al.* A double-blind, placebo-controlled study of sertraline in the prevention of depression in stroke patients. *Psychosomatics* (2003) 44(3): 216–221.

Robert G. Robinson
USA
2005

Part I

Introduction

Recent trends in the epidemiology of stroke

Stroke like other illnesses has a dynamic evolution as a result of increasing knowledge and availability of healthcare around the world. In the 1970s, much of the epidemiological literature documented the declining incidence of stroke from 1945 to 1974. The annual incidence of stroke for both men and women between 1945 and 1949 was 190 per 100,000 population in the Rochester, Minnesota area. In 1970–1974, the rate had dropped to 104 per 100,000 population. During this time, the rates had dropped in all age categories, but were particularly dramatic in the very old. For example, in 1964, the average annual rates for those 55 to 59 years and those 80 years or older were 209 and 2932 per 100,000 persons respectively or a ratio of 1:14. By 1974, the average annual rates for these age groups had declined to 205 and 1287 per 100,000 or a ratio of 1:6. For both men and women the annual incidence rates increased with increasing age from 55 through 80 (Garraway *et al.* 1979).

In Japan, the incidence of cerebral infarction declined by 34% and that of cerebral hemorrhage by 29% between the periods 1961–1966 and 1972–1976 (Ueda *et al.* 1981). This decline was thought to be primarily the result of improved control of hypertension. Beginning in approximately 1980, however, the annual incidence of stroke appeared to increase. In Sweden, there was a 38% increase in the incidence in stroke among women from 1975–1978 to 1983–1985 (Terent 1989). This increasing incidence of stroke has continued throughout the 1990s. Pessah-Rasmussen *et al.* (2003) examined the incidence of stroke in the city of Malmö, Sweden between 1989 and 1998. During this period, the age standardized incidence was 647 per 100,000 person years for men and 400 per 100,000 person years for women. The annual increase, however, was 3.1% in men and 2.9% in women. Among men, that were 50–59, 60–69, and 70–79 years of age, the age standardized stroke incidence increased annually by 4.8%, 4.5%, and 2.1%, respectively. Among women, the corresponding values were 7.3%, 1.8%, and 2.8% (Fig. 1.1(a, b)).

Community based longitudinal studies performed in Minnesota (Brown *et al.* 1996) and Massachusetts (Derby *et al.* 2000), however, found that stroke incidence rates were unchanged in the USA during the past two decades. Nevertheless, in the

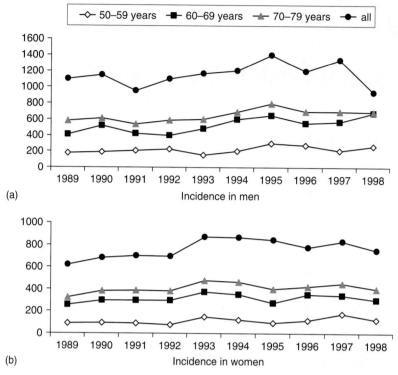

Figure 1.1   (a) Time trends in stroke incidence in Malmö, Sweden, 1989–1998, in men; (b) time trends in stroke incidence in Malmö, Sweden, 1989–1998, in women (reprinted with permission from Pessah-Rasmussen *et al.* 2003).

USA, there are approximately 600,000 new or recurrent strokes occurring each year and, among those who survive, according to the American Heart Association, 70% are left with sufficient disability to limit vocational capacity.

Explanations for the increasing incidence of stroke found in several studies may be related to decreasing mortality from ischemic heart disease, thus theoretically increasing the population at risk for stroke. Other possible reasons for the increasing stroke incidence may be worsening of the cardiovascular risk factors. For example, treatment of hypertension continues to be a challenge in daily practice with only a 50% success rate in treated patients in the USA (Weber 1998). In addition, the increasing number of immigrants to all of the industrialized countries of the West may have contributed to the increasing incidence of stroke.

This increasing incidence of stroke in some countries, which has lasted for approximately two decades, however, has been accompanied by a decline in stroke mortality. Howard *et al.* (2001) analyzed mortality data in the USA between 1968 and 1996. Jefferson County in Alabama, for example, declined from 600 deaths due to stroke per 100,000 population in 1968 to 280 in 1996. Queens County in New York

City declined from 350 per 100,000 in 1965 to 100 in 1996. In Malmö, Sweden, (Pessah-Rasmussen *et al.* 2003) found that although the mortality rates among men were unchanged from 1989 to 1998 among women there was a significant decline from 12.3% in 1989 to 2.0% in 1998 (odds ratio (OR): 0.89; 95% confidence interval (CI): 0.8–0.95). The decrease in stroke mortality appears to be related to declines in case fatality in the first few weeks after stroke onset. The changes in case fatality within the first 2 weeks following stroke may be related to changes in disease severity or to changes in stroke care. For instance, a large change in fatality was noted in the Malmö study to be related to the opening of a specialized stroke unit. Furthermore, the same factors that affect stroke incidence may also affect stroke severity.

The continuing decline in stroke mortality would be expected to influence the prevalence of stroke survivors in the community. Muntner *et al.* (2002) reported that in the USA, age-, race-, and sex-adjusted prevalence of stroke increased from 1.41% in 1971–1975 to 1.87% in 1988–1994. This represented an average increase of 7.5% for each 5-year period during this time. The prevalence of stroke among US population 60–74 years old increased from 4.2% to 5.2% during the study period. In the USA, the number of stroke survivors was 1.5 million in 1973, 2.0 million in 1978 and 2.4 million in 1991. At the present time the American Heart Association estimates that the prevalence of stroke in the USA is 4 million.

Men with Japanese heritage participating in the Honolulu heart study were compared to non-Japanese heritage men participating in the Framingham, Massachusetts study for risk factors associated with stroke (Rodriguez *et al.* 2002). In both cohorts, hemorrhagic and thromboembolic stroke were consistently elevated in the presence of hypertension and cigarette smoking. In addition, diabetes and body mass index increased the risk of thromboembolic stroke in both samples, while diabetes increased the risk of hemorrhagic stroke only in the Framingham study. Alcohol intake and low total cholesterol were associated with hemorrhagic stroke in Honolulu but not in Framingham. Similarly, the finding from the World Health Organization monitoring of trends and determinants of cardiovascular disease (WHO-Monica project) found that among 35–64 year old people in 15 populations across 9 countries, that systolic blood pressure showed a strong association with stroke trends in women but not in men. In women, 38% of the variation in stroke event trends was explained by changes in systolic blood pressure. However, combining trends in systolic blood pressure, daily cigarette smoking, serum cholesterol, and body mass index explained only a small fraction of the variation in stroke event trends for the entire population (Tolonen *et al.* 2002). These differences from studies that have found an association of stroke with the usual factors of cardiovascular disease may be due to the fact that the Monica study examined only patients up to age 65 and did not differentiate between first episode of stroke and recurrent strokes.

Just as stroke incidence rates have stopped declining and have been increasing in some studies, the stroke mortality rates are also expected to begin climbing in the next decade.

Elkins and Johnston (2003) estimated that the number of deaths would increase from 139,000 in 2002 to 275,000 in 2032 while the total US population would increase by only 27% in the same time period. These projected mortality rates, however, may be affected by continuing advances in stroke care. Although a detailed description of the advances in stroke care are beyond the scope of this text, the past decade has noted some dramatic improvements in the acute care of patients following stroke. The use of tissue plasminogen activator (TPA) as well as mechanical intravascular removal of thromboembolic infarcts has dramatically improved the outcome of patients who are able to receive treatment within 3 h following an acute stroke. Perhaps one of the most exciting advances in stroke research, however, has been the identification of neuronal regeneration after stroke (Liu *et al.* 1998; Arvidsson *et al.* 2002). Arvidsson *et al.* (2002) have shown that in a rat model of stroke, induced by temporary occlusion of the middle cerebral artery, stroke not only leads to a marked increase in the proliferation of neural progenitor cells in the subventricular zone but also to the migration of these recently regenerated neuroblasts into the damaged striata. Two weeks after the stroke, some of the migrating neuroblasts had differentiated into mature neurons and 5 weeks after the stroke, 42% of the population of cells had differentiated into the dominant type of striatal neuron. Thus, some of the new neurons had locally differentiated into the phenotype of neurons that had been destroyed in the ischemic striatum. None of the new cells, however, were found in damaged cerebral cortex and about 80% of the newly arrived neurons had died within 6 weeks after the stroke. Thus, only 0.2% of the dead striatal neurons were replaced through neurogenesis. Although it will be a challenge to create an environment within ischemic brain tissue to facilitate neuronal migration and differentiation, this newly discovered potential of neuronal regeneration after brain ischemia may represent an important new avenue to achieve functional brain reconstruction and recovery. Furthermore, pharmacological stimulation including antidepressant medications has been shown in animal models to induce neurogenesis. Neurogenesis has been reported primarily in two regions: the subventricular zone and the subgranular zone of the hippocampal dentate gyrus (Gage 2000). Thus, the findings that both cerebral ischemia and antidepressant medications lead to neurogenesis suggest an exciting new area for research and the potential for novel treatments of poststroke physical and cognitive impairments as well as emotional disorders.

In summary, stroke continues to represent one of the major public health problems in the world. It is the third leading cause of death in the industrialized countries of the world and the leading cause of disability and long-term functional impairment. Stroke is the second leading cause of nursing home placement, second only to dementia. The amount of healthcare resources devoted to the care of patients with stroke is obviously enormous. Recent advances in the acute care of stroke has led to increased survival but also to increased prevalence of long-term disability. There is a long way to go in eliminating or treating the impairments associated with stroke and advances in pharmacological treatment as well as neurogenesis may provide a whole new avenue for advancement in the care of patients with stroke. This book will be devoted to the assessment and care of the emotional disorders associated with stroke and their impact on long-term survival and recovery. Through mechanisms of neurotransmitter replacement, neuroreceptor regeneration and neurogenesis, we may be on the verge of a whole new era in the treatment of patients suffering from the neuropsychiatric consequences of stroke.

REFERENCES

Arvidsson, A., Collin, T., Kirik, D., *et al.* Neuronal replacement from endogenous precursors in the adult brain after stroke. *Nat Med* (2002) 8(9):963–970.

Brown, R. D., Whisnant, J. P., Sicks, J. D., *et al.* Stroke incidence, prevalence, and survival: secular trends in Rochester, Minnesota, through 1989. *Stroke* (1996) 27(3):373–380.

Derby, C. A., Lapane, K. L., Feldman, H. A., *et al.* Trends in validated cases of fatal and nonfatal stroke, stroke classification, and risk factors in southeastern New England, 1980 to 1991: data from the Pawtucket Heart Health Program. *Stroke* (2000) 31(4):875–881.

Elkins, J. S., and Johnston, S. C. Thirty-year projections for deaths from ischemic stroke in the United States. *Stroke* (2003) 34:2109–2113.

Gage, F. H. Mammalian neural stem cells. *Science* (2000) 287(5457):1433–1438.

Garraway, W. M., Whisnant, J. P., Furlan, A. J., *et al.* The declining incidence of stroke. *N Engl J Med* (1979) 330:449–452.

Howard, G., Howard, V. J., Katholi, C., *et al.* Decline in US stroke mortality: an analysis of temporal patterns by sex, race, and geographic region. *Stroke* (2001) 32(10):2213–2220.

Liu, J., Solway, K., Messing, R. O., *et al.* Increased neurogenesis in the dentate gyrus after transient global ischemia in gerbils. *J Neurosci* (1998) 18(19):7768–7778.

Munter, P., Garret, E., Klag, M. J., *et al.* Trends in stroke prevalence between 1973 and 1991 in the US population 25 to 74 years of age. *Stroke* (2002) 33:1209–1213.

Pessah-Rasmussen, H., Engstrom, G., Jerntorp, I., *et al.* Increasing stroke incidence and decreasing case fatality, 1989–1998. A study from the Stroke Register in Malmö, Sweden. *Stroke* (2003) 34:913–918.

Rodriguez, B. L., D'Agostino, R. B., Abbott, R. D., *et al.* Risk of hospitalized stroke in men enrolled in the Honolulu heart program and the Framingham study. A comparison of incidence and risk factor effects. *Stroke* (2002) 33:230–237.

Terent, A. Survival after stroke and transient ischemic attacks during the 1970s and 1980s. *Stroke* (1989) 20:1320–1326.

Tolonen, H., Mähönen, M., Asplund, K., *et al.* Do trends in population levels of blood pressure and other cardiovascular risk factors explain trends in stroke event rates? Comparisons of 15 populations in 9 countries within the WHO MONICA Stroke Project. *Stroke* (2002) 33:2367–2375.

Ueda, K., Omae, T., Hirota, Y., *et al.* Decreasing trend in incidence and mortality from stroke in Hisayama residents, Japan. *Stroke* (1981) 12:154–160.

Weber, M. A. Unsolved problems in treating hypertension: rationale for new approaches. *Am J Hypertens* (1998) 11(10):145S–149S.

2

Historical perspective

A historical perspective of the neuropsychiatric disorders associated with stroke must logically begin with a discussion of the word "stroke." Although many clinicians do not like the term "stroke," it has become so ingrained in both the public and professional literature that it will likely remain the primary word used to describe this cerebrovascular disorder.

One of the problems with the word "stroke" is that it has multiple meanings. A stroke of luck or a tennis stroke have very different meanings from the catastrophic medical disorder. Originally the term was used in medicine to describe being struck down by an illness, especially one which rendered the victim unconscious or paralytic (Millikan *et al.* 1987). The use of the word stroke to indicate apoplexy (*plexus* meaning stroke and *apo* meaning from) began in the 17th century. The recognition, however, of apoplexy as an important medical condition is evident from the writings of Hippocrates (460–370 BC). He noted that unaccustomed attacks of numbness and anesthesia were a sign of impending apoplexy and that when patients, who were not febrile, complained of headache, noises in the head, vertigo, slowness of speech, or numbness of the hands, there was a high likelihood that they would become epileptic or suffer from apoplexy (Millikan *et al.* 1987). It was not until the development of the microscope by Leeuwenhoek (1632–1723), however, that an understanding of the nature of stroke occurred. Bichat (1771–1802) was the first to describe cerebral softening and Rostan (1823) identified that brain softening found in victims of apoplexy was not due to inflammation. Hughlings-Jackson (1875) wrote that cerebral softening was always focal, "it is localized by vessels, mostly arteries." Information about the physiology of the cerebral circulation, however, began with the observations of Monro (1783). He reported that the volume of blood in the brain was constant and that blood was continually flowing in through arteries and out through veins. Hughlings-Jackson also noted that the middle cerebral artery, or some of its branches, were almost always the vessels occluded. Furthermore, Hughlings-Jackson distinguished between cerebral softening due to arterial disease and cerebral softening due to embolism.

The earliest reports of emotional disorders related to stroke were descriptions of patients by neurologists and psychiatrists. Disturbances of language function have frequently been associated with emotional disorders because aphasia is a common and easily recognized behavioral manifestation of dominant hemisphere brain damage. Furthermore, speech is intimately associated with emotions and thoughts. Pierre Paul Broca, a surgeon and anthropologist (1861) described a single case of aphasia in a patient who was able to utter only one syllable "tan." At autopsy the patient was found to have a large lesion of the left hemisphere including the posterior aspect of the inferior frontal gyrus which has been named Broca's area (Fig. 2.1). Carl Wernicke (1874) proposed that aphasia was the result of impairment in elementary psychic processes which were localized in different brain areas. Wernicke described the first patients with impairment in verbal comprehension with lesions involving the temporal occipital–parietal junction of the left hemisphere which has become known as Wernicke's area.

Broca (1878) also first described an area of cortex which he called the limbus cortex that surrounded the midbrain. This included phylogenetically older areas of cortex such as the inferior temporal lobe, hippocampal gyri, cingulate cortex, and

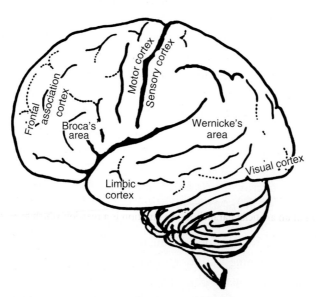

Figure 2.1   Schematic lateral view of the brain indicating functional brain regions. Broca's and Wernicke's areas play an important role in the production and comprehension of language. The anterior basal portion of the temporal cortex is part of the limbic circuit and the frontal association cortex plays an important role in coordinating motor and cognitive functions of the frontal lobe. The motor, sensory, and visual corticis have topographic and columnar organization for focal motor, sensory, and visual functions.

inferior frontal cortex. He noted that all mammals had this large cerebral convolution which formed a ring or limbus around the lower brain stem structures. Limbus cortex has given rise to the term "limbic system." In 1937, Papez (1937) suggested, based purely on anatomical observations (i.e., the older phylogenetic age of the limbic cortex and its circular anatomical organization), that this limbus cortex or limbic system formed the anatomical basis for emotion (this proposal will be discussed more fully in Chapter 3).

Some of the earliest writings about the cerebral basis of emotion, however, were published by Hughlings-Jackson (1915). Hughlings-Jackson, widely regarded as the father of English neurology, was appointed to the National Hospital in 1862. Jackson was the first to identify that brain lesions were associated with a duality of symptoms. That is, brain lesions produced both a loss of specific function as well as a positive symptom such as a movement disorder or a mental process not previously seen. He explained this emergence of "positive symptoms" as a result of removal of higher controls normally inhibiting these functions. This culminated in his view that there was a hierarchy in the organization of the nervous system with the prefrontal cortex mediating the highest level of mental function.

Similar to his concept of duality of symptoms associated with brain injury, Hughlings-Jackson conceptualized language as an expression of brain function existing in two forms. Language was either intellectual (conveying content) or emotional (expressing feelings). He proposed that these components might be separated by disease. This was the first suggestion that emotional expression was distinct from spoken language and that stroke might produce disorders of emotion without producing disorders of language function.

Adolph Meyer (1904), on the other hand, conceptualized emotion, as he did psychopathology, as a response to multifaceted influences including both physiological and mental processes that he referred to as psychobiology (Lewis 1957):

> In the concept of emotion one is able to see most clearly the basic psychobiological premise of the unity of "mental" and "bodily" functions. Emotion as, in fact, the middle ground serves as a striking refutation of an artificial parallelism. An emotion is a reaction which by its very nature covers the entire range of human reactivity, including in the response the non-conscious vasomotor and other organic changes as well as the conscious feelings of rage, joy, etc. In fact, it is in the emotion, permeating and coloring as it does the entire psychobiological activity that one has most definitively and convincingly the feeling of self.

Based in part on his background in neuropathology, Adolph Meyer became very interested in focal brain injury associated with trauma. He stated, "considering the meager knowledge of unmistakably reliable facts of etiology in mental disease, traumatism would seem to furnish unusually clean-cut conditions of interference with the mechanisms of motor sensory plasticity. The first question is: has the localization of the injury, as such, anything to do with the production of specific symptoms? An examination in detail of the many cases in which laceration has occurred in different regions of the brain affords some reason to believe that purely intellectual and emotional disorders can be directly connected with the localization of the injury. Lesions of the left frontal lobe were all accompanied by some mental aberration or deficiency apart from stupor and, in 10 cases, with lesions of both frontal lobes that 8 showed specific mental disturbance." He identified delirium, dementia, and aphasia as disorders which he attributed to the direct result of brain injury. In keeping with his psychobiological view of most mental "reactions," however, he saw disorders such as manic-depressive illness and paranoiac conditions as arising from a combination of head injury (specifically citing left frontal lobe and cortical convexities) as well as family history of psychiatric disorder and other premorbid vulnerabilities such as a personal history of prior psychiatric disorder.

Bleuler (1951) described the long-term nature of depressions following stroke when he stated that "melancholic moods lasting for months and sometimes longer appear frequently." Another example of the psychiatric perspective is that of Post (1962) who in his classic empirical study of 100 elderly patients with depression remarked that the association of brain ischemia with a first episode of depressive disorder was so common that it suggested the causes of atherosclerotic disease and depression may be "etiologically linked."

Early 20th century neurologists, on the other hand, described disorders which were associated with specific lesion locations, such as frontal lobe or parietal lobe syndromes, or behavioral disorders which were unique to brain injury. Babinski (1914), for example, described patients with stroke who would not acknowledge the existence of an obvious motor deficit. These patients were said to have "anosognosia" (*gnosia* meaning knowledge and *anos* meaning without). When confronted with their physical impairment, patients with anosognosia simply denied that anything was wrong. Babinski also noted that they frequently displayed indifference to their impairments or an inappropriate level of cheerfulness. These disorders of recognition of impairment and inappropriate affect are often associated with right hemisphere lesions.

Another example of an emotional disorder which is unique to brain injury is the catastrophic reaction. Goldstein (1939) described the catastrophic reaction as the abrupt onset of emotional symptoms of frustration, depression, and embarrassment. Lasting from a few seconds to a few minutes, the catastrophic reaction is characterized by a display of emotion (shouting, swearing, pounding fists, and throwing things) followed by return to the previous calm emotional state. Mixing explanation with description, Goldstein (1939) described the catastrophic reaction as "a sudden outburst of emotion provoked by a cognitive task which is based on the inability of the organism to cope when faced with a serious defect in physical and cognitive functions." "Survival," he wrote, "becomes paramount, in a pathologically changed organism. Survival may be normal and ordered or disordered and inconsistent." He referred to this latter type of survival, embedded in physical and mental shock, as "catastrophic."

Another emotional disorder, felt to be unique to patients with brain injury, is the indifference reaction. This disorder was first described by Hecaen *et al.* (1951) and Denny-Brown *et al.* (1952) and is associated with right hemisphere lesions. Gainotti (1972) described the indifference reaction as indifference towards failures, lack of interest in family and friends, making foolish, inappropriate jokes, and minimization of physical disability. The indifference reaction was also noted to be frequently associated with severe perceptual deficits and impairment in orientation.

The final emotional disorder that is unique to brain injury is pathological laughter or crying. Although pathological laughter and crying can occur with a variety of lesions, Ironside (1956) described a particular type of disorder in which pathological laughter or crying is a prominent feature, that is pseudobulbar palsy. This disorder is associated with bilateral and often multiple lesions affecting the corticobulbar pathways at any level above the pons. These upper motor neuron lesions produce dysphagia, dysarthria, and paralysis of the voluntary facial muscles. Patients with pseudobulbar palsy may also have uncontrollable episodes of crying or sometimes laughter which usually last only a few seconds but may be totally disconnected from their mental state. Sudden noises or non-emotional conversation may trigger an episode of crying or laughter and lead to embarrassment and social withdrawal.

Beginning in the early 1960s, most reports about poststroke emotional symptoms attributed them to understandable psychological responses to the associated impairments. For example, Ullman and Gruen (1960) reported that stroke was particularly stressful to the organism, as Goldstein had suggested, because the organ governing the emotional response to injury had itself been damaged. Adams and Hurwitz (1963) reported that discouragement and frustration caused by disability could themselves impede recovery from stroke. Fisher (1961) described depression associated with cerebrovascular disease as reactive and understandable because "the brain is the most cherished organ of humanity." Thus, depression was empathically understood and, therefore, explained as a natural emotional reaction to a decrease in self-esteem produced by the combination of a life-threatening injury, the associated physical and intellectual disability, and the resulting loss of independence.

A few investigators, such as Post (1962), however, impressed by the frequency of the association between brain injury and emotional disorders, hypothesized the existence of direct causal connections between stroke and depression. The first systematic study, however, which examined emotional reactions in patients with stroke and other forms of brain damage was conducted by Gainotti (1972). Depressive catastrophic reactions were found more frequently among 80 patients with left hemisphere brain damage, particularly those with aphasia, than among 80 patients with right hemisphere brain injury. Patients with right hemisphere lesions, however, were noted to have an increased frequency of indifference reactions. The indifference reaction was also associated with neglect for the opposite half of the body and space. Gainotti agreed with Goldstein's explanation that the catastrophic reaction was a psychological response to severe physical disability. The indifference reaction, on the other hand, was not as easy to explain. Gainotti suggested that denial of illness and disorganization of the non-verbal type of synthesis may have been responsible for this emotional symptom.

Another systematic study conducted prior to the 1980s was done by Folstein *et al.* (1997), in which 20 patients between 1 and 2 months following stroke were compared to 10 patients with hip fracture or severe arthritis for frequency of depressive disorder as defined by having 8 or more of 13 depressive symptoms on a semi-structured mental state exam. Although the physical impairment in both groups was comparable (and matched in a subgroup), the stroke patients had a 45% frequency of depression compared to 10% in the orthopedic group. The authors concluded that, "mood disorder is a more specific complication of stroke than simply a response to motor disability."

Thus, explanations for the cause of emotional disorders produced by stroke have followed two lines of reasoning. One line suggested that brain injury may provoke specific emotional disorders, mediated through pathophysiological responses of the brain to injury. The other line of reasoning emphasized that emotional disorders were an understandable psychological response to the loss of ego integrity produced by brain injury. McHugh and Slavney (1998) have termed these differences as "perspectives of psychiatry." Each perspective is based on different, underlying assumptions and methods of reasoning. Poststroke emotional disorders are usually viewed from either the "disease perspective" in which the brain injury provokes a pathophysiological response which leads to clinical symptoms or from the "life story perspective" in which a person becomes vulnerable based on their life experience and in the midst of a stressful life event they develop an empathically understandable psychological disorder. These different perspectives have led to many of the continuing controversies and uncertainties about emotional disorders following stroke. Some clinicians, for example, using the life story perspective, wonder whether the depressive disorders associated with stroke are "real" depressions or whether they represent an entirely different category from major depressions seen in patients with unipolar or bipolar mood disorders (Gainotti *et al.* 1999). Similarly, empathic life story reasoning has led some health care professionals to speculate that these depressions should be encouraged or at least tolerated as a way of promoting the patient's "adjustment" and acceptance of the limitations imposed by the stroke. Baker and Baker (1976), for example, state in their discussion of Broca's aphasia that the patient's recognition of their deficit can be considered a more favorable prognostic finding in a patient who is depressed and apathetic. "We have seen patients who make no gain in aphasia therapy until some degree of depression appears, at which time benefit from the program can be noted." On the other hand, most health care workers now target emotional disorders such as depression for vigorous therapeutic intervention. Numerous studies (see Chapter 18) have demonstrated that depressed patients do not recover physically, cognitively, or in language function as well as comparable patients who are not depressed.

Although these differences in underlying assumptions about the cause of emotional disorders accompanying stroke can be viewed as obstacles to progress, they also represent fuel for research since it is only through systematic empirical research that these controversies can be resolved and a clear understanding of the nature, cause, and treatment of emotional disorders following stroke can be gained.

In summary, for more than 100 years, clinicians have recognized that emotional disorders accompany stroke. The clinical disorders produced by brain injury have fallen into two major categories. One category has included disorders in which the brain injury is viewed as a cause of emotional disorders which are also seen in patients without brain injury. These disorders are sometimes called symptomatic or secondary disorders. Examples of these disorders include depression, mania, anxiety disorders, and personality disorders. Another category of emotional disorders that occur after brain injury includes those that are unique to brain injury, including the catastrophic reaction, the indifference reaction, anosognosia or denial of illness, aprosodia (the inability to comprehend or express emotion), and the pathological display of emotion. The causes of these disorders are also viewed from two perspectives, one a direct result of pathophysiological changes produced by brain injury termed the disease perspective or alternatively as empathically understood psychological responses to impairment and/or loss in a vulnerable individual termed the life story perspective. Both of these concepts and etiological viewpoints continue to be endorsed by different groups of investigators as well as practicing clinicians.

REFERENCES

Adams, G. F., and Hurwitz, L. M. Mental barriers to recovery from strokes. *Lancet* (1963) 2:533–537.

Babinski, J. Contribution a l'etude des troubles mentaux dans l'hemiplegie organique cerebrale (anosognosie). *Rev Neurol (Paris)* (1914) 27:845–848.

Baker, A. B., and Baker, L. H. *Clinical Neurology*, Vol. 1. Harper & Row, Hagertown, Maryland, 1976.

Bleuler, E. P. *Textbook of Psychiatry*. MacMillan, New York, 1951.

Broca, P. Sur la faculte du langage article, suuivi d/une observation d'amphemie. *Bull Anatom Soc (Paris)* (1861) 2:330–357.

Broca, P. Anatomie comparee de circonvolutions cerebrales le grand lobe limbique et al scissure limbique dans la serie des mammiferes. *Rev Antropol* (1878) 1:385–498.

Denny-Brown, D., Meyer, J. S., and Horenstein, S. The significance of perceptual rivalry resulting from parietal lesions. *Brain* (1952) 75:434–471.

Fisher, S. H. Psychiatric considerations of cerebral vascular disease. *Am J Cardiol* (1961) 7:379–385.

Folstein, M. F., Mairberger, R., and McHugh, P. R. Mood disorders as a specific complication of stroke. *J Neurol Neurosurg Psychiatr* (1997) 40:1018–1020.

Gainotti, G. Emotional behavior and hemispheric side of the brain. *Cortex* (1972) 8:41–55.

Gainotti, G., Azzoni, A., and Marra, C. Frequency, phenomenology and anatomical-clinical correlates of major post-stroke depression. *Br J Psychiatr* (1999) 175:163–167.

Goldstein, K. *The Organism: A Holistic Approach to Biology Derived from Pathological Data in Man*. American Books, New York, 1939.

Hecaen, H., deAjuriaguerra, J., and Massonet, J. Les troubles visoconstructifs para lesion parieto occipitale droit. *Encephale* (1951) 40:122–179.

Hughlings-Jackson, J. A lecture on softening of the brain. *Lancet* (1875) 2:335–339.

Hughlings-Jackson, J. On affections of speech from disease of the brain. *Brain* (1915) 38:106–174.

Ironside, R. Disorders of laughter due to brain lesions. *Brain* (1956) 79:589–609.

Lewis, N. D. C. *A Science of Man*. Charles C. Thomas Publisher, Springfield, Illinois, 1957.

McHugh, P. R., and Slavney, P. R. *Perspectives of psychiatry*. Johns Hopkins University Press, Baltimore, London, 1998.

Meyer, A. The anatomical facts and clinical varieties of traumatic insanity. *Am J Insanity* (1904) 60:373–442.

Millikan, C. H., McDowell, F., and Easton, J. D. *Stroke*. Lea & Feiger, Philadelphia, 1987.

Monro, A. *Observations on the Structure and Functions of the Nervous System*. W. Crrech, Edinburgh, 1783.

Papez, J. W. A proposed mechanism of emotion. *Arch Neurol Psychiatry* (1937) 38:725–743.

Post, F. *The Significance of Affective Symptoms in Old Age*. Vol. Maudsley Monograph #10. Oxford University Press, London, 1962.

Rostan, L. *Recherches dur le Ramollissement du Cherveau*. Bechet Jeune, Paris, 1823.

Ullman, M., and Gruen, A. Behavioral changes in patients with stroke. *Am J Psychiatry* (1960) 117:1004–1009.

Wernicke, C. *The Aphasic Symptom-Complex*. Cohn and Weigert, Breslan, 1874.

3

Brain organization and cerebral basis of emotion

As described in Chapter 2, as early as the 19th century Hughlings-Jackson (1875) recognized that symptoms associated with brain lesions may produce both loss of normal function as well as emergence of new, sometimes abnormal symptoms. These new symptoms may arise from the effect of injury on distant uninjured brain areas leading to the release of normally "inhibited" functions or the loss of normally "activated" functions. Thus, this chapter will review brain anatomy, particularly the limbic region, to help readers understand the basis of emotional disorders following brain ischemia.

Schematic drawings of the brain from lateral, coronal, and axial views are shown in Fig. 3.1. Although on initial inspection of the brain, the two hemispheres appear to be symmetrical, it has been demonstrated since the early 1800s that the human brain is functionally asymmetrical. Broca (1861) reported that disruption of language commonly occurred following left hemisphere brain injury while disturbances of language rarely resulted from right hemisphere injury. Subsequent investigations identified anatomical asymmetries associated with this lateralized language function. In a classic paper, Geschwind and Levitsky (1968) reported that the planum temporale, a structure on the dorsal surface of the temporal lobe was significantly larger in the left compared with the right hemisphere. Galaburda *et al.* (1978) have subsequently identified a number of additional structural brain asymmetries, including a longer and wider occipital pole in the left hemisphere and a wider frontal pole in the right hemisphere.

As mentioned previously, language is usually mediated predominantly by the left or dominant hemisphere. Language, however, includes a broad range of functions such as reading, writing, comprehension, expression and repetition of language, naming objects, appropriate syntax, grammatical use of language, and virtually any reasoning task that requires words. The non-dominant right hemisphere, on the other hand, mediates functions such as recognition of shapes, appreciation of the relative position of objects in space, musical ability, and facial recognition. Thus, the brain is both anatomically and functionally lateralized. In trying to understand

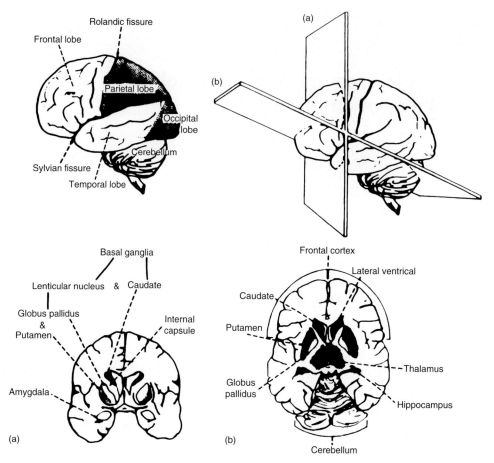

Figure 3.1   Anatomy of the human brain. (a) and (b) views of the brain are taken from the planes indicated on the whole brain.

the brain structures which subserve emotion, differences in hemispheric structure as well as localization of function must be taken into account for their possible effect on the nature and type of emotion.

The anterior regions of the frontal lobes appear to be important in drive, attention, motivation, inhibition of socially inappropriate behavior, temporal (time) organization as well as sequencing, and recognition of organizational themes. There are three general regions of the frontal lobe that are recognized as having different functional roles: the medial portion (including the anterior cingulate), the lateral area, and the orbitofrontal region. Injury to the dorso- and ventrolateral prefrontal cortex is characterized by cognitive executive function deficits as well as depressive disorder. Orbitofrontal injury is characterized by marked personality change with disinhibition, irritability, and unconcern. Medial-frontal injury is characterized by lack of drive and motivation.

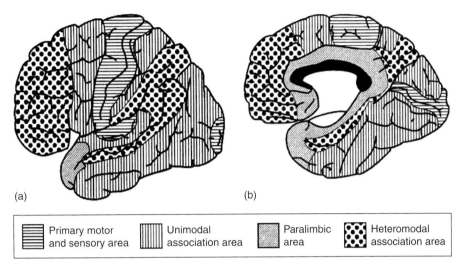

Figure 3.2   Distribution of primary and association cortex on lateral (a) medial and (b) view of the brain (modified from Coffey and Cummings (ed.). *Textbook of Geriatric Neuropsychiatry,* APA Press, Washington DC, 1994, used with permission).

The Wisconsin card sorting test, generally regarded as a measure of frontal lobe function, examines a person's ability to organize a series of cards by different criteria such as color, number, or shape. The neocortex is differentiated into primary motor and sensory areas as well as unimodal and heteromodal association areas. The distribution of these regions is shown in Fig. 3.2. Primary sensory areas subserve vision, hearing, and somatic sensations and are located in the parietal, temporal, and occipital cortex. Primary motor cortex subserves movement and is located in the posterior portion of the frontal lobe. The association cortex is the largest functional brain region occupying more than three-quarters of the neocortex (Mesulam 1985). The unimodal association areas subserve a second level of information processing after primary sensory cortex. These areas serve modality-specific information processing and are located in the temporal, parietal, and occipital cortices (Fig. 3.2). The unimodal auditory area, for example, is located in the posterior and superior parietotemporal junction. Lesions produce a modality-specific loss of language and comprehension (i.e., fluent aphasia).

The heteromodal association cortex mediates the highest level of information processing. In humans, there is general agreement that the inferior parietal lobule and prefrontal cortex are heteromodal association areas. Lesions of these areas produce complex behavioral or cognitive deficits which transcend unimodal sensory impairments. Prefrontal lesions, for example, produce deficits in motor programming, memory retrieval, set shifting, abstraction, and judgment.

Thus, the cognitive and behavioral processes of the human brain can be divided into a regional neuroanatomy of the cerebral cortex. Processing of sensory information proceeds from primary to association to integrative regions. Cerebral infarctions, depending upon their location, produce characteristic syndromes of behavioral, cognitive, and emotional deficits.

Subcortical brain regions are organized in approximately an anterior to posterior sequence (Fig. 3.1). These are the basal ganglia, the diencephalon, the midbrain, and the brain stem/cerebellum. The basal ganglia is the most anterior subcortical region and is composed of three gray matter nuclei: the caudate, putamen, and globus pallidus. These nuclei are primarily involved in the control of involuntary movements. The internal capsule runs through the basal ganglia separating the caudate and the putamen. The internal capsule contains a collection of myelinated nerve fibers, primarily involved in movement, which begin in the cortex and extend to the spinal cord. Injury to the internal capsule results in an inability to voluntarily move the opposite side of the body. Injury to the basal ganglia may produce movements disorders, such as tremor, rigidity, or sudden involuntary movements.

The diencephalon is composed of the inferiorly located hypothalamus and the superiorly located thalamus. The hypothalamus is involved in a wide range of functions including regulation of the autonomic nervous system (i.e., blood pressure control, heart rate, vasodilatation, sweating, etc.), control of pituitary secretions, regulation of body temperature, and probably emotions. The thalamus relays impulses of all types from lower brain areas to the cerebral cortex, and it receives sensory information from all cortical areas. The thalamus may also play a role in attention and concentration by making certain cortical sensory areas more receptive to sensory input than other areas.

The midbrain and lower brain stem contain the cranial nerve nuclei, as well as the reticular formation. These midbrain and brain stem nuclei control eye movement, facial musculature, tongue movement, neck muscle movement, taste, smell, autonomic functions, vision, and the vocal cords. The brain stem reticular formation plays an important role in fundamental functions such as maintenance of consciousness, sleep/wake cycling, rhythmic breathing, and heart rate.

The other major structure deep in the brain is the cerebellum. The cerebellum is a large structure attached to both the midbrain and brain stem. It resembles in some ways the cerebral cortex, although the cerebellar cortex is indented by parallel folds as compared to the cerebral cortex which is ridged by deep gyri running in all directions. The function of the cerebellum is primarily related to the coordination of movements, maintenance of an upright posture, and the ability to recognize and compensate for bodily position in space. Conscious perception and initiation of movement, however, do not occur in the cerebellum. The cerebellum interacts with motor and sensory nerves from cortical, subcortical, and spinal cord regions.

The specific areas of brain whose injury leads to loss of a particular function are said to be the "the locus" of that function (see Fig. 2.1). So, for example, injury to Broca's area will lead to an impairment in the production of speech. Injury to Broca's area leaves the patient either mute or able to express only a few simple words. Broca's area is, therefore, said to be a locus for the expression of verbal language. Many other brain areas, however, also contribute to the production of speech. Thus, "localization" of function to a specific brain area is merely a short-hand way of indicating that the normal expression of that function requires this area of brain to be intact. Injury to other areas of the brain, however, can also disrupt the same behavior, such as subcortical damage producing language dysfunction. True localization will ultimately require the identification of neuronal circuits or neuronal networks which receive input from other brain areas and mediate the physical and psychological expression of a particular behavior.

How emotion is mediated by the brain and which areas are directly involved have long been a matter of debate, speculation, and experimental investigation. It is perhaps the failure to localize emotion in the same way that language was "localized" to the left frontal, temporal, and parietal cortex that has led some investigators to conclude that emotion is not primarily mediated by one brain area but is an expression of the "whole brain." The inability of early investigators to find an anatomical basis for emotion led Freud to develop his detailed theories of mind function. Freud reasoned that the inability to find a particular type of emotional disorder associated with injury to a specific area of the brain was an indication that the relationship between brain and mind was so complicated that, within the foreseeable future, it was not possible to propose a comprehensive theory of emotion based on underlying brain function. Thus, the mind and the principles that Freud proposed for its regulation were separated from those associated with brain function and the beginnings of modern psychoanalytic theory were born.

Seventy or eighty years after the theories were proposed by Freud, our understanding of the relationship between brain and mind remains a major challenge confronting modern neuroscience. As mentioned in Chapter 2, the brain structures that have most frequently been associated with emotion, however, are the "limbic structures" (Fig. 3.3).

Papez (1937) proposed that several of these limbic structures are particularly important in emotion. These limbic structures which compose the "Papez circuit" form a tight circular pathway, starting in the hippocampus (a structure which plays an important role in memory), extending through the fornix to the mamillary bodies (also important in memory), and to the anterior nucleus of the thalamus (important in sensory processing), with radiation to the cingulate cortex and back to the hippocampus (Fig. 3.3). This circuit has connections to both memory and sensory areas of the brain.

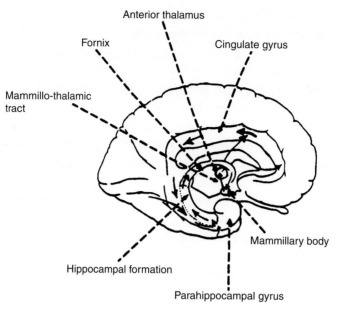

Figure 3.3   Papez circuit.

Cortical limbic structures are three-layered as opposed to the six-layered neo-cortex. All of the limbic structures are connected to the hypothalamus and through indirect connection with the amygdala and hippocampus. The hippocampus, as indicated previously, plays a major role in memory while the amygdala is related to control of aggression and affective response to incoming sensations. The amygdala also modulates anxiety, associations between stimuli and reinforcement, and formation of emotional memory. The parahippocampal gyrus (which includes the entorhinal cortex) is a meeting point where sensory information integrates with brain activity in higher cortical regions. Thus, sensory information first reaches the cortex at unimodal primary sensory areas. It is then projected to secondary sensory areas and then to multi-modal association cortex. These cortical regions project to the parahippocampal gyrus providing integrated sensory information. This integrated information goes to the hippocampus and amygdala which receive inputs from the hypothalamus and other limbic structures.

The cingulate gyrus appears to be involved in highly complex mammalian functions including maternal behavior, play, pain, and attention. This structure has been surgically interrupted as a treatment for obsessive compulsive disorder, pain, and depression.

The basal ganglia includes the caudate nucleus, putamen, and globus pallidus. The striatum refers to the caudate and the putamen. The caudate is a large nucleus that runs along the length of the lateral ventricles and is continuous anteriorly with

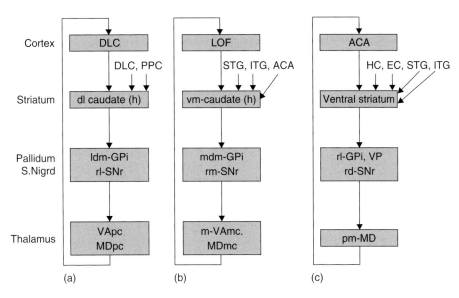

Figure 3.4   The three (a–c) circuits relevant to behavior are shown. Injury to the dorsolateral prefrontal circuit produces executive dysfunction, damage to the orbitofrontal circuit causes disinhibition, and dysfunction of the medial frontal circuit produces apathy. VA: ventral anterior nucleus; MD: medial dorsal nucleus; DLC: dorsolateral prefrontal cortex; PPC: posterior parietal cortex; STG: superior temporal gyrus; ITG: inferior temporal gyrus; ACA: anterior cingulate area; HC: hippocampal cortex; EC: entorhinal cortex; Gpi: internal segment of globus pallidus; Vapc: ventralis anterior pars parvocellularis; MDpc: medialis dorsalis pars parvocellularis; pm: posteromedial; LOF: lateral orbital frontal (modified from Cummings. Frontal subcortical circuits and human behavior. *Arch Neurol* 50: 875). Copyright © 1993 American Medical Association. All Rights reserved.

the putamen. Medially, within the head of the caudate nucleus, is the nucleus accumbens. Nucleus accumbens and some adjacent dopamine rich nuclei are often termed the ventral or limbic striatum. The extended amygdala outputs to the ventral striatum are thought to influence emotional motor behavior.

The basal ganglia mediate cognitive and language functions as well as emotion and motor processes. Five cortical–subcortical circuits have been described (Alexander *et al.* 1986) that link specific cortical regions with basal ganglia and thalamus. The five loops originate in the supplementary motor cortex, the frontal eye fields, dorsal lateral prefrontal cortex, the orbital frontal cortex, and the anterior cingulate cortex, respectively. The three behaviorally and emotionally relevant circuits involve the dorsal lateral prefrontal cortex, the orbital frontal cortex, and the anterior cingulate cortex and are schematically shown in Fig. 3.4. Each circuit has sequential connections between the frontal and/or temporal lobes, caudate or putamen, globus pallidus, and substania nigra and thalamus with connections back to the frontal lobes. There are also indirect pathways connecting the subthalamic nucleus, the globus pallidus externa, and the globus pallidus interna. The ventral striatum flows to the ventral pallidum and to the thalamus. The ventral pallidum is also called the substantia innominata, an area rich in acetyl choline containing neurons.

One of the best known demonstrations of emotional dysfunction resulting from lesions to limbic structures is the Klüver–Bucy syndrome (1937). Bilateral removal of the anterior temporal lobe including the amygdala and hippocampus in monkeys produces a marked charge in aggressiveness with docile animals becoming bold and aggressive animals becoming tame. In addition, some animals with the Klüver–Bucy syndrome demonstrate disinhibited sexual behavior, unprovoked irritability, hyperresponsiveness to visual stimuli, and an altered means of exploring their environment by putting objects in their mouth. Similar kinds of unusual or exaggerated emotionally related behavior have also been found in humans following injury to these limbic brain areas.

Recent data on normal emotion has come from studies of emotional induction in subjects undergoing functional imaging of regional brain activity. Pardo *et al.* (1993), for example, asked normal volunteers to recall a sad event from their past. This was correlated with increased blood flow in the inferior (particularly left) frontal cortex. Mayberg *et al.* (1995) also used sad memories to induce sadness and found relative decreases in blood flow in the inferior frontal, temporal cortex as well as other limbic and paralimbic regions. George *et al.* (1995) used a combination of recall and visual stimulation with mood-congruent facial expression to induce happiness or sadness in normal women. There were increases in blood flow found in the medial prefrontal and left lateral prefrontal cortices, the left anterior cingulate, left thalamus, and basal ganglia with sad memories and decreases in the right midtemporal and right prefrontal cortices associated with happiness. Our studies of emotion induced by pictures of faces or scenes of happiness, sadness, or fear/disgust in normal elderly subjects found that sadness led to increased blood flow in the ventral prefrontal and temporal cortexes, and thalamus compared with neutral or happy stimuli.

These studies, although providing the first direct evidence of limbic involvement in the experience of emotion, have left many unresolved questions. Each study has found increases or decreases in blood flow in different limbic structures associated with emotion. There are also reports of gender-related differences in blood flow in limbic structures (Gur *et al.* 1995). This suggests that men and women may process emotion differently and have differences in baseline (resting) emotional tone. There is much work still needed to identify the structures involved in each emotion as well as the mechanism of its production in consciousness.

The issue of how the brain recovers from injury is also essential in understanding the course of poststroke emotional disorders. For many years, clinicians and neuroscientists have been trying to discover the mechanism by which patients recover from impairments following brain injury. Various mechanisms have been proposed to explain behavioral recovery after brain injury (Feeney and Sutton 1987). Some functional imaging studies have found that behaviors such as language are taken over by other uninjured brain areas not normally involved in that behavior or, alternatively, that brain areas which normally contribute to the behavior take over more of that behavioral function. Other theories have proposed that new behaviors are learned to compensate for the loss of function produced by the brain damage or that recovery from temporary shock and transient shutdown in non-injured brain areas may result in apparent recovery of function.

It is not known why some functions recover more readily than others, although brains of younger patients, particularly children, have repeatedly been shown to be more capable of recovery than the brains of elderly patients. Young children can often apparently completely recover from severe deficits after brain injury including hemispherectomy while this is rarely the case in older patients.

Perhaps the most intriguing new finding related to recovery from stroke is the identification of neuronal regeneration following stroke (Liu *et al.* 1998; Arvidsson *et al.* 2002). As indicated in Chapter 1, Arvidsson *et al.* 2002 demonstrated that temporary occlusion of the middle cerebral artery in rats led to the proliferation of neural progenitor cells in the subventricular zone. These cells migrated to the injured striatum and matured to the dominant type of striatal neuron. Furthermore, injection of nerve growth factor (NGF) increased the number of new neurons by ten-fold and led to improved recovery of learning skills (Nakatomi *et al.* 2002). Although 80% of newly arrived neurons died within 6 weeks of stroke, inflammation may be responsible (Monje *et al.* 2003). It is unclear if therapeutic drugs may be as potent as nerve growth factors in stimulating neural proliferation, but antidepressants (Santarelli *et al.* 2003), the cholesterol lowering statins (Chen *et al.* 2003), and even Viagra (Zhang *et al.* 2002) have all been shown to induce the growth of new neurons primarily in the subventricular zone and the subgranular zone of the hippocampal dentate gyrus (Gage 2000) (see Chapter 2).

In summary, the cerebral basis of emotion appears to involve both limbic and paralimbic structures. A great deal of interest has been focused on the dorsal lateral, orbital frontal, and cingulate circuits involving the striatum and the thalamus, and how they may mediate depression and other emotional syndromes. Future research may identify how these structures as well as neuronal response to injury may lead to poststroke emotional disorders and their natural course of recovery.

REFERENCES

Alexander, G. E., DeLong, M. R., and Strick, P. L. Parallel organization of functionally segregated circuits linking basal ganglia and cortex. *Annu Rev Neurosci* (1986) 9:357–381.

Arvidsson, A., Collin, T., Kirik, D., *et al.* Neuronal replacement from endogenous precursors in the adult brain after stroke. *Nat Med* (2002) 8(9):963–970.

Broca, P. Sur la faculte du langage article, suuivi d/une observation d'amphemie *Bulletin Anatomical Society (Paris)* (1861) 2: 330–357.

Chen, J., Zhang, Z. G., Li, Y., *et al.* Statins induce angiogenesis, neurogenesis, and synaptogenesis after stroke. *Ann Neurol* (2003) 53(6):743–751.

Cummings, J. Frontal-subcortical lesions and human behavior. *Arch Neurol* (1993) 50:873–880.

Cummings, J. L., and Coffey, C. E. Geriatric neuropsychiatry. In C. E. Coffey and J. L. Cummings, eds., *Textbook of Geriatric Neuropsychiatry.* Washington, DC: American Psychiatric Press, Inc., 1994, p. 75.

Feeney, D. M., and Sutton, R. L. Pharmacotherapy for recovery of function after brain injury. *Crit Rev Neurobiol* (1987) 3:135–197.

Gage, F. H. Mammalian neural stem cells. *Science* (2000) 287(5457):1433–1438.

Galaburda, A. M., LeMay, M., Kemper, T. L., *et al.* Right–left asymmetries in the brain: structural differences between the hemispheres may underlie cerebral dominance. *Science* (1978) 199:852–856.

George, M. S., Ketter, T. A., Parekh, P. I., *et al.* Brain activity during transient sadness and happiness in healthy women. *Am J Psychiatr* (1995) 152:341–351.

Geschwind, N., and Levitsky, W. Human brain: left–right asymmetries in temporal speech region. *Science* (1968) 161:186–187.

Gur, R., Mozley, L., Mozley, P., *et al.* Sex differences in regional cerebral glucose metabolism during a resting state. *Science* (1995) 267:528–531.

Klüver, H., and Bucy, P. C. Psychic blindness and other symptoms following bilateral temporal lobectomy in rhesus monkeys. *Am J Physiol* (1937) 119:352–353.

Liu, J., Solway, K., Messing, R. O., *et al.* Increased neurogenesis in the dentate gyrus after transient global ischemia in gerbils. *J Neurosci* (1998) 18(19):7768–7778.

Mayberg, H. S., Liotti, M., Jerabek, P. A., *et al.* Induced sadness: a PET model of depression. *Hum Brain Mapp* (1995) Suppl 1: 396.

Mesulam, M.-M. *Principles of Behavioral Neurology.* Davis, Philadelphia, 1985.

Monje, M. L., Toda, H., and Palmer, T. D. Inflammatory blockade restores adult hippocampal neurogenesis. *Science* (2003) 302(5651):1760–1765.

Nakatomi, H., Kuriu, T., Okabe, S., *et al.* Regeneration of hippocampal pyramidal neurons after ischemic brain injury by recruitment of endogenous neural progenitors. *Cell* (2002) 110(4):429–441.

Papez, J. W. A proposed mechanism of emotion. *Arch Neurol Psychiatry* (1937) 38:725–743.

Pardo, J. V., Pardo, P. J., and Raichle, M. D. Neural correlates of self-induced dysphoria. *Am J Psychiatr* (1993) 150:713–719.

Santarelli, L., Saxe, M., Gross, C., *et al.* Requirement of hippocampal neurogenesis for the behavioral effects of antidepressants. *Science* (2003) 301(5634):805–809.

Zhang, R., Wang, Y., Zhang, L., *et al.* Sildenafil (Viagra) induces neurogenesis and promotes functional recovery after stroke in rats. *Stroke* (2002) 33(11):2675–2680.

4

Vascular anatomy and classification of stroke

The arterial supply to the brain consists of four large vessels – two (right and left) internal carotid arteries and two vertebral arteries (Fig. 4.1). The brain itself is perfused by two kinds of arteries, large-diameter arteries that lead from the inferior portion of the brain over the lateral surfaces of the cerebral hemispheres, brain stem, and cerebellum, and penetrating arteries that branch from these large surface arteries and enter the brain parenchyma to supply specific areas. There are also interconnecting arteries at the base of the brain that form the circle of Willis (Fig. 4.2).

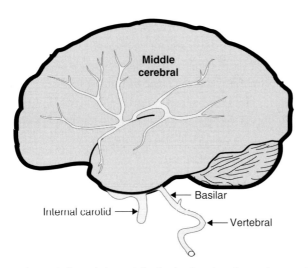

Figure 4.1   Schematic lateral view of the brain showing the major arterial vessels. The internal carotid gives rise to the anterior and middle cerebral arteries. The vertebral–basilar arteries constitute the posterior circulation including the posterior cerebral hemispheres, brain stem, cerebellum, and medial subcortical structures.

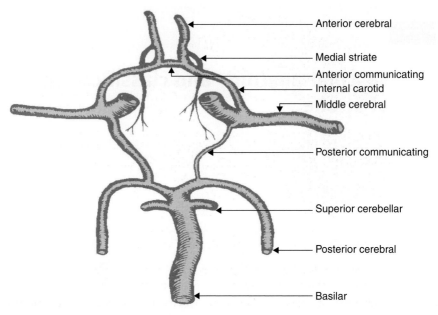

Anterior cerebral

Medial striate

Anterior communicating

Internal carotid

Middle cerebral

Posterior communicating

Superior cerebellar

Posterior cerebral

Basilar

Figure 4.2   The circle of Willis connecting the anterior internal carotid circulation with the posterior circulation. The posterior communicating arteries lie at the base of the brain and allow internal carotid artery to supply some posterior cerebral brain regions (modified from R. G. Clark, *Clinical Neuroanatomy and Neurophysiology*, FA Davis, Philadelphia, 1975, with permission).

Carotid system

The carotid arteries supply anterior portions of the brain. The right common carotid artery branches from the innominate artery while the left common carotid artery branches directly from the aortic arch. These vessels course upward in the neck and bifurcate approximately at the angle of the jaw to form the internal and external carotid arteries. The internal carotid artery then passes up to the base of the skull and through the carotid canal. It traverses the cavernous sinus after entering the skull and sends tiny branches to the eye and the optic nerve as well as the pituitary, trigeminal nerve, and middle ear.

The posterior communicating artery is the next branch and runs posteriorly connecting with the posterior cerebral artery (Fig. 4.2). The anterior choroidal artery supplies portions of the hippocampus, caudate nucleus, and amygdala as well as portions of the basal ganglia (Fig. 4.3). The internal carotid artery then bifurcates into two main branches: the middle cerebral artery and the anterior cerebral artery (Fig. 4.2). These two arteries provide the blood supply for all of the anterior cerebral hemispheres.

The anterior cerebral arteries course forward into the interhemispheric fissure just above the optic chiasma and then pass upward and around the corpus callosum over the medial surface of the cerebral hemispheres (Fig. 4.4). These branches

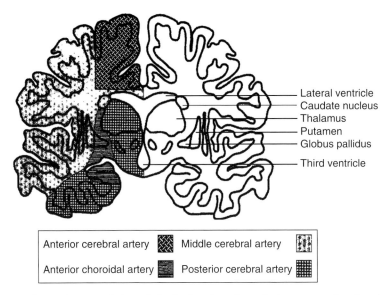

Figure 4.3   A schematic coronal view of the brain taken through the temporal and parietal cortex and thalamus. The overlapping regions subserved by anterior and middle cerebral arteries (internal carotid circulation) and posterior cerebral arteries (posterior circulation) are demonstrated.

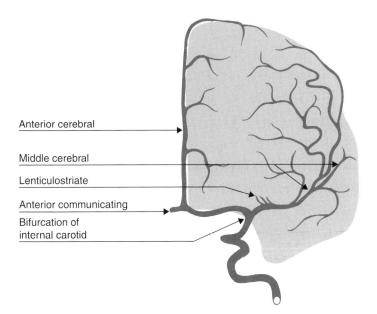

Figure 4.4   The anterior and middle cerebral artery circulation demonstrating the medial course of the anterior cerebral artery along the interhemispheric separation and the lenticulostriate arteries which penetrate the brain to provide circulation to the basal ganglia (modified from R. G. Clark, *Clinical Neuroanatomy and Neurophysiology*, FA Davis, Philadelphia, 1975, with permission).

supply blood to the anterior medial and superior portions of the frontal lobes. A large branch of the anterior cerebral artery, called the medial striate or Heubner's artery, penetrates the brain substance and often supplies the internal capsule and anterior portions of the basal ganglia.

The anterior communicating artery connects the two anterior cerebral arteries (Fig. 4.4). Penetrating branches of the anterior cerebral artery may reach the anterior thalamus and anterior portions of the basal ganglia.

The middle cerebral artery courses laterally along the base of the hemisphere emerging through the Sylvian fissure where its branches spread over the lateral surface of the cerebral hemispheres (Fig. 4.1). The middle cerebral artery usually divides into two or three large branches which course over the cerebral hemispheres and give rise to as many as 20 penetrating branches. These are called the lenticulostriate arteries which supply the lateral portion of the basal ganglia, the lateral portion of the thalamus, and the posterior limb of the internal capsule (Fig. 4.4).

The middle cerebral artery supplies the bulk of the cerebral hemispheres, including the motor and sensory cortex for the hand, arm, shoulder, face, tongue, and portion of the leg (Fig. 4.1). Most strokes occur within the distribution of the middle cerebral artery and occlusion may cause varying degrees of weakness and sensory loss in the shoulder, arm, hand, face, and lower extremity on the opposite side of the body. When the dominant cerebral hemisphere (usually the left hemisphere) is damaged by middle cerebral artery occlusion, speech may be impaired. Occlusion of the penetrating branches of the middle cerebral artery gives rise to a variety of clinical syndromes, depending on the size of the artery and the specific area of brain infarcted.

Vertebral–basilar system

The posterior portion of the brain is supplied by the vertebral system. The vertebral arteries arise from the subclavian arteries and ascend through the vertebral canal and the foramen magnum to enter the skull. At the rostral end of the medulla, they unite to form the basilar artery which courses the full length of the pons to the midbrain (Fig. 4.2). Connections between the posterior circulation (i.e., the vertebral–basilar system) and the anterior circulation (i.e., the carotid system) occur by way of the posterior communicating arteries. The basilar–vertebral arteries supply the brain stem and cerebellum. The vertebral–basilar system supplies both midline brain stem structures as well as circumferential arteries which pass around the brain stem and supply the dorsal portions of the brain stem.

The posterior–inferior cerebellar artery is usually the last branch of each vertebral artery while the anterior–inferior cerebellar artery arises from the basilar artery. The superior cerebellar artery arises close to the rostral end of the basilar artery and supplies large portions of the cerebellar hemispheres. The posterior cerebral arteries become the terminal branches of the basilar artery (Fig. 4.2). The two posterior cerebral arteries encircle the brain stem and supply branches to the cerebellar peduncles, the geniculate bodies, posterior portions of the thalamus, the medial portion of the occipital lobes, and the inferior–medial portion of the temporal lobes (Fig. 4.3). The most distal branches supply the calcarien cortex (primary visual cortex).

Venous system

The venous drainage consists of a superficial system and a deep system. Both of these venous drainage systems enter into a collecting system of large channels called sinuses which in turn drain into the internal jugular veins that leave the skull through the jugular foramina and eventually empty into the superior vena cava.

The superficial venous system consists of surface veins that carry blood into the superior saggital sinus, the cavernous sinus, and the transverse and petrosal sinuses.

The deep venous system generally empties into large veins in the interventricular foramen of Monroe, several veins join to form the internal cerebral vein which joins the inferior saggital sinus. The inferior saggital sinus also collects blood from basal areas of the preoptic region and hypothalamus. The superior saggital sinus courses over the brain between the hemispheres, the inferior saggital sinus forms the straight sinus, while the transverse sinus is located in the fixed lateral margin of the tentorium cerebella. The cavernous sinuses are paired venous spaces in the dura on either side of the sella turcica receiving blood from the orbit by way of the thalamic veins.

The most clinically important abnormalities of the venous system include thrombolic occlusion of the superior saggital sinus which may impair acceptance of cerebral spinal fluid. Thrombosis of the transverse sinus may be caused by disease of the temporal bone. Occlusion of the deep cerebral veins may be caused by hemorrhage of deep cerebral structures. Infections may enter the brain through the venous system, such as sepsis within the orbit or nasal bacteria entering the cavernous sinus leading to swelling of orbital brain tissue.

Classification of cerebrovascular disease

There are many ways to classify the wide range of disorders that are called stroke. On the one hand, cerebrovascular disease can be understood as an anatomical–pathological process of the blood vessels that have been discussed. This would lead to a classification based on the etiologies of underlying anatomical–pathological processes. Such a classification would include an extensive list of diseases, including those with infectious, connective tissue, neoplastic, hematological, pharmacological, and traumatic causes. Alternatively, a classification of stroke could be based on the mechanism by which these vascular pathological processes manifest themselves. For example, the interactive effects of systemic hypertension and atherosclerosis on the resilience of large arteries, integrity of vessel lumens, and production of end-organ ischemia might be one mechanistic classification of stroke. Another might be the formation of aneurysm dilatations or vascular disease or the effect of cardiac arrhythmias on the propagation of thromboemboli.

From the perspective of schematizing the emotional disorders associated with stroke, however, probably the most pragmatic way of classifying cerebrovascular disease is not to focus on the anatomical–pathological process or the interactive mechanisms but to examine the means by which parenchymal changes in the brain occur (Table 4.1). Using this classification, the first major category is ischemia which occurs in about 80–85% of patients with symptomatic cerebrovascular disease. Ischemia may occur either with or without infarction of parenchyma, and includes transient ischemic attacks (TIAs), atherosclerotic thrombosis, cerebral embolism, and small lacunar infarction. The second major category is hemorrhage which occurs in about 15–20% of patients with symptomatic cerebrovascular disease. Hemorrhage may cause either direct parenchymal damage by extravasation of blood into the surrounding brain tissues as in intracerebral hemorrhage (ICH),

Table 4.1. Classification of cerebrovascular disease

Ischemic disorders
- Infarction
  1. Atherosclerotic thrombosis
  2. Cerebral embolism
  3. Lacunae
  4. Other causes: arteritis (e.g., infectious or connective tissue disease), cerebral thrombophlebitis, fibromuscular dysplasia, and venous occlusions
- TIAs

Hemorrhagic disorders
- Intraparenchymal hemorrhage
  1. Primary (hypertensive) ICH
  2. Other causes: hemorrhagic disorders (e.g., thrombocytopenia and clotting disorders) and trauma
- Subarachnoid or intraventricular hemorrhage
  1. Ruptured saccular aneurysm or AVM
  2. Other causes
- SDH or epidural hematoma

or indirect damage by hemorrhage into the ventricles, subarachnoid space, extra-dural area, or subdural area. These changes result in a common mode of expression, defined by Adams and Victor (1985) as a sudden, non-convulsive, focal neurological deficit – or stroke.

Expanding on this categorization (i.e., the means by which parenchymal changes occur), there are four major categories of ischemic cerebral infarction. These include atherosclerotic thrombosis, cerebral embolism, lacunae, and other more rare conditions. Studies of the incidence of cerebrovascular disease (e.g., Wolf *et al.* 1977) found that the ratio of infarcts to hemorrhages is about 5:1. Atherosclerotic thrombosis and cerebral embolism each account for approximately one-third of all strokes.

Atherosclerotic thrombosis

Atherosclerotic thrombosis is often the result of a dynamic interaction between hypertension and atherosclerotic deposition of hyaline-lipid material in the walls of peripheral, coronary, and cerebral arteries. Risk factors in the development of atherosclerosis include hyperlipidemia, diabetes mellitus, hypertension, and cigarette smoking. Atheromatous plaques tend to propagate at the branchings and curves of the internal carotid artery, in the carotid sinus, in the cervical part of the vertebral arteries and their junction to form the basilar artery, in the posterior cerebral arteries as they wind around the midbrain, and in the anterior cerebral arteries as they curve over the corpus callosum. These plaques may lead to stenosis of one or more of these cerebral arteries or to complete occlusion. TIAs, defined as periods of transient focal ischemia associated with reversible neurological deficits, almost always indicate that a thrombotic process is occurring. Only rarely is embolism or ICH preceded by transient neurological deficits. Thrombosis of virtually any cerebral or cerebellar artery can be associated with TIAs.

TIAs, therefore, although not listed among the main causes of stroke, may precede, accompany, or follow the development of stroke or may occur by themselves without leading to complete occlusion of a cerebral or cerebellar artery. Most commonly, TIAs have a duration of 2–15 min, with a range from a few seconds to up to 12–24 h. Since the neurological examination between successive episodes of this thrombotic process shows entirely normal findings, the existence of permanent neurological deficits indicates that infarction has occurred. The progression of events leading to the completed thrombotic stroke, however, can be quite variable.

Cerebral embolism

Cerebral embolism, which accounts for approximately one-third of all strokes, is usually caused by a fragment breaking away from a thrombus within the heart and traveling up the carotid artery. Less commonly, the source of the embolism may be from an atheromatous plaque within the lumen of the carotid sinus or from the distal end of a thrombus within the internal carotid artery, or it may represent a fat, tumor, or air embolus within the internal carotid artery. The causes of thrombus formation within the heart can include cardiac arrhythmias, congenital heart disease, infectious processes (e.g., syphilitic heart disease, rheumatic valvular disease, and endocarditis), valve prostheses, postsurgical complications, or myocardial infarction with mural thrombus. Of all strokes, those due to cerebral embolism develop most rapidly. In general, there are no warning episodes; embolism can occur at any time. A large embolus may occlude the internal carotid artery or the stem of the middle cerebral artery producing a severe hemiplegia. More often, however, the embolus is smaller and passes into one of the branches of the middle cerebral artery, producing infarction distal to the site of arterial occlusion, characterized by a pattern of neurological deficits consistent with the vascular distribution, or producing a transient neurological deficit that resolves as the embolus fragments and travels into smaller, more distal arteries.

Lacunae

Lacunae, which account for nearly one-fifth of all strokes, are the result of occlusion of small penetrating cerebral arteries. They are infarcts that may be so small as to produce no recognizable deficits, or, depending on their location, they may be associated with pure motor or sensory deficits. There is a strong association between lacunae and both atherosclerosis and hypertension, suggesting that lacunar infarction is the result of the extension of the atherosclerotic process into small-diameter vessels.

Hemorrhage

Intracranial hemorrhages, which account for about one-seventh of all strokes, is the fourth most frequent cause of stroke. The main causes of intracranial hemorrhage that present as acute strokes include ICH, usually associated with hypertension; rupture of saccular aneurysms or arteriovenous malformations (AVMs); a variety of hemorrhagic disorders of assorted etiology; and trauma-producing hemorrhage. Primary (hypertensive) ICH occurs within the brain tissue. The extravasation of blood forms a roughly circular or oval-shaped mass that disrupts and displaces the parenchyma. Adjacent tissue is compressed, and seepage into the ventricular system usually occurs, producing bloody spinal fluid in more than 90% of cases. ICH can range in size from massive bleeds of several centimeters in diameter to petechial hemorrhages of a millimeter or less, most commonly occurring within the putamen, in the adjacent internal capsule, or in various portions of the white matter underlying the cortex. Hemorrhages of the thalamus, cerebellar hemispheres, or pons are also common. Severe headache is generally considered to be a constant accompaniment of ICH, but this occurs in only about 50% of cases.

The prognosis for ICH is grave, with 70–75% of patients dying within 1–30 days (Adams and Victor 1985).

Aneurysms and AVMs

Ruptured aneurysms and arterial venous malformations (AVMs) are the next most common type of cerebrovascular disease after thrombosis, embolism, lacunae, and ICH. Aneurysms are usually located at arterial bifurcations and are presumed to result from developmental defects in the formation of the arterial wall; rupture occurs when the intima bulges outward and eventually breaks through the adventitia. AVMs consist of a tangle of dilated vessels that form an abnormal communication between arterial and venous systems. They are developmental abnormalities consisting of embryonic patterns of blood vessels. Most AVMs are clinically silent but will ultimately bleed. Hemorrhage from aneurysms or AVMs may occur within the subarachnoid space, leading to an identifiable presentation as a bleeding vessel anomaly, or may occur within the parenchyma, leading to hemiplegia or even death.

Subdural and epidural hematomas

Although it could be contended that subdural hematomas (SDH) and epidural hematomas do not represent forms of cerebrovascular disease, nonetheless their behavior as vascular space-occupying lesions that produce many of the signs and symptoms of stroke warrants a brief description here.

Chronic SDHs are frequently (60%), but not exclusively, caused by head trauma, followed by a gradual progression of signs and symptoms during the subsequent days to weeks. Traumatic chronic SDH may be caused by tears of bridging veins in the subdural space. Non-traumatic causes include ruptured aneurysms or AVMs of the pial surface or rapid deceleration injuries. The most common symptom of chronic SDH is headache as well as a variety of neuropsychiatric manifestations which parallel the gradual increase in intracranial pressure. These include confusion, inattention, apathy, memory loss, drowsiness, and coma. Chronic SDH is also one of the many conditions in the differential diagnosis of treatable causes of dementia. Fluctuations in the level of consciousness predominate over any focal or lateralizing signs, which may include hemiparesis, hemianopsia, cranial nerve abnormalities, aphasia, or seizures. Chronic SDH may continue to expand if left unchecked, or may reabsorb spontaneously.

Acute SDH and epidural hematomas, although frequently manifested by similar changes in level of consciousness and focal neurological deficits (as in chronic SDH), are associated with severe head trauma. They may occur simultaneously or in combination with cerebral laceration or contusion, and progress rapidly over a period of a few hours to days, rather than days to weeks. Epidural hematomas usually follow temporal or parietal skull fracture that causes a laceration or avulsion of the middle meningeal artery or vein or a tear of the dural venous sinus; acute SDH is usually caused by the avulsion of bridging veins or laceration of pial arteries. Both conditions produce loss of consciousness or a brief period of lucidity followed by a loss of consciousness, hemiparesis, cranial nerve palsies, and death, usually secondary to respiratory compromise, if the hematoma is not emergently evacuated.

Other types of cerebrovascular disease

One of the other causes of cerebrovascular disease is fibromuscular dysplasia, which leads to narrowed arterial segments caused by degeneration of elastic tissue, disruption and loss of the arterial muscular coat, and an increase in fibrous tissue. Inflammatory diseases of the arterial system can also lead to stroke; these include meningovascular syphilis, pyogenic or tuberculous meningitis, temporal arteritis, and systemic lupus erythematosus.

There are many other less common causes of cerebrovascular disease that have not been cited here due to lack of space. It appears obvious, however, that examining the many causes and types of cerebrovascular disease in relation to specific neuropsychiatric disorders is a very formidable task. Few studies have compared the emotional disorders associated with thromboembolic stroke to those associated with hemorrhagic (Robinson *et al.* 1983a). In general, our studies have included lesions caused by both ischemia and hemorrhage and have found that the associated mood disorders are similar, depending on the size and location of the lesion and the time elapsed since injury. This issue, however, has never been systematically investigated. As indicated previously, the type or pattern of neuronal damage may be different, depending on the cause of the cerebrovascular disease. Resultant neuropsychiatric disorders may also vary depending on the nature of the vascular disorder.

In summary, whether emotional changes are directly or indirectly produced by stroke, they are ultimately dependent upon the brain's structural and vascular anatomy. The most frequent location for cerebral infarctions is the distribution of the middle cerebral artery. Thrombosis or emboli which occlude the large-diameter vessels on the lateral surface of the brain produce the largest lesions. Posterior circulation lesions affecting the brain stem or penetrating arterial lesions affecting subcortical structures usually produce small focal or lacunar lesions.

Classification of cerebrovascular disease may be based on either the cerebral vessels occluded, the cause of the vessel disease or the means by which tissue damage occurs. I have outlined a classification of stroke based on the cause of tissue damage. The most frequent type of stroke is thromboembolic infarction followed by ICH. These vascular disorders lead to permanent damage of cerebral tissue and the physical and cognitive impairments produced by stroke.

As discussed in Chapter 3, emotional disorders are thought to be associated with dysfunction in the limbic system. Limbic structures are supplied by anterior cerebral (i.e., orbitofrontal cortex), posterior cerebral (i.e., thalamus and the medial portion of temporal lobe) as well as penetrating branches of the middle cerebral arteries (i.e., septum, accumbens, as well as portions of temporopolar cortex and orbital–frontal cortex). Thus, strokes which lead to emotional disorders may occur within any of the anterior, middle, or posterior cerebral arteries, and may occur in large surface arteries or deep penetrating arteries. The infarct may be large or small depending upon the artery affected and may be either hemorrhagic or ischemic in nature. Vascular anatomy and stroke classification give us a basis for understanding where and how the stroke occurred but do not predict the likelihood of an emotion disorder which may be a consequence.

REFERENCES

Adams, R. D., and Victor, M. *Principles of Neurology.* McGraw-Hill, New York, 1985.

Robinson, R. G., Kubos, K. L., Starr, L. B., *et al.* Mood changes in stroke patients: relationship to lesion location. *Compr Psychiatr* (1983) 24:555–566.

Wolf, P. A., Dawber, T. R., Thomas, H. E., *et al.* Epidemiology of stroke. In R. A. Thompson and J. R. Green, eds., *Advances in Neurology.* Raven Press, New York, 1977, 5–19.

Part II

Poststroke depression

5

Diagnosis of depression

Method of diagnosis

For a number of years the generally accepted method for research diagnoses of psychiatric disorders has been to conduct a structured or semi-structured mental status interview to elicit the presence and duration of symptoms of the disorder and apply these to Diagnostic and Statistical Manual (DSM) or International Classification of Diseases (ICD) criteria for that disorder. The current DSM-IV TR (American Psychiatric Association 2000) has identified a category of disorders which are judged by the clinician to be the consequence of a general medical condition. The DSM-IV diagnostic criteria for mood disorders due to stroke or other medical disorders are shown in Table 5.1. At the present time, although there is some debate in the literature as to the most appropriate way to diagnose depression in patients with brain injury, this is the accepted criteria and method for diagnosis in psychiatry.

There are a number of structured and semi-structured interviews for diagnosis in psychiatry and investigators of poststroke depression have utilized a wide variety of these instruments. Eastwood *et al.* and we have recently used the Schedule for Affective Disorders and Schizophrenia (SADS) (Eastwood *et al.* 1989; Robinson 2000). Morris *et al.* (1990) used the Composite Index of Diagnostic Interviews (CIDI). Throughout most of our studies, we and other investigators have used the Present State Examination (PSE) (Robinson and Price 1982; House *et al.* 1990; Pohjasvaara *et al.* 1998), which is a semi-structured interview that we have modified to elicit all of the specific symptoms required for a DSM-IV diagnosis of mood or anxiety disorder. The full spectrum of instruments is shown in Table 6.1 on the prevalence of poststroke depression. Although some authors have expressed a preference for one interview over another, a comparison of diagnostic instruments has not been conducted in poststroke mood disorders.

Although the use of a structured or semi-structured psychiatric interview has clearly been the accepted method for systematic elicitation of symptomology, a

Table 5.1. DSM-IV diagnostic criteria

Mood disorder due to a general medical condition, mood-incongruent delusions of
hallucinations, or disorganized speech
The essential feature is a prominent and persistent mood that is judged to be due to the direct
physiological effects of a general medical condition
Subtypes
  I. With depressive features – predominant mood is depressed but full criteria for a major
      depressive episode are not met
  II. With major depressive-like episode
     A. At least five of the following symptoms present during at least a 2-week period.
        At least one of the symptoms is either (1) depressed mood or (2) loss of interest or
        pleasure
        1. Depressed mood most of the day
        2. Markedly diminished interest or pleasure
        3. Significant weight loss or weight gain
        4. Insomnia or hypersomnia
        5. Psychomotor agitation or retardation
        6. Fatigue or loss of energy
        7. Feelings of worthlessness or excessive or inappropriate guilt
        8. Diminished ability to think or concentrate
        9. Recurrent thoughts of death
     B. Distress or impairment in social, occupation, or other functioning
     C. Not bereavement
  III. With manic features – predominant mood is elevated euphoric or irritable
  IV. With mixed features – the symptoms of both mania and depression are present but neither
      predominates

surprising number of studies have utilized a cutoff score on a depression rating
scale for an approximation to the diagnosis of depression (Sinyor *et al.* 1986; Collin
et al. 1987; Wade *et al.* 1987; Andersen *et al.* 1994; Kotila *et al.* 1998; Desmond *et al.*
2003). The consistency of findings in mood disorders following stroke would
undoubtedly be improved by the consistent use of structured or semi-structured
psychiatric interviews and standardized criteria for depression rather than a cutoff
point on a rating scale.

Applicable diagnostic categories

In Chapter 7, I will discuss the controversy over the specificity of symptoms in
patients with medical illness and alternative suggestions for diagnosis. This chapter,

however, will be devoted to the methodology and criteria used for diagnosis of poststroke depression or poststroke mania. The diagnostic category "mood disorder due to stroke" has four subtypes: the first is mood disorder due to stroke with depressive features; the second is with major depressive-like episode; the third is with manic features; and the fourth is with mixed features.

The first subtype (i.e., with depressive features) only requires the presence of a predominantly depressed mood but lacks full criteria for major depression. The obvious problem with this diagnosis and the reason we have not used it is that a patient with depressed mood alone and no other symptoms could be diagnosed using these criteria. The lack of specific depressive symptoms as well as number of symptoms required for diagnosis make this such a loose category as to not be useable for research investigations. Similar problems arise in subtypes three and four (i.e., mood disorder due to stroke with manic features or mood disorder due to stroke with mixed features). There are no specific symptoms required for these diagnoses and patients with either an elevated or irritable mood and no other symptoms or patients with alternating depressed and irritable mood could be diagnosed with manic or mixed features using these criteria.

Due to these problems with diagnostic subtypes one, three, and four, we have recently been using DSM-IV research criteria for minor depression. Minor depression is a term taken from research diagnostic criteria (RDC) (Feighner *et al.* 1972) to designate a subsyndromal form of major depression requiring at least two but less than five symptoms of major depression. Before DSM-IV had been published, we had used the symptom criteria, but not the duration criteria, from DSM-III dysthymic disorder for the diagnosis of minor depression. By using the term "minor" rather than "dysthymic," we tried to emphasize that these depressions were not long-term chronic depressions, but simply a less severe form of depressive disorder. The frequency of each of the symptoms for all acute stroke patients that we have examined with major or minor depression based on interviews using the PSE and DSM-IV symptom criteria are shown in Table 5.2. Spalletta *et al.* (2005) has recently reported on the same comparison among 50 patients with major depression, 62 with minor depression, and 88 non-depressed patients. Symptoms were elicited using the Structured Clinical Interview for DSM-IV patient (SCID-P). Results showed that χ^2 analysis found that the three groups differed significantly in the frequency of every symptom. After Bonferroni correction, only feelings of guilt failed to distinguish the three groups. Post-hoc analysis showed that patients with minor depression had significantly higher frequency of depressed mood, decreased interest, loss of energy, insomnia, and psychomotor disturbance compared with non-depressed patients.

The following are two case histories that demonstrate in Case A, major depressive disorder and in Case B, minor depressive disorder.

Table 5.2. Frequency of DSM-IV symptoms

N (%)	Initial Evaluation			
	A Not depressed n = 250	B Minor depression n = 66	C Major depression* n = 80	p < 0.05
Depressed mood	2 (0.8)	63 (95.5)	80 (100.0)	A < B, A < C
Loss of interest	2 (0.8)	10 (15.2)	41 (51.3)	A < B, B < C, A < C
Appetite/weight loss	48 (19.2)	16 (24.2)	49 (61.3)	B < C, A < C
Insomnia	66 (26.4)	22 (33.3)	63 (78.8)	A < B, B < C, A < C
Psychomotor disturbance	101 (40.4)	44 (66.7)	74 (92.5)	A < B, B < C, A < C
Loss of energy	89 (35.6)	33 (50.0)	68 (85.0)	A < B, B < C, A < C
Feelings of guilt	36 (14.4)	16 (24.2)	47 (58.8)	A < B, B < C, A < C
Decreased concentration	60 (24.0)	20 (30.3)	54 (67.5)	B < C, A < C
Suicidal ideation	2 (0.8)	2 (3.0)	18 (22.5)	B < C, A < C

* All symptoms are significantly more frequent in major depression compared to no depression.

Case A

When Dr. R. recounted her stroke, she remembered feeling, almost instanta-
neously, an inability to understand what people were saying to her. She was in her
early 50s and had just returned from a year of teaching and research abroad. As
a distinguished historian, she had just completed a sabbatical year and was sought
after by many universities. Although her father had died in his 50s of a heart attack,
there was no family history of stroke. Her mother, a retired school teacher and hospital administrator was in good health in her 70s. It was a devastating symptom for
someone whose life depended upon her ability to use language.

After the onset of her stroke, a series of other symptoms rapidly developed over
the next few minutes. She was unable to move her right-side, she had lost sensation
on that side of her body, she was unable to see in her right visual field, and she was
unable to speak.

The first time I saw her was 3 years later. After 3 months in a rehabilitation hospital, her physical and speech recovery had been an enormous uphill battle. A year
later she began having seizures. Two years after the stroke, while trying to walk, she
fell down the stairs and sustained a traumatic brain injury including a subdural
hematoma. She again was admitted to hospital and underwent surgery to evacuate
the hematoma. Three years after the original stroke, although she was able to understand all but the most complicated sentences, she was unable to speak a coherent
sentence, to read or to write.

Depression began almost immediately after the stroke. She had recurrent episodes of depression that would last for many months. Eventually, the depression would begin to show some improvement, but then relapse. When I saw her, the depression was readily evident. She had crying spells in my office, admitted to feelings of hopelessness and expressed feelings that life was not worth living. The profoundness of her depression, however, was matched by her intense preoccupation with recovering her ability to read and write. For many months she had been focused on the idea that she was going to read and write again. Although this preoccupation with recapturing her lost identity was understandable, the obstacles were almost insurmountable. During this current episode of depression, for the first time, she had refused to go to speech therapy, lost interest in virtually all activities, became socially and emotionally withdrawn, lost interest in sex, felt like a worthless person, had difficulty concentrating, cried frequently, and felt there was no hope that she would ever recover.

Case B

At the time I first saw Mr. B., he had been depressed for 7 months. He was 59 years old and had been married for 34 years. He had been raised on a farm and still lived in a rural area. He had completed 2 years of college and worked for many years as a state auditor. He had suffered rheumatic heart disease as a child and at 39 had undergone electrical cardioversion to convert his heart from atrial fibrillation to normal sinus rhythm. As a result of the rheumatic heart disease, at age 50 he underwent open heart surgery for replacement of the mitral valve. After the surgery, he took anticoagulants and diuretic medications. His stroke occurred during sleep. He woke up disoriented to both time and place. He also noted ringing in his ears and difficulty seeing on the right side.

When I saw Mr. B., he did not look profoundly depressed but reported that his low mood began within a few days after the stroke. The depression was more severe on some days than it was on others but it had continued at some level for the past 7 months. Although the patient's father had died 2 months after his stroke, his grief did not seem to be excessive or to be a cause of his prolonged depression. Mr. B. reported symptoms of anxiety, tension, restlessness, worry, low energy, and loss of interest in activities that he previously enjoyed such as eating out or shopping. He also felt hopeless but did not report a change in his appetite, sleep, or ability to concentrate.

In addition to these symptoms of depression, Mr. B. was preoccupied by fears of having another stroke. Although he had returned to work, he was frightened that his performance would not be up to his supervisor's standards and that he would be forced to take a disability retirement.

Mr. B.'s depression responded to psychotherapeutic treatment. Talking about his concerns, reassurance about his capacity to make appropriate decisions and recognizing that he had an unfounded and exaggerated fear of complete loss of control of his life were enough to improve his depression without antidepressant medication.

Reliability and validity of diagnoses

The use of diagnostic criteria in psychiatry ultimately requires both demonstration of reliability as well as validity. We examined the use of a rating scale or a screening instrument, the Center for Epidemiological Studies-Depression Scale (CES-D), for diagnosis of poststroke depression compared with diagnoses based on standard PSE interview and DSM-III diagnostic criteria (Parikh *et al.* 1988). This study compared diagnoses in 80 patients who were interviewed using both the CES-D and the PSE with diagnosis based on DSM-III criteria. Using a cutoff point of 21 or greater on the CES-D, the specificity, sensitivity, and positive predictive value (PPV) of the CES-D for the diagnosis of major or minor depression was 94% specificity, 72% sensitivity, and 85% PPV using the PSE interview and DSM-III criteria as the gold standard (Parikh *et al.* 1988). The optimal CES-D score, however, was 16 which had a sensitivity of 90%, a specificity of 86%, a PPV of 80%, and a negative predictive value of 93%. The Spearman correlation between CES-D score and diagnosis of major, minor, or no depression was rho -0.53, $p < 0.001$ in-hospital. Thus, although an optimal number may be selected for an instrument to screen for poststroke depression, there are always patients with depression who are missed as well as patients without depression who are included in the sample. Thus, the diagnosis of poststroke depression for both accuracy and consistency across the literature should be based on a structured or semi-structured interview and DSM-IV criteria.

Aben *et al.* (2002) recently examined the reliability and validity of diagnoses comparing self-rated and interview-rated scales for the diagnosis of poststroke depression utilizing 202 stroke patients examined 1 month after their first ever ischemic stroke. Determining optimal cutoff values, the sensitivity of the self-rated scales varied between 80% and 90% while the specificity was approximately 60% compared with the gold standard of a structured interview (i.e., SCID-I-R) (First *et al.* 1996) and DSM-IV diagnostic criteria. The best rating scale was the observer rated Hamilton depression rating scale (HDRS) which had a sensitivity of 78.1% and a specificity of 74.6%. Interestingly, the instruments had higher sensitivity and specificity in men compared with women. Thus, even using optimal cutoff scores, severity rating scales are not satisfactory substitutes for diagnostic criteria.

The issue of reliability for elicitation of symptoms using structured or semi-structured interviews is discussed in Chapter 7, Phenomenology and specificity of depressive symptoms. Once the symptoms are elicited, an algorithm can be selected to determine whether the patient meets the DSM-IV diagnostic criteria for major or minor depression. We have used this technique for the investigation of the validity of distinguishing minor depression from major depression. The question which gives rise to this study is whether or not depressive disorder following stroke should be seen as a continuum or whether there are distinct forms of major and minor depression. The concept of subsyndromal depressive disorder has received increasing attention and numerous studies have provided validation for the distinction between major and minor depression (Judd *et al.* 1998). The previously cited study by Spalletta *et al.* (2005) found that the frequency of decreased concentration, psychomotor disturbance decreased interest/pleasure, weight/appetite decrease, and suicidal ideation were all significantly greater in the 50 patients with poststroke major depression compared with 62 patients with minor depression.

Our validation study of major versus minor poststroke depression included 301 consecutive admissions to the University of Maryland Hospital in Baltimore with acute stroke (Paradiso and Robinson 1999). All patients who had a computed tomography (CT) or magnetic resonance imaging (MRI) verified single first ever lesion of either the left ($n = 64$) or right ($n = 77$) hemisphere that was compatible with their acute stroke symptoms were selected. Thirty patients (22%) had a DSM-IV diagnosis of minor depression, 24 (17%) had a DSM-IV diagnosis of mood disorder due to stroke with major depressive-like episode, and 87 patients (62%) were non-depressed.

Results demonstrated that a previous personal history of psychiatric disorder was significantly more frequent among patients with major depression (30.4%) versus minor depression (3.4%) ($p < 0.02$). In addition, significantly more patients with major depression had lesions whose anterior border was less than 40% of the anterior-posterior (AP) distance on CT scan (83.3%) compared to the patients with minor depression (56.7%) ($p < 0.05$). In addition, minor depression was significantly associated with a greater frequency of left hemisphere lesions and younger age when compared with control patients. Thirty-one of 87 control patients (35.6%) had a left hemisphere lesion compared with 20 of 30 (66.7%) with minor depression. Furthermore, the posterior border of the lesion was farther from the frontal pole in patients with minor depression compared with control subjects (i.e., 67.7% $\pm$ 22.0 SD of total AP measurement for minor depression versus 54.3 $\pm$ 21.0 SD for control subjects, $p < 0.02$). No differences were found in lesion volume. In addition, there was a significant positive correlation between Ham-D and distance of both the anterior (Spearman's rho $= 0.18, p < 0.05$), and posterior (Spearman's rho $= 0.27, p < 0.005$) border of the lesion from the frontal pole for patients with minor depression, or no depression (Fig. 5.1).

When patients with major depression were compared to patients with minor depression, only 4 of 24 patients (16.7%) with major depression had posterior lesions (anterior border greater than 40% of AP distance) compared to 14 of 30

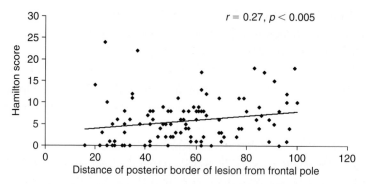

Figure 5.1   Scatterplot of the relationship between the distance of the posterior border of the lesion
from the frontal pole (as a percentage of the overall A–P distance) and the severity of
depression symptoms as measured by the Ham-D among patients with minor *poststroke*
depression or no mood disorder ($r = 0.27$, $p < 0.005$) reprinted with permission from
Paradiso and Robinson (1999).

patients (43.3%) with minor depression ($p = 0.03$). Finally, among patients with
major depression, 17 of 24 (71%) also met DSM-IV symptom criteria for generalized anxiety disorder (GAD), while only 7 of 84 (8%) of non-depressed patients,
and 9 of 30 (30%) with minor depressions had associated GAD. The patients with
minor depression had significantly more GAD diagnoses than control patients and
significantly less GAD diagnoses than patients with major depression ($p < 0.006$).

In addition to this study which was specifically aimed at distinguishing patients
with minor depression from those with major depression, we will show in Chapter 14
that, in contrast to patients with major depression, patients with minor depression
do not demonstrate a cognitive impairment related to depression.

Other diagnostic categories

Besides major and minor depression, the other diagnostic category, which may
sometimes be applicable to patients with poststroke depression, is adjustment disorder with depressed mood or adjustment disorder with mixed anxiety and
depressed mood. These diagnoses using DSM-IV criteria are based on the existence of depressed mood, tearfulness, or feelings of hopelessness with or without
nervousness, worry, or jitteriness occurring within 3 months of the onset of an
identified source of social stress. These depressive symptoms must be accompanied
either by stress in excess of what would be expected from exposure to the stressor
or by significant impairment in social or occupational functioning. The symptoms
must not represent bereavement, exacerbation of a preexisting axis I or axis II disorder, or be present for more than 6 months after termination of the stressor.

If the psychosocial stressor may be seen as the loss of job or social role which may result from the cognitive or physical impairments produced by stroke, this diagnosis may be appropriate. Several investigators have used this category for diagnosing patients with depression following stroke (House *et al.* 1991). The diagnosis of adjustment disorder does not require any specific symptoms. Furthermore, judgments about whether the distress is in excess of what would be expected or whether the depression *per se* has led to social or occupational impairment are often difficult determinations to make in patients with physical and mental impairments following stroke. Another difficult judgment is when the stressor is gone. Since we know that depressions last more than 6 months, the stressor would have to be seen as extended beyond the acute stroke period, but how long? The lack of specificity of symptomatology and the ambiguity of defining criteria make this an unappealing research diagnosis. Most researchers, therefore, have chosen to distinguish major depression and frequently minor depression associated with stroke. I believe that adjustment disorders or dysthymic disorders with duration of depressive symptoms for greater than 2 years are only rarely applicable to patients with poststroke mood disorders. The consistency of diagnosis would be improved if poststroke depression diagnoses were restricted to major or minor depressive disorder.

In summary, the diagnosis of poststroke depression should be based on the use of a structured or semi-structured psychiatric interview to elicit symptoms of depression and the DSM-IV diagnostic criteria for mood disorder due to stroke with major depressive like episode or minor depression. We have demonstrated that there are significant differences between patients with major depression and minor depression in the frequency of personal history of psychiatric disorder as well as distance of the anterior border of the lesion from the frontal pole and Spalletta has shown differences in the frequency of five of the nine symptoms of major depression. Patients with minor depression during the acute poststroke period tend to have posterior lesions of the left hemisphere while patients with major depression tend to have anterior left hemisphere lesions. In addition, depression related cognitive impairment is associated with major depression but not minor depression. Although additional studies will be needed to validate the diagnosis of both major and minor depression in the stroke population, at least the process has begun of demonstrating that there are clinical variables, symptom frequency, and pathological variables which distinguish major depression from minor depression.

Ultimately the validation of diagnostic categories requires that a specific etiology, pathophysiology of the disorder be identified. Since this level of validation has not been established for any of the psychiatric disorders, studies aimed at showing differences among diagnostic criteria in terms of clinical presentation, longitudinal course, clinical correlates, pathological correlates, and response to treatment have been used to validate diagnostic categories in psychiatry. Several investigations have been able to demonstrate differences between major and minor depression as outlined in this chapter and have provided some initial validation for the importance of distinguishing major and minor depression.

REFERENCES

Aben, I., Verhey, F., Lousberg, R., *et al.* Validity of the Beck depression inventory, Hospital anxiety and depression scale, SCL-90, and Hamilton depression rating scale as screening instruments for depression in stroke patients. *Psychosomatics* (2002) 43(5):386–393.

American Psychiatric Association. *Diagnostic and Statistical Manual of Mental Disorder-DSM-IV-TR.* American Psychiatric Association 2000, Washington, DC.

Andersen, G., Vestergaard, K., Riis, J. O., *et al.* Incidence of post-stroke depression during the first year in a large unselected stroke population determined using a valid standardized rating scale. *Acta Psychiatr Scand* (1994) 90:190–195.

Collin, S. J., Tinson, D., and Lincoln, N. B. Depression after stroke. *Clin Rehabil* (1987) 1:27–32.

Desmond, D. W., Remien, R. H., Moroney, J. T., *et al.* Ischemic stroke and depression. *J Int Neuropsychol Soc* (2003) 9(3):429–439.

Eastwood, M. R., Rifat, S. L., Nobbs, H., *et al.* Mood disorder following cerebrovascular accident. *Br J Psychiatr* (1989) 154:195–200.

Feighner, J. P., Robins, E., Guze, S. B., *et al.* Diagnostic criteria for use in psychiatry research. *Arch Gen Psychiatr* (1972) 26:57–63.

First, M. B., Donovan, S., and Frances, A. Nosology of chronic mood disorders. *Psychiatr Clin North Am* (1996) 19(1):29–39.

House, A., Dennis, M., Warlow, C., *et al.* The relationship between intellectual impairment and mood disorder in the first year after stroke. *Psychol Med* (1990) 20:805–814.

House, A., Dennis, M., Mogridge, L., *et al.* Mood disorders in the year after first stroke. *Br J Psychiatr* (1991) 158:83–92.

Judd, L. L., Akiskal, H. S., Maser, J. D., *et al.* A prospective 12-year study of subsyndromal and syndromal depressive symptoms in unipolar major depressive disorders. *Arch Gen Psychiatr* (1998) 55(8):694–700.

Kotila, M., Numminen, H., Waltimo, O., *et al.* Depression after stroke. Results of the FINNSTROKE study. *Stroke* (1998) 29:368–372.

Morris, P. L. P., Robinson, R. G., and Raphael, B. Prevalence and course of depressive disorders in hospitalized stroke patients. *Int J Psychiatr Med* (1990) 20:349–364.

Paradiso, S., and Robinson, R. G. Minor depression after stroke. An initial validation of the DSM-IV construct. *Am J Geriatr Psychiatr* (1999) 7(3):244–251.

Parikh, R. M., Eden, D. T., Price, T. R., *et al.* The sensitivity and specificity of the Center for Epidemiologic Studies depression scale as a screening instrument for post-stroke depression. *Int J Psychiatr Med* (1988) 18:169–181.

Pohjasvaara, T., Leppavuori, A., Siira, I., *et al.* Frequency and clinical determinants of poststroke depression. *Stroke* (1998) 29:2311–2317.

Robinson, R. G. Stroke. In E. C. Lauterbach, ed., *Psychiatric Management in Neurological Disease*. American Psychiatric Association, Washington DC, 2000, 219–247.

Robinson, R. G., and Price, T. R. Post-stroke depressive disorders: a follow-up study of 103 out-patients. *Stroke* (1982) 13:635–641.

Sinyor, D., Amato, P., and Kaloupek, P. Post-stroke depression: relationship to functional impairment, coping strategies, and rehabilitation outcome. *Stroke* (1986) 17:112–117.

Spalletta, G., Ripa, A., and Caltagirone, C. Symptom profile of DSM-IV major and minor depressive disorders in first-ever stroke patients. *Am J Geriatr Psychiatr* (2005) 13(2):108–115.

Wade, D. T., Legh-Smith, J., and Hewer, R. A. Depressed mood after stroke, a community study of its frequency. *Br J Psychiatr* (1987) 151:200–205.

6

Prevalence of depressive disorders

The prevalence of poststroke depression has been assessed in a large number of patients who have been examined in various settings throughout the world. Since the first edition of this text, large numbers of patient populations have been added to the literature and pooling of the data has provided prevalence rates based on more than 6000 patients. There are at least three factors which have complicated the determination of prevalence rates. The first is the setting in which patients were examined. Community studies have generally reported somewhat lower prevalence rates than studies done in hospital outpatient settings. Community studies have generally included many patients who had very mild or frequently no motor sensory or other neurological symptoms associated with their stroke. Thus, some of these patients have such minimal brain injury that they would not be expected to have stroke-induced depression. On the other hand, patients with more severe motor sensory or other physical symptoms of stroke who have been hospitalized would be expected to have more severe brain damage and higher rates of depression reflecting the association between severity of depression and severity of physical impairments associated with stroke.

The second factor which has complicated prevalence studies of poststroke depression is the number of patients who are excluded from studies of poststroke depression. Patients with hemorrhagic rather than ischemic stroke, decreased level of consciousness, fatigue, prior stroke, other brain injury, comorbid physical illness, atypical strokes due to collagen disease, or other systemic illness, comprehension deficits due to fluent aphasias or global aphasias have been excluded from some studies or all studies of poststroke depression. Although some investigators have tried to estimate the frequency of depression in some of these patients based on behavioral observations (Egelko et al. 1989; Damecour and Caplan 1991), no reliable method has been devised to examine patients who are unable to reliably respond to a verbal interview. Examiner judgments about whether a patient is depressed depending upon observation of behavior such as difficulty falling asleep, waking up early in the morning, not eating, losing weight, frequent tearfulness, social withdrawal, or acts of self harm are often unreliable. In addition, making a diagnosis of depression based on only observed behavior would require that these new diagnostic criteria be validated. Based on observations in patients without comprehension deficits we know that symptoms, such as insomnia, decreased appetite, decreased energy, can occur in patients who deny depressed mood (Fedoroff *et al.* 1991). Furthermore, although some of these patients with comprehension deficits who may have improved in some of these symptoms (e.g., insomnia) after receiving antidepressants, the diagnosis of depressive disorder still remains uncertain. Until we have a laboratory test for depression or some other non-verbal means of diagnosing depression, it will be impossible to know for sure if the patient who cannot provide reliable responses to questions about their subjective mental state has a depressive disorder. Therefore, as a result of patient exclusions in all studies of poststroke depression, prevalence estimates must be understood as rates based on the limited stroke population that was examined.

Based on our findings in patients with mild comprehension deficits, however, patients with comprehension deficits do not appear to have a significantly greater frequency of depression than those without comprehension deficits (Robinson and Benson 1981; Starkstein and Robinson 1988; Herrmann *et al.* 1993) (see Chapter 15). Therefore, it is likely that the prevalence rate for poststroke depression are not dramatically distorted by the absence of patients with comprehension impairments or patients with decreased level of consciousness but this issue remains uncertain.

The third factor which has led to variability in reported prevalence rates for poststroke depression is the use of cutoff scores on depression rating scales for the diagnosis of depression. As can be seen in Table 6.1. There are many studies which have used cutoff scores on a depression rating scale rather than a structured interview and established diagnostic criteria such as the Diagnostic and Statistical Manual (DSM-IV) or International Classification of Diseases (ICD-10). As discussed in Chapter 5, a cutoff score only approximates a diagnosis and prevalence rates should be determined using standardized diagnostic criteria.

The "prevalence" rates from studies reported in the literature are shown in Table 6.1 divided by the setting in which patients were examined. The lowest prevalence rates for depressive disorder were found in patients studied in community settings. Prevalence rates in acute hospitals, rehabilitation hospitals, and outpatient settings have been quite similar. The mean prevalence for major depression in community studies was 14% while the prevalence rate for minor depression was 9%. In acute hospital or rehabilitation hospital studies, the mean prevalence rate of major depression was 19% and minor depression was 30%. In outpatient settings which have varied between 3 months and 3 or more years followings stroke, the mean prevalence rate for major depression was 24% and for minor depression was 24%.

Table 6.1. Prevalence studies of poststroke depression

Investigators	Patient population	N	Criteria	Major (%)	Minor (%)	Total (%)
Wade et al. (1987)	Community	379	Cutoff score	11		22
House et al. (1991)	Community	89	PSE-DSM-III	11	12	23
Burvill et al. (1995)	Community	294	PSE-DSM-III	15	8	23
Kotila et al. (1998)	Community	321	Cutoff score			44
Hayee et al. (2001)	Community	161	Cutoff BDE, 3 months			41
		156	Cutoff BDE 12 months			42
Stewart et al. (2001)	Community	287	Cutoff score, GDS			19
Desmond et al. (2003)	Community	421	Cutoff, struct Ham-D			11
Pooled data means for community studies		2108		14.1	9.1	25.9
Robinson et al. merged data (1983–1990)	Acute hospital	278	PSE-DSM-IV	27	20	47
Ebrahim et al. (1987)	Acute hospital	149	Cutoff score			23
Shima et al. (1994)	Hospital (1–2 months)			9		9
Gonzalez-Torrecillas et al. (1995)	Hospital	130	SADS, RDC	26	11	37
Astrom et al. (1993)	Acute hospital	80	DSM-III	25	NR	25*
Herrmann et al. (1993)	Acute hospital	21	RDC	24	14	38
Andersen et al. (1994)	Acute hospital or outpatient	285	HDRS cutoff	10	11	21
Kauhanen et al. (1999)	Stroke unit (3 months)	106	DSM-III-R	9	44	53
Palomaki et al. (1999)	Hospital	100	DSM-III-R	6		6
Gainotti et al. (1999)	Acute or Rehabilitation Hospital	153	PSDRS	31	NR	31
Aben et al. (2002)	Acute hospital	190	SCID & DSM-IV	23	16	39
Singh et al. (2000)	Acute hospital (3 months)	81	Cutoff score, Zung, MADRS	26	27	53
Berg et al. (2003)	Acute hospital (2 weeks)	89	Cutoff BDI			27
House et al. (2001)	Acute hospital	448	ICD 10	22	NR	22+
Pooled data means for acute hospital studies		2178		22.1	17.3	31.6

Study	Setting	N	Diagnostic method			
Folstein et al. (1977)	Rehabilitation hospital	20	PSE & items			45
Finklestein et al. (1982)	Rehabilitation hospital	25	Cutoff score			48
Sinyor et al. (1986)	Rehabilitation hospital	64	Cutoff score			47
Finset et al. (1989)	Rehabilitation hospital	42	Cutoff score			36
Eastwood et al. (1989)	Rehabilitation hospital	87	SADS-RDC	10	40	50
Morris et al. (1990)	Rehabilitation hospital	99	CIDI-DSM-III	14	21	35
Schubert et al. (1992)	Rehabilitation hospital	18	DSM-III-R	28	44	72
Schwartz et al. (1993)	Rehabilitation hospital	91	DSM-III	40	NR	40*
Robinson (2000)		95	DSM-IV	14	28	42
Cassidy et al. (2004)	Rehabilitation hospital	50	DSM-IV	20	NR	20+
Pooled data for rehabilitation hospital studies		591		19.3	30.4	40.8+
Pooled data for acute and rehabilitation hospital studies		2769		21.6	20.0	33.6
Kauhanen et al. (1999)	Outpatient (1 year)	92	DSM-III-R	16	26	42
Palomaki et al. (1999)	Outpatient (12 months)	44	DSM-III-R	11	NR	11
	(18 months)	44	DSM-III-R	16	NR	16
Gainotti et al. (1999)	Outpatient <2 months	58	DSM-III-R	27	NR	27+
	2–4 months	52	DSM-III-R	27	NR	27
	>4 months	43	DSM-III-R	40	NR	40+
Pohjasvaara (1998)	Outpatient	277	SCAN DSM-IV	26	14	40
Feibel et al. (1982)	Outpatient (6 months)	91	Nursing evaluation			26
Robinson and Price (1982)	Outpatient (6 months–10 years)	103	Cutoff score			29
Robinson et al. (1983–1990)	Merged data (3 months)	77	DSM-IV	17	27	44
	(6 months)	79	DSM-IV	20	27	47
	(12 months)	70	DSM-IV	10	24	34
	(24 months)	66	DSM-IV	24	15	39
Herrmann et al. (1998)	Outpatient	150	MDRS, Zung			27
Singh et al. (2000)	Outpatient (1 year)	136	Cutoff score MDRS, Zung			22
Kim et al. (2000)	Outpatient (2–4 months)	148	DSM-IV, BDI, PSE-I	18	NR	18

Table 6.1. (*Continued*)

Investigators	Patient population	N	Criteria	Major (%)	Minor (%)	Total (%)
Collin *et al.* (1987)	Outpatient	111	Cutoff score			42
Astrom *et al.* (1993)	Outpatient (3 months)	77	DSM-III	31	NR	31*
	(1 year)	73	DSM-III	16	NR	16*
	(2 years)	57	DSM-III	19	NR	19*
	(3 years)	49	DSM-III	29	NR	29*
Castillo *et al.* (1995)	Outpatient (3 months)	77	PSE-DSM-III	20	13	33
	(6 months)	80	PSE-DSM-III	21	21	42
	(1 year)	70	PSE-DSM-III	11	16	27
	(2 years)	67	PSE-DSM-III	18	17	35
Pooled data for outpatient studies		2191		24.0	23.9	31.5+
Pooled data for all studies		7068		21.7	19.5	30.6

Note: BDI: Beck depression inventory; CIDI: composite international diagnostic interview; DSM: diagnostic and statistical manual; HDRS: Hamilton depression rating scale; ICD: international classification of diseases; MADRS: Montgomery aspery depression rating scale; NR: not reported. *Because minor depression was not included, these values may be low; PSDRS: poststroke depression rating scale; PSE: present state examination; RDC: research diagnostic criteria; SADS: schedule for affective disorders and schizophrenia; SCAN: schedules for clinical assessment in neuropsychiatry. SCID: structured clinical interview for DSM-IV.

When these estimates of the prevalence of poststroke depression are combined with the annual incidence of stroke in the USA, of approximately 500,000 new strokes and 100,000 recurrent strokes per year (see Chapter 1), the major impact of poststroke depression can be appreciated. Based on an acute poststroke survival rate of approximately 75%, 220,000 new cases of poststroke depression would occur in the acute or rehabilitation hospital setting each year in the USA.

These new cases of poststroke major and minor depression are then compounded by the fact that these depressions last an average of almost 1 year for major depression (a minority of cases last 3 years or more) and minor depression may last from a few months to 2 or more years or develop into major depression. In addition, many patients develop late-onset depression several months after the brain injury. We have found that the risk period for developing poststroke depression lasts for at least 2 years and Astrom *et al.* (1993) reported that the prevalence of major depression increased between 2 and 3 years poststroke from 19% to 29%.

Based on 2 years of follow-up data on 357 patients that we examined with acute stroke, combining four acute and rehabilitation hospital studies, 19.9% had major and 17.6% developed minor depression during the acute stroke period, while another 16.3% developed major depression and 37.4% developed minor depression during the first year, 8.3% developed major depression and 10.4% developed minor depression during the second year after stroke. Thus, if patients who died or were lost to follow-up are excluded, 44.5% of patients developed a major depression and 65.4% developed a minor depression some time during the 2 years of follow-up. At any one time point the mean prevalence rates for major and minor depression were 14.6% and 18.3% and, based on the 158 patients seen at 1 or 2 years follow-up, 37.3% had never developed a known depression.

Based on a prevalence estimates by the American Heart Association, there are 4.4 million stroke survivors in the USA. Using our worldwide mean outpatient depression rates, there would be 2.1 million patients at any one time with poststroke depression, almost half of these cases being major depression. It is likely that 3 million of these patients would have been depressed at some time since their initial stroke. Thus, there are millions of people worldwide who are afflicted with these depressive disorders. The financial impact of these depressive disorders has never been studied but the enormity of the problem is obvious from these statistics.

In summary, depression appears to be the most common and the most severe emotional disorder associated with stroke. Furthermore, the consistent findings that poststroke depression is associated with impaired recovery in cognitive function (see Chapter 14), impaired recovery in activities of daily living (see Chapter 13), and increased mortality (see Chapter 19) supports the conclusion that among all the emotional disorders following stroke, depression produces the most severe consequences for patients.

REFERENCES

Aben, I., Verhey, F., Lousberg, R., *et al.* Validity of the Beck depression inventory, Hospital anxiety and depression scale, SCL-90, and Hamilton depression rating scale as screening instruments for depression in stroke patients. *Psychosomatics* (2002) 43(5):386–393.

Andersen, G., Vestergaard, K., Riis, J. O., *et al.* Incidence of post-stroke depression during the first year in a large unselected stroke population determined using a valid standardized rating scale. *Acta Psychiatr Scand* (1994) 90:190–195.

Astrom, M., Adolfsson, R., and Asplund, K. Major depression in stroke patients: a 3-year longitudinal study. *Stroke* (1993) 24:976–982.

Berg, A., Psych, L., Palomaki, H., *et al.* Poststroke depression – an 18-month follow-up. *Stroke* (2003) 34(1):138–143.

Burvill, P. W., Johnson, G. A., Jamrozik, K. D., *et al.* Prevalence of depression after stroke: the Perth Community Stroke Study. *Br J Psychiatr* (1995) 166:320–327.

Cassidy, E., O'Connor, R., and O'Keane, V. Prevalence of post-stroke depression in an Irish sample and its relationship with disability and outcome following inpatient rehabilitation. *Disabil Rehabil* (2004) 26(2):71–77.

Castillo, C. S., Schultz, S. K., and Robinson, R. G. Clinical correlates of early-onset and late-onset poststroke generalized anxiety. *Am J Psychiatr* (1995) 152:1174–1179.

Collin, S. J., Tinson, D., and Lincoln, N. B. Depression after stroke. *Clin Rehabil* (1987) 1:27–32.

Damecour, C. L., and Caplan, D. The relationship of depression to symptomatology and lesion site in aphasic patients. *Cortex* (1991) 27:385–401.

Desmond, D. W., Remien, R. H., Moroney, J. T., *et al.* Ischemic stroke and depression. *J Int Neuropsychol Soc* (2003) 9(3):429–439.

Eastwood, M. R., Rifat, S. L., Nobbs, H., *et al.* Mood disorder following cerebrovascular accident. *Br J Psychiatr* (1989) 154:195–200.

Ebrahim, S., Barer, D., and Nouri, F. Affective illness after stroke. *Br J Psychiatr* (1987) 151:52–56.

Egelko, S., Simon, R. E., Gordon, W. A., *et al.* First year after stroke: tracking cognitive and affective deficits. *Arch Phys Med Rehabil* (1989) 70:297–302.

Fedoroff, J. P., Lipsey, J. R., Starkstein, S. E., *et al.* Phenomenological comparison of major depression following stroke, myocardial infarction or spinal cord lesion. *J Affect Disord* (1991) 22:83–89.

Feibel, J. H., and Springer, C. J. Depression and failure to resume social activities after stroke. *Arch Phys Med Rehabil* (1982) 63:276–278.

Finklestein, S., Benowitz, L. I., Baldessarini, R. J., *et al.* Mood, vegetative disturbance, and dexamethasone suppression test after stroke. *Ann Neurol* (1982) 12:463–468.

Finset, A., Goffeng, L., Landro, N. I., *et al.* Depressed mood and intra-hemispheric location of lesion in right hemisphere stroke patients. *Scand J Rehabil Med* (1989) 21:1–6.

Folstein, M. F., Maiberger, R., and McHugh, P. R. Mood disorder as a specific complication of stroke. *J Neurol Neurosurg Psychiatr* (1977) 40:1018–1020.

Gainotti, G., Azzoni, A., and Marra, C. Frequency, phenomenology and anatomical-clinical correlates of major poststroke depression. *Br J Psychiatr* (1999) 175:163–167.

Gonzalez-Torrecillas, J. L., Mendlewicz, J., and Lobo, A. Effects of early treatment of poststroke depression on neuropsychological rehabilitation. *Int Psychogeriatr* (1995) 7(4):547–560.

Hayee, M. A., Akhtar, N., Haque, A., *et al.* Depression after stroke-analysis of 297 stroke patients. *Bangladesh Med Res Counc Bull* (2001) 27(3):96–102.

Herrmann, M., Bartles, C., and Wallesch, C.-W. Depression in acute and chronic aphasia: symptoms, pathoanatomical-clinical correlations and functional implications. *J Neurol Neurosurg Psychiatr* (1993) 56:672–678.

Herrmann, N., Black, S. E., Lawrence, J., *et al*. The Sunnybrook stroke study. A prospective study of depressive symptoms and functional outcome. *Stroke* (1998) 29:618–624.

House, A., Dennis, M., Mogridge, L., *et al*. Mood disorders in the year after first stroke. *Br J Psychiatr* (1991) 158:83–92.

House, A., Knapp, P., Bamford, J., *et al*. Mortality at 12 and 24 months after stroke may be associated with depressive symptoms at 1 month. *Stroke* (2001) 32(3):696–701.

Kauhanen, M., Korpelainen, J. T., Hiltunen, P., *et al*. Poststroke depression correlates with cognitive impairment and neurological deficits. *Stroke* (1999) 30(9):1875–1880.

Kim, J. S., and Choi-Kwon, S. Poststroke depression and emotional incontinence: correlation with lesion location. *Neurology* (2000) 54(9):1805–1810.

Kotila, M., Numminen, H., Waltimo, O., *et al*. Depression after stroke. Results of the FINNSTROKE study. *Stroke* (1998) 29:368–372.

Morris, P. L. P., Robinson, R. G., and Raphael, B. Prevalence and course of depressive disorders in hospitalized stroke patients. *Int J Psychiatr Med* (1990) 20:349–364.

Palomaki, H., Kaste, M., Berg, A., *et al*. Prevention of poststroke depression: 1 year randomised placebo controlled double blind trial of mainserin with 6 month followup after therapy. *J Neurol Neurosurg Psychiatr* (1999) 66:490–494.

Pohjasvaara, T., Leppavuori, A., Siira, I., *et al*. Frequency and clinical determinants of poststroke depression. *Stroke* (1998) 29:2311–2317.

Robinson, R. G. Stroke. In E. C. Lauterbach, ed., *Psychiatric Management in Neurological Disease*. American Psychiatric Association, Washington DC, 2000, 219–247.

Robinson, R. G., and Benson, D. F. Depression in aphasic patients: frequency, severity and clinical-pathological correlations. *Brain Lang* (1981) 14:282–291.

Robinson, R. G., and Price, T. R. Poststroke depressive disorders: a follow-up study of 103 outpatients. *Stroke* (1982) 13:635–641.

Schubert, D. S. P., Taylor, C., Lee, S., *et al*. Physical consequences of depression in the stroke patient. *Gen Hosp Psychiatr* (1992) 14:69–76.

Schwartz, J. A., Speed, N. M., Brunberg, J. A., *et al*. Depression in stroke rehabilitation. *Biol Psychiatr* (1993) 33:694–699.

Shima, S., Kitagawa, Y., Kitamura, T., *et al*. Poststroke depression. *Gen Hosp Psychiatr* (1994) 16(4):286–289.

Singh, A., Black, S. E., Herrmann, N., *et al*. Functional and neuroanatomic correlations in poststroke depression: the Sunnybrook Stroke Study. *Stroke* (2000) 31:637–644.

Sinyor, D., Amato, P., and Kaloupek, P. Post-stroke depression: relationship to functional impairment, coping strategies, and rehabilitation outcome. *Stroke* (1986) 17:112–117.

Starkstein, S. E., and Robinson, R. G. Aphasia and depression. *Aphasiology* (1988) 2:1–20.

Stewart, R., Prince, M., Richards, M., *et al*. Stroke, vascular risk factors and depression – cross-sectional study in a UK Caribbean-born population. *Br J Psychiatr* (2001) 178:23–28.

Wade, D. T., Legh-Smith, J., and Hewer, R. A. Depressed mood after stroke, a community study of its frequency. *Br J Psychiatr* (1987) 151:200–205.

Phenomenology and specificity of depressive symptoms

Phenomenology refers to the study of the structure of observable events. In the study of poststroke depression, phenomenology refers to the study of signs and symptoms which constitute the basis for the diagnosis of depression. Since depression occurs in the context of an acute medical illness, one might naturally wonder whether these depressions are like depressions in patients without acute illness or whether the acute medical illness interferes with our ability to diagnose depression using standard diagnostic techniques.

As indicated in the first edition of this text, we have conducted several studies examining the phenomenology of poststroke depression compared with the signs and symptoms of depression in patients without brain injury. We have also examined the frequency of specific symptoms of poststroke depression compared with stroke patients who are not depressed to examine whether these symptoms may reflect physical illness or depressive disorder. The only other investigators who have specifically examined the phenomenology of poststroke depression are Spalletta *et al.* (2005) and Gainotti *et al.* (1997, 1999). In Chapter 5, I compared the findings of Spalletta *et al.* (2005) with our findings and showed that both studies found, among patients with poststroke major depression, the frequency of virtually every symptom was significantly greater than non-depressed stroke patients (Table 5.2).

The first study to examine the phenomenology with poststroke depression was conducted by our group examining frequency of depressive symptoms among a group of 43 patients with poststroke major depression to a group of 43 age comparable patients with depression without any known brain pathology (Lipsey *et al.* 1986). The mean ± SD ages were 58 ± 14 for poststroke depression and 58 ± 19 for functional depression. The frequency of males was 44% versus 37%, respectively; whites, 51% versus 77%; married, 35% versus 42%; and Hollingshead Class IV or V, 86% versus 63%. None of the demographic differences was statistically significant. Using the present state examination (PSE), both groups showed almost identical profiles of symptoms including symptoms that were not part of the diagnostic criteria for major depression (Fig. 7.1).

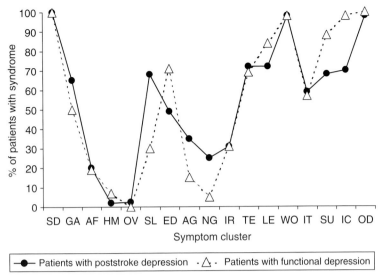

Figure 7.1   Patients with major depression following acute stroke (N = 43) were compared to age
comparable patients hospitalized for functional primary depression (N = 43). The
symptom clusters are "syndromes" derived from the semi-structured interview of the PSE.
SD: simple depression; GA: general anxiety; AF: affective flattening; HM: hypomania; OV:
overactivity; SL: slowness; ED: special features of depression; AG: agitation; NG: self-
neglect; IR: ideas of reference; TE: tension; LE: lack of energy; WO: worrying; IT: irritability;
SU: social unease; IC: loss of interest and concentration; and OD: other symptoms of
depression. Patients with primary and poststroke depressions showed the same frequency
of all syndromes except SL (stroke patients showed a higher frequency) and IC (primary
depression patients showed a higher frequency) (reprinted with permission from Lipsey
et al. 1986).

The only symptom clusters (i.e., groups of related symptoms clustered into
"syndromes" according to the criteria established for the PSE) (Wing *et al.* 1974)
that were significantly different between patients with functional major depression
and those with poststroke major depression were slowness (SL), which was more
frequent in the stroke patients and loss of interest and concentration (IC), which
was more frequent in the functional depression group (Fig. 7.1).

The fact that the symptom profiles only differed in 2 of 18 possible categories
suggests that major depression following stroke is probably quite similar to the primary depressive disorders (i.e., no brain injury) in the elderly.

Gainotti *et al.* (1997, 1999) also published studies comparing the phenomenology of poststroke depression with major depression in patients without brain
injury. The diagnosis of poststroke depression was made using the scale devised by
Gainotti *et al.* (1997) entitled the poststroke depression rating scale (PSDS). The

PSDS consists of 10 sections examining the following symptoms: (1) depressed mood, (2) guilt feelings, (3) thoughts of death or suicide, (4) vegetative disorders, (5) apathy and loss of interest, (6) anxiety, (7) catastrophic reactions, (8) hyper emotionalism, (9) anhedonia (i.e., inability to enjoy pleasant experiences), and (10) diurnal mood variation. The section on diurnal mood variation is scored -2, if there is both an unmotivated cause for depression and prominent increased severity of depression in the early morning. A score of $+2$, on the other hand, represents a clearly motivated cause for depression with the depression worsening during situations that bring out handicaps and disabilities. Inter-rater reliability between a neurologist's and a psychiatrist's use of the PSDS was examined in 33 stroke patients who were independently examined on the same day in the morning and early afternoon. Spearman rho correlation coefficients for each of the 10 sections ranged from 0.92 for depressed mood to 0.62 for diurnal mood variation (Gainotti et al. 1997). Using the PSDS, another group of 120 patients were examined using the PSDS and added to the original 33 (Gainotti et al. 1999). Dividing patients by time since stroke, 58 patients were examined within the first 2 months after stroke, 52 patients were examined between 2 and 4 months poststroke, and 43 were examined more than 4 months poststroke. These patients were compared with 30 patients hospitalized for major depression without known brain injury (i.e., primary depression). Statistical analysis of the mean scores obtained on each section of the PSDS showed a significantly higher score for patients with primary major depression compared to patients with poststroke major depression on depressed mood, feelings of guilt, suicidal thoughts, and anhedonia, while the patients with poststroke major depression had significantly higher scores on anxiety, catastrophic reactions, hyper emotionalism, and diurnal mood variations compared to the patients with primary depression. Furthermore, when Gainotti et al. examined time since stroke, there were no statistically significant differences in mean scores on the PSDS on any of the 10 sections among patients who were less than 2 months, 2–4 months, and greater than 4 months poststroke. Validity of the PSDS was examined by correlating scores on the Hamilton depression (Ham-D) rating scale with scores on the PSDS for a few symptoms including depressed mood, guilt feelings, suicidal thoughts, vegetative disorders, anhedonia, and anxiety. Spearman rho scores ranged from 0.41 for guilt feelings to 0.88 for vegetative disorders.

Does the demonstration by Gainotti et al. of differences between patients with primary depression and poststroke depression in a number of symptom areas, indicate that the PSDS constitutes a better way of diagnosing poststroke depression? To answer that question, I believe that each of the findings needs to be considered. First, the increased frequency of symptoms such as catastrophic reactions, hyper emotionalism, emotion lability, anxiety, or diurnal variation among patients with poststroke depression that are not used in the diagnosis of major depressive disorder must be shown to be an integral part of the syndrome of poststroke depression. In fact, the existing data on catastrophic reactions (Chapter 37), hyper emotionalism (Chapter 41), and anxiety (Chapter 30) demonstrate that these are comorbid disorders. Anxiety, catastrophic reactions, and emotional lability are all common disorders in patients with poststroke major depression. However, catastrophic reactions, anxiety, and pathological emotions also occur frequently in patients without poststroke depression. Furthermore, the duration of these disorders and the clinical and pathological correlates are almost always different than those of poststroke major depression. Thus, these disorders are comorbid disorders rather than integral components of poststroke major depressive disorder. Similarly, the fact that diurnal variation was scored based on whether the patient attributes their depression to the stroke-related disabilities only indicates that patients with poststroke depression tend to attribute their depression to their impairments regardless of whether or not this is truly the cause. The fact that there were no significant differences between patients with primary depression and poststroke depression in the frequency of vegetative symptoms and apathy (i.e., low energy) suggests similarities between these two kinds of depressive disorder. The second major finding was that depressed mood, anhedonia, feelings of guilt, and suicidal thoughts had higher mean scores among primary depression compared with poststroke depression patients. This finding may have been the result of comparing patients who were hospitalized for endogenous depression with patients who were being treated for stroke not depression. These selection criteria inevitably lead to more severe depressions in the endogenous depression compared to the poststroke depression group.

Finally, an assessment of the Gainotti *et al.* data must address the issue that the PSDS are clearly in conflict with the well-established criteria for the diagnosis of major depression in Diagnostic and Statistical Manual of Mental Disorder-IV Text Revised (DSM-IV-TR: American Psychiatric Association 2000). The addition of symptoms such as catastrophic reactions and hyper emotionalism would clearly change the phenomenology of major depression as we know it. Altering the symptoms that are widely accepted as criteria for major depression must be validated as defining a specific population of patients with a unique disorder. Validation of this new form of poststroke depressive disorder requires demonstration of a predictable duration of the disorder, specific associated clinical and pathological correlates, and responses to treatment that are not found when standard criteria are used. Our data presented here, Spalletta's data in Chapter 5, and the data of others in Chapter 8 on the course of depression, Chapter 23 on the treatment of poststroke depression, biological markers in Chapter 20, and the role of abnormalities of serotonergic function in Chapter 21 on the mechanism of poststroke depression, all suggest similarities rather than differences between endogenous and poststroke depression. It is possible, of course, that poststroke depression may have different mechanisms, and a different course than primary depression, but these differences have yet to be demonstrated. The large literature on primary depression in the elderly (Alexopoulos *et al.* 1997a, b; Krishnan *et al.* 1997) has shown that depression in the elderly is frequently associated with vascular ischemia seen as hyperintensities on MRI. These and other findings such as decreased frequency of family history of depression in the elderly (Hickie *et al.* 1995) suggest more similarities than differences in poststroke and primary major depression. I believe that the majority of current data supports the interpretation that poststroke depression is a form of major depression which is provoked in some patients by injury to strategic areas of the brain and others by social or psychological factors which involve the same final common pathways and pathophysiological changes as primary depression in the elderly. The next section will examine the specificity of symptoms used in the diagnosis of depressive disorder in patients with acute medical illnesses such as stroke. Since physical illnesses, such as stroke, may produce symptoms such as fatigue, weight loss, or sleep disturbance which are also used for the diagnosis of depression, we wanted to determine which "depressive" symptoms occurred as commonly in non-depressed as in depressed patients. Alternatively, we also wanted to determine whether the medical condition might have been masking depressive symptoms that would result in a failure to diagnose depression. It is well known that some types of brain injury can lead to unawareness of deficit (i.e., anosognosia) (Starkstein *et al.* 1993) (see Chapter 36) and a severe physical illness can lead to a denial of illness. This analysis, however, was different than the comparisons shown in Chapter 5 where patients with diagnosed depressions were compared for symptom frequency.

Using a combination of Baltimore plus Iowa patients who were hospitalized with an acute stroke, there were 125 who acknowledged the presence of a depressed mood for most of the time since stroke (no other symptom of depression was required). They were compared with 270 acute stroke patients without a depressed mood. The group with depressed mood was younger than the group without mood disturbance (57.4 ± 15 years versus 62.8 ± 13 years, respectively, $p = 0.0004$). They also had more impairment, as shown by their scores on the mini-mental state exam (MMSE) (22 ± 6 versus 24 ± 6, $p = 0.036$) and activities of daily living scale (i.e., Johns Hopkins functioning inventory or JHFI) (7.5 ± 5.4 versus 5.4 ± 4.8, $p = 0.0001$). Otherwise, there were no significant differences in the demographic characteristics or the level of impairment between the depressed and non-depressed groups. In order to examine a spectrum of depressive symptoms and not just the symptoms used in DSM-IV diagnostic criteria, we selected a number of psychological and vegetative depressive symptoms identified by Davidson and Turnbull (1986) as characteristic of depressive disorder.

The frequencies of each psychological and autonomic (i.e., vegetative or physiological) symptoms of depression were then compared between depressed and non-depressed groups (Table 7.1). All symptoms except social withdrawal were significantly more frequent among patients with a depressed mood than in patients without a depressed mood ($p < 0.001$).

The 125 patients with depressed mood had a significantly greater mean number of autonomic symptoms than the 270 patients without mood disturbance (3.2 ± 1.9 versus 1.2 ± 1.3) ($p < 0.001$). The depressed patients also had significantly more psychological symptoms than the non-depressed patients (4.0 ± 2.9 versus 1.2 ± 1.6) ($p < 0.001$). The frequency distributions for the total number of autonomic and

Table 7.1. Autonomic and psychological symptoms in acute stroke patients with and without depressed mood

Symptom	Depressed mood ($n = 125$) N (%)	Non-depressed mood ($n = 270$) N (%)	χ^2	P value*
Autonomic				
Anxiety	46 (37)	22 (8)	49.2	0.0001
Anxious foreboding	42 (34)	21 (8)	39.5	0.0001
Morning depression	81 (65)	19 (7)	147.3	0.0001
Weight loss	47 (39)	40 (15)	25.8	0.0001
Delayed sleep	50 (40)	37 (14)	32.5	0.0001
Subjective anergia	84 (67)	102 (38)	30.1	0.0001
Early awakening	41 (33)	41 (15)	14.0	0.0002
Loss of libido	33 (27)	30 (11)	14.0	0.0002
Psychological				
Worrying	80 (64)	52 (19)	75.4	0.0001
Brooding	47 (38)	21 (8)	49.7	0.0001
Loss of interest	47 (38)	6 (2)	88.4	0.0001
Hopelessness	41 (48)	25 (9)	31.7	0.0001
Suicidal plans	55 (44)	3 (1)	125.1	0.0001
Social withdrawal	19 (15)	29 (11)	1.5	0.2146
Self-depreciation	30 (24)	21 (8)	18.6	0.0001
Lack of self-confidence	36 (29)	22 (8)	27.0	0.0001
Simple ideas of reference	40 (32)	40 (15)	14.8	0.0001
Guilty ideas of reference	26 (21)	20 (7)	13.8	0.0002
Pathological guilt	28 (23)	23 (9)	13.7	0.0002
Irritability	54 (43)	35 (13)	42.3	0.0001

*Bonferroni corrected $p < 0.001$.

psychological symptoms are shown in Fig. 7.2. These bar graphs also show a smooth exponential decline in the percentage of non-depressed patients with psychological or vegetative symptoms of depression. Less than 5% of the non-depressed patients had three or more depressive symptoms. Depressed patients, on the other hand, appeared to have a biphasic distribution of symptoms. There were peaks in the percent of patients who had two symptoms or greater than five symptoms. This may suggest that there are two groups of depressions that differ in their number of associated psychological and autonomic symptoms.

The adequacy of DSM-IV criteria for major depression in this group of medically ill patients was assessed first by determining whether major depression was over diagnosed. There were 79 of the 395 patients who were assigned a DSM-IV

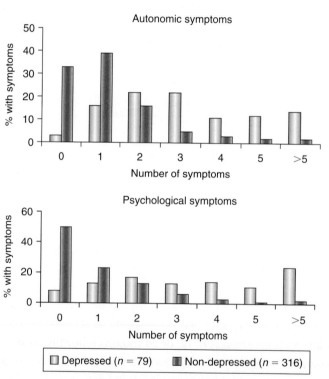

Figure 7.2   The percent of patients hospitalized with acute stroke who acknowledge autonomic (vegetative) symptoms (top panel) depression (see Table 7.1 for list of symptoms). Patients without depressed mood do acknowledge some vegetative and psychological symptoms of depression but significantly fewer than the depressed mood patients (3.6 ± 2.1 SD versus 1.0 ± 1.1, $p = 0.001$ for autonomic symptoms and 4.1 ± 2.8 SD versus 0.9 ± 1.2, $p = 0.001$ for psychological symptoms). Of the 29 patients with five or more autonomic symptoms, 27 had major and two had minor depression.

diagnosis of major depression. Since vegetative or autonomic symptoms (e.g., sleep disturbance) would be the symptoms expected to occur as a non-specific result of an acute medical illness, we adjusted diagnostic criteria to account for the mean rate (i.e., 1.0) of autonomic symptoms in the non-depressed patients. One extra autonomic or psychological symptom (taken from the list of symptoms in Table 7.1) was required in addition to the symptoms required by DSM-IV (i.e., patients had to have one additional depressive symptom beyond the minimum five symptoms required for major depression). This requirement changed the diagnosis from major depression to no major depression in only 3 of 79 patients. Requiring two extra symptoms changed the diagnosis in seven patients. Thus, the rate of major depression according to standard DSM-IV criteria was 20%. This rate of depression declined by 1% if one additional symptom was required and it declined by 2.5% if two additional symptoms were required. This finding suggests that standard DSM-IV criteria will not substantially over diagnose major depression in patients with acute stroke even though they have some "depressive" symptoms that may result from acute stroke or hospitalization rather than depression.

Cohen-Cole and Stoudemire (1987) reported that four approaches have been used to assess depression in the physically ill. These approaches are the "inclusive approach" in which depressive diagnostic symptoms are counted regardless of whether they may be related to physical illness (Rifkin et al. 1985), the "etiological approach" in which a symptom is counted only if the diagnostician feels it is not caused by the physical illness (Rapp and Vrana 1989), the "substitutive approach" of Endicott (1984) in which other psychological symptoms of depression replace the vegetative symptoms and the "exclusive approach" in which symptoms are removed from the diagnostic criteria if they are not found to be more frequent in depressed than non-depressed patients (Bukberg et al. 1984).

We examined the longitudinal course of the specificity of depressive symptoms among patients with depression following stroke compared to non-depressed patients who were examined at 3, 6, 12, or 24 months following stroke. Among 395 patients with acute stroke described in the previous study, 142 patients were followed up for examination at 3, 6, 12, or 24 months following stroke. The patients who were not included in the follow-up had either died, could not be located or follow-up was not planned. Of 142 patients with follow-up, 60 (42%) reported the presence of a depressed mood (depressed group) while they were in hospital and the remaining 82 patients were non-depressed (Paradiso et al. 1997). There were no significant differences in the background characteristics between the depressed and non-depressed group except that the depressed group was significantly younger ($p = 0.006$) and had a significantly higher frequency of personal history of psychiatric disorder ($p = 0.04$).

The frequency of psychological and vegetative symptoms in hospital and at each of the follow-up visits is shown in Figs 7.3 and 7.4. Throughout the 2-year follow-up, depressed patients showed a higher frequency both of vegetative and psychological symptoms compared with the non-depressed patients. The only symptoms which were not more frequent in the depressed compared to non-depressed patients were: weight loss and early awakening at the initial evaluation; weight loss, delayed sleep, and early morning awakening at 3 months; weight loss and early morning awakening at 6 months; weight loss, early morning awakening, anxious foreboding, and loss of libido at 1 year; and weight loss and loss of libido at 2 years (Fig. 7.3). Among the psychological symptoms, the depressed patients had a higher frequency of most psychological symptoms throughout the 2-year follow-up (Fig. 7.4). The only psychological symptoms that were not significantly more frequent in the depressed than in the non-depressed group were suicidal plans, simple ideas of reference and pathological guilt at 3 months, pathological guilt at 6 months, pathological guilt, suicidal plans, guilty ideas of reference and irritability at 1 year, and pathological guilt and self-depreciation at 2 years (Fig. 7.4).

We examined the effect of using each of the proposed alternative diagnostic methods for poststroke depression using DSM-IV criteria (Paradiso *et al.* 1997). The initial diagnoses were based on the inclusive criteria (i.e., symptoms that the patients acknowledged were included as positive even if there was some suspicion that the symptom may have been related to the physical illness). During the in-hospital evaluation, 27 patients (19%) met DSM-IV diagnostic criteria for major depression. We then modified DSM-IV diagnostic criteria by requiring five or more specific symptoms (i.e., we excluded weight loss and early morning awakening from DSM-IV diagnostic criteria because they were not significantly more frequent in the depressed than non-depressed patients). Of 27 patients with major depression, three were excluded. Compared to diagnoses based solely on the existence of five or more specific symptoms for the diagnosis of DSM-IV major depression, diagnoses based on unmodified symptoms (i.e., early awakening and weight loss included) had a specificity of 98% and a sensitivity of 100%.

We then modified DSM-IV criteria to examine the substitutive approach (i.e., all vegetative symptoms were eliminated and the presence of four symptoms plus depressed mood was required for the diagnosis of major depression). Using this approach, none of the original 27 patients with major depression were excluded. Finally, there were four patients who presented with four or more specific symptoms of major depression but denied the presence of a depressed mood. These cases may represent "masked" depression.

At 3-month follow-up, use of the exclusive approach, which requires only specific symptoms (i.e., weight loss, insomnia, and suicidal ideation were eliminated) led to one of 12 patients (16%) with major depression being excluded. Using

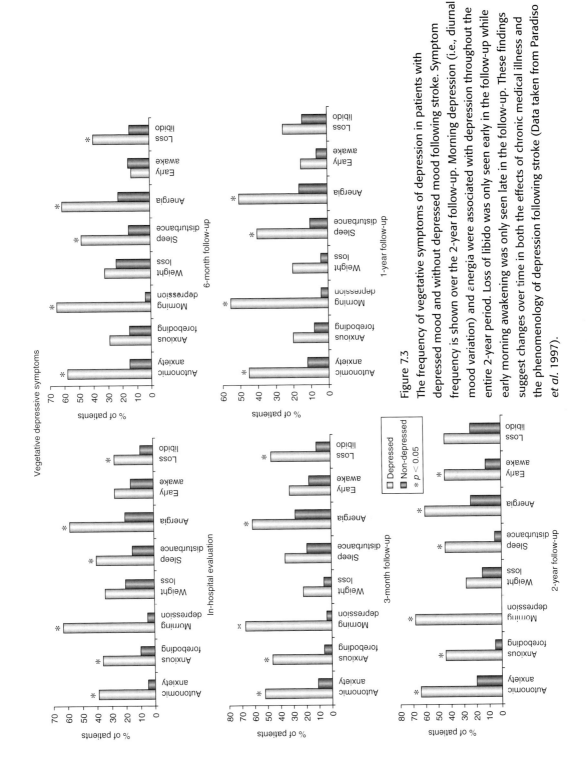

Figure 7.3

The frequency of vegetative symptoms of depression in patients with depressed mood and without depressed mood following stroke. Symptom frequency is shown over the 2-year follow-up. Morning depression (i.e., diurnal mood variation) and anergia were associated with depression throughout the entire 2-year period. Loss of libido was only seen early in the follow-up while early morning awakening was only seen late in the follow-up. These findings suggest changes over time in both the effects of chronic medical illness and the phenomenology of depression following stroke (Data taken from Paradiso et al. 1997).

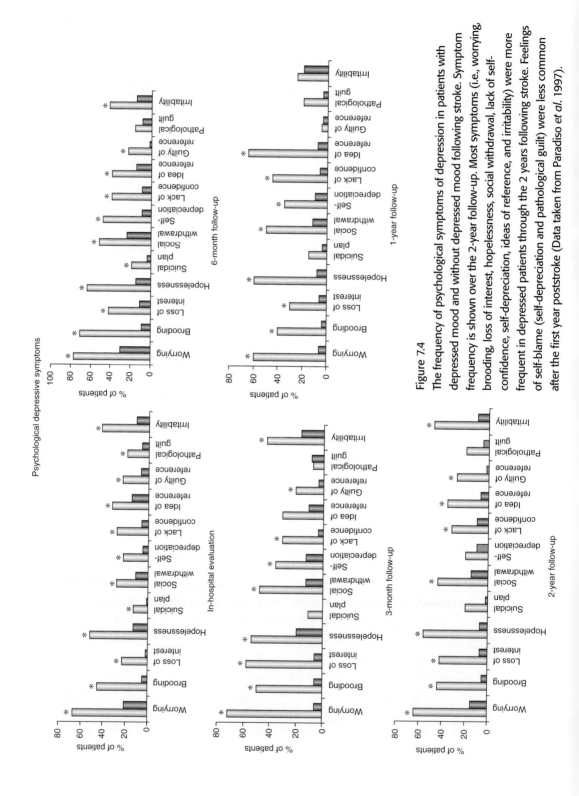

Figure 7.4

The frequency of psychological symptoms of depression in patients with depressed mood and without depressed mood following stroke. Symptom frequency is shown over the 2-year follow-up. Most symptoms (i.e., worrying, brooding, loss of interest, hopelessness, social withdrawal, lack of self-confidence, self-depreciation, ideas of reference, and irritability) were more frequent in depressed patients through the 2 years following stroke. Feelings of self-blame (self-depreciation and pathological guilt) were less common after the first year poststroke (Data taken from Paradiso et al. 1997).

diagnoses based on specific symptoms as the gold standard, unmodified DSM-IV criteria had 100% sensitivity and 97% specificity. Using the substitutive approach requiring depression plus four psychological symptoms, none of the 12 patients would have been excluded. There was one patient who had four or more specific symptoms of depression but denied the presence of a depressed mood.

At 6-month follow-up, the exclusive approach (i.e., weight loss and insomnia were excluded) resulted in 3 out of 15 patients no longer meeting the criteria for major depression. Using the specific symptoms as the gold standard, the unmodified DSM-IV criteria (i.e., using unmodified criteria and not differentiating between depression related to physical-illness-related symptoms) had 100% sensitivity and 95% specificity. Using the substitutive approach, none of the 15 patients with major depression would have been excluded. There were two patients who presented with four or more specific symptoms of major depression but denied the presence of depressed mood.

At 1-year follow-up, the exclusive approach (weight loss, difficulty concentrating, and suicidal ideation were excluded) resulted in three out of seven patients no longer meeting diagnostic criteria. Using specific symptom diagnosis as the gold standard, unmodified DSM-IV criteria had 100% sensitivity and 95% specificity. The substitutive approach resulted in none of the seven patients being excluded. There were two patients who presented with four or more specific symptoms of major depression but who denied the presence of a depressed mood.

At 2-year follow-up, the exclusive approach (i.e., weight loss was excluded) resulted in 2 out of 16 patients with major depression being excluded. Unmodified DSM-IV criteria had 100% sensitivity and 96% specificity. The substitutive approach excluded none of the 16 patients and one patient who presented with four or more symptoms of major depression denied the presence of depressed mood.

Kathol *et al.* (1990) concluded that the substitutive approach was the best approach given our current knowledge. However, the inclusive approach had a 100% sensitivity and 95+% specificity compared with the exclusive (only specific symptoms) approach. Moreover, our 2-year study of the specificity of depressive symptoms found that three vegetative symptoms (autonomic anxiety, morning depression, and subjective anergia) were significantly more frequent in depressed than non-depressed patients at all time points throughout the 2-year period. The vegetative symptom of loss of libido was no longer significantly more common in depressed than non-depressed patients after 6 months and similarly, self-depreciation was no longer more common after 1 year. In contrast, early morning awakening was more frequent in the depressed group only at 2-year follow-up. Weight loss was the only symptom that was not significantly more frequent in depressed than non-depressed patients over the entire 2-year period. Autonomic symptoms of anxiety, anxious foreboding, and worrying were significantly associated with depression throughout the entire first 2 years following stroke. In the present study, the sensitivity of unmodified DSM-IV criteria consistently showed a sensitivity of 100% and a specificity that ranged from 95% to 98% compared to criteria only using specific symptoms. Thus, one could reasonably conclude that modifying DSM-IV criteria because of the existence of an acute medical illness is probably unnecessary.

These findings also suggest that the nature of poststroke depression may be changing over time. Since the symptoms that were specific to depression changed over time, this may reflect an alteration in the underlying etiology of poststroke depression associated with early onset depression compared to the late or chronic poststroke period. Early onset depression was found to be characterized by anxious foreboding, loss of libido, and feelings of guilt which may have been more biologically determined, while symptoms such as early morning awakening and social withdrawal, which were found to be significantly different in depressed compared with non-depressed patients only during the 1- or 2-year follow-up may characterize forms of depression that are related to psychosocial or other factors.

Another question we tried to address (Fedoroff *et al.* 1991) was whether major depression might be under diagnosed because some patients were unable or unwilling to acknowledge their depressed mood. To answer this question, we determined how many patients would have met diagnostic criteria for major depression except they had not denied having a depressed mood. In the initial study of 395 patients in-hospital, there were 19 such patients. The background characteristics of these patients, compared to those of the patients who met the standard DSM-IV criteria for major depression (i.e., they acknowledged a depressed mood) are shown in Table 7.2. There were no significant differences in background characteristics between the groups with major depression and major depression without depressed mood. The mean scores for the major depression and no depressed mood groups on the MMSE were 22 ± 6 ($\pm$SD) and 23 ± 7, respectively, and on the JHFI they were 8 ± 6 ($\pm$SD) and 8 ± 5, respectively. These scores were not significantly different. However, the 77 patients who met all of the criteria for major depression had more severe depressive symptoms as measured by the mean Ham-D score compared with patients without a depressed mood (18 ± 7 versus 15 ± 5) (NS). In addition, there was a significantly higher frequency of right hemisphere lesions in the patients with no depressed mood compared to those in the group with major depression (Table 7.2).

Although a number of explanations might be proposed to understand these findings, one explanation is that these 19 patients had an inability to recognize their depressed mood as well as other symptoms of depression such as hopelessness or guilt. These patients, therefore, had less severe depressions. This failure to recognize depressive symptoms is associated with right hemisphere lesions. Future

Table 7.2. Characteristics of acute stroke patients who met all DSM-III criteria for major depression or all DSM-III criteria except depressed mood

Characteristic	Met all criteria (n = 77)		Met all criteria except depressed mood (n = 19)	
	N	%	N	%
Male	40	52	8	42
Black	28	36	6	32
Married	37	48	10	53
Hollingshead social Class I–III	19	25	6	32
Lesion location				
Left hemisphere	27	38	3	18
Right hemisphere*	30	42	13	76
Other (multiple, brain stem, or cerebellar)	15	21	1	6

*The difference between groups was significant (Fisher's exact $p = 0.0142$).

studies may examine the longitudinal course of these patients or their response to treatment to determine whether they are truly masked depressions.

    In summary, the phenomenology of major depressive disorder in patients with stroke appears to be similar to that found in patients with primary mood disorders. In addition, the presence of an acute cerebral infarction does not appear to lead to a significant number of incorrectly diagnosed cases of depression. Perhaps 1–2% of cases may be over diagnosed based on symptoms that result from physical illness. On the other hand, a small percentage of patients may be under diagnosed based on their failure to acknowledge having a depressed mood. Although these problems of evaluating depressive symptoms in acutely ill-stroke patients may lead to a small proportion of patients being over diagnosed or under diagnosed, the presence of an acute physical illness does not appear to necessitate the development of an entirely new method for diagnosing major depression in this population.

REFERENCES

Alexopoulos, G. S., Meyers, B. S., Young, R. C., *et al.* Vascular depression hypothesis. *Arch Gen Psychiatr* (1997a) 54:915–922.

Alexopoulos, G. S., Meyers, B. S., Young, R. C., *et al.* Clinically defined vascular depression. *Am J Psychiatr* (1997b) 154:562–565.

American Psychiatric Association. *Diagnostic and Statistical Manual of Mental Disorder-DSM-IV-TR.* American Psychiatric Association, Washington, 2000.

Bukberg, J., Penman, D., and Holland, J. C. Depression in hospitalized cancer patients. *Psychosom Med* (1984) 46:199–212.

Cohen-Cole, S. A., and Stoudemire, A. Major depression and physical illness: special considerations in diagnosis and biologic treatment. *Psychiatr Clin North Am* (1987) 10:1–17.

Davidson, J., and Turnbull, C. D. Diagnostic significance of vegetative symptoms in depression. *Br J Psychiatr* (1986) 148:442–446.

Endicott, J. Measurement of depression in patients with cancer. *Cancer* (1984) 53(Suppl):2243–2248.

Fedoroff, J. P., Lipsey, J. R., Starkstein, S. E., *et al.* Phenomenological comparison of major depression following stroke, myocardial infarction or spinal cord lesion. *J Affect Disord* (1991) 22:83–89.

Gainotti, G., Azzoni, A., Razzano, C., *et al.* The post-stroke depression rating scale: a test specifically devised to investigate affective disorders of stroke patients. *J Clin Exp Neuropsychol* (1997) 19(3):340–356.

Gainotti, G., Azzoni, A., and Marra, C. Frequency, phenomenology and anatomical-clinical correlates of major post-stroke depression. *Br J Psychiatr* (1999) 175:163–167.

Hickie, I., Scott, E., Mitchell, P., *et al.* Subcortical hyperintensities on magnetic resonance imaging: clinical correlates and prognostic significance in patients with severe depression. *Biol Psychiatr* (1995) 37:151–160.

Kathol, R. G., Noyes, R., Williams, J., *et al.* Diagnosing depression in patients with medical illness. *Psychosomatics* (1990) 31:434–440.

Krishnan, K. R. R., Hays, J. C., and Blazer, D. G. MRI-defined vascular depression. *Am J Psychiatr* (1997) 154:497–501.

Lipsey, J. R., Spencer, W. C., Rabins, P. V., *et al.* Phenomenological comparison of functional and post-stroke depression. *Am J Psychiatr* (1986) 143:527–529.

Paradiso, S., Ohkubo, T., and Robinson, R. G. Vegetative and psychological symptoms associated with depressed mood over the first two years after stroke. *Int J Psychiatr Med* (1997) 27:137–157.

Rapp, S. R., and Vrana, S. Substituting nonsomatic for somatic symptoms in the diagnosis of depression in elderly male medical patients. *Am J Psychiatr* (1989) 146:1197–1200.

Rifkin, A., Reardon, G., Siris, S., *et al.* Trimipramine in physical illness with depression. *J Clin Psychiatr* (1985) 46[2 (Sec 2)]:4–8.

Spalletta, G., Ripa, A., and Caltagirone, C. Symptom profile of DSM-IV major and minor depressive disorders in first-ever stroke patients. *Am J Geriatr Psychiatr* (2005) 13(2):108–115.

Starkstein, S. E., Fedoroff, J. P., Price, T. R., *et al.* Neuropsychological deficits in patients with anosognosia. *Neuropsychiatr Neuropsychol Behav Neurol* (1993) 6:43–48.

Wing, J. K., Cooper, J. E., and Sartorius, N. *The Measurement and Classification of Psychiatric Symptoms: An Instructional Manual for the PSE and CATEGO Programs.* Cambridge University Press, New York, 1974.

8

Natural course of depression

Given the number of effective treatments that are available for poststroke depression (see Chapter 20), it is increasingly difficult to conduct studies on the natural course of this disorder. Several studies, however, were conducted prior to publication of the current treatment studies. In addition, most of these pretreatment studies examined the course of poststroke depression in the setting of "usual care." Thus, in these studies, a minority of patients were treated with antidepressants by their primary care physician. Since effective treatment, however, must produce more rapid improvement of symptoms than would naturally occur over time, it is essential to study the natural course of poststroke depressive disorders. Our data on the natural course of depressive disorder is based on longitudinal studies in which patients received "usual care" and the vast majority were not given antidepressant treatment. We have studied the natural course of poststroke depression in two studies and several other groups have conducted similar investigations (Morris *et al.* 1990; House *et al.* 1991; Astrom *et al.* 1993a; Burvill *et al.* 1995; Pohjasvaara *et al.* 2001).

Our first longitudinal study of acute stroke patients was reported in 1983 (Robinson *et al.* 1983). A consecutive series of 103 patients admitted to the hospital with acute stroke, and diagnosed for depression using diagnostic and statistical manual (DSM-III) criteria were prospectively studied over a 2-year period. We have recently examined diagnostic outcomes using DSM-IV criteria in a larger group of 215 patients (i.e., the 103 previously described patients, who were re-diagnosed with DSM-IV criteria, plus a new group of 112 patients). These data have not previously been published. Follow-up was obtained for 142 of these patients (3 months $n = 75$, 6 months $n = 78$, 12 months $n = 69$, 24 months $n = 70$).

The diagnostic outcomes are displayed in Fig. 8.1. Diagnoses included DSM-IV "mood disorder due to stroke with major depression-like episode" or "minor depression" (research criteria) which required depression or anhedonia plus one other major depression symptom but fewer than the five total symptoms (see Chapter 5). The findings from this larger group were generally consistent with those found in the initial group of 103. Of the 27 patients (19% of the overall group) with major depression in-hospital, 18% had no depressive diagnosis at 3 months, (38% still had major depression, and 44% had developed minor depression). Major depression, nevertheless, continued to persist in about half of the cases during the first 6 months (i.e., at 6 months, 47% of the original 27 patients still had major depression). There was a marked decrease in frequency of major depression, however, between 6 and 12 months poststroke. At 12 months, only 11% of the original group still had major depression and at 24 months, none of the original group had major depression. In contrast, the 2-year outcome for in-hospital minor depression showed a more persistent rate of major and minor depression (Fig. 8.1). Although more than half of the minor depressions had remitted by 3-month follow-up, about a quarter of the patients had developed major depression. Throughout the 2-year follow-up more than half of the patients with in-hospital minor depression continued to have either major or minor depression. In fact, at 24-month follow-up, a significantly higher frequency of depression (major or minor) was found in patients with in-hospital minor depression (i.e., 65% had major or minor depression) than among patients with in-hospital major depression (i.e., only 22% had minor depression [$p < 0.01$]). In addition, about one third of the non-depressed patients developed major or minor depression at follow-up (Fig. 8.1). Thus, our new data indicate that major poststroke depression has a mean duration of 5.6 months, while minor depression has a mean duration of 9.4 months. Furthermore, a significant number of non-depressed patients developed major or minor depression after the acute stroke period. Of the 79 patients not depressed at the initial evaluation, 11 (13.9%) developed major depression, and an additional 18 (22.8%) developed minor depression (Fig. 8.1).

Morris *et al.* (1990) evaluated 56 patients in an Australian rehabilitation hospital at 8 weeks poststroke and again at 15 months. Only 2 of 7 major depressions (29%) and 2 of 14 minor depressions (14%) persisted throughout that entire time period (Fig. 8.2). The mean duration of major depression was 39.0 ± 31.8 (SD) weeks based on patients' reports of the time of remission, while the mean duration of minor depression was 12.2 ± 18.2 (SD) weeks.

House *et al.* (1991) examined a community sample of 128 patients, who were identified by their family physician as having had a first stroke. The present state examination was conducted on 89 patients at 1 month poststroke, on 119 patients at 6 months (i.e., 30 patients were seen for the first time at 6 months) and 112 patients at 12 months poststroke. Although the diagnostic status of the 10 patients (11%) with major depression at 1 month was not reported at 6 months, two patients continued to have major depression at both 6 months and 1 year. Using the

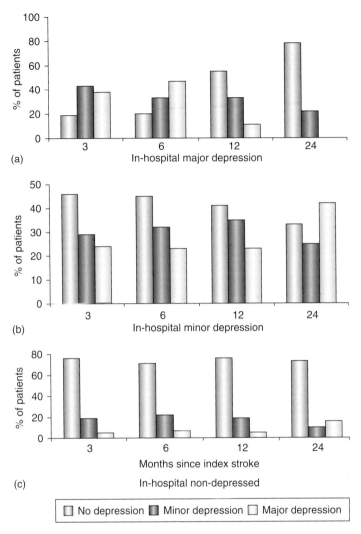

Figure 8.1   Diagnostic outcome at 3, 6, 12, and 24-month follow-up for 142 patients based on their
in-hospital diagnoses of DSM-IV major depression ($n = 27$). DSM-IV minor depression
($n = 36$) or no mood disorder ($n = 79$). Among the patients with in-hospital major
depression (a) note the increase in the non-depressed group at 12 and 24 months. This is
not seen in the minor depression patients (b) About 25% of the initially non-depressed
patients (c) were found to have a depressive diagnosis at follow-up.

Beck depression inventory (BDI) as a measure of depression, 6 of 14 patients who
scored 13 or more at 1 month continued to score 13 or more at 6-month follow-up.

Burvill *et al.* (1995) conducted psychiatric interviews using a modified version
of the present state exam at 4 months following stroke in 248 patients as part of
a community based study of stroke. At 12 months following stroke, 234 of these

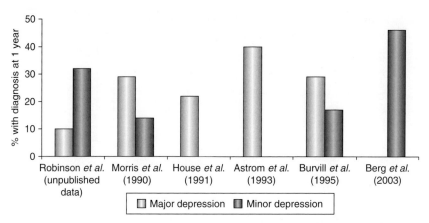

Figure 8.2   The percent of patients with an initial assessment diagnosis of major poststroke
depression who continued to have a diagnosis of major depression, or had changed to
a diagnosis of minor depression at 1-year follow-up. Note the number of chronic cases
varies between studies probably reflecting a mixture of etiologies among the group with
in-hospital major poststroke depression. The mean frequency of persistent major
depression at 1-year follow-up across all studies was 26%.

patients were reassessed. Of 42 patients with major depression at 4 months, 29%
continued to have major depression at 1-year follow-up and 17% now had minor
depression (10% had developed agoraphobia, and 9% anxiety or emotional lability). Only 35% were without a diagnosis (Fig. 8.2). Among patients with minor
depression at 4 months, 27% continued to have minor depression and 14% now
had major depression at 1 year. Only 46% had no diagnosis.

Astrom *et al.* (1993b) also examined 80 patients with a first stroke and followed
them for three years. At the initial in-hospital evaluation, 19 of 76 patients (25%)
who could be assessed had major depression. One year later, 10 of 25 patients
(40%) who developed major depression in-hospital or at 3 months continued to
have major depression. Furthermore, 8 of these 10 patients survived to the 3-year
follow-up, and 6 (75%) of them continued to be depressed. The latest study was
done by Berg *et al.* (2003) in which 46% of patients with Beck depression scores
above 9 at the acute or 2 month evaluation continued to have these scores at 12- or
18-months follow-up. As shown in Fig. 8.2, all of the longitudinal studies have
found that most major depressions spontaneously improve by 1 year following
stroke. However, using pooled data from across all of the studies cited, 26% of
patients with acute poststroke major depression continued to have major depression 1 year later while 41% of patients with acute poststroke minor depression
continued to have minor or major depression at 1-year follow-up. Thus, the
duration of depression was greater than a year in a substantial number of patients
and the duration of major depression in some patients was more than 3 years.

Another question related to the course of depression following stroke is whether these depressions may recur after treatment or spontaneous remission? The answers to questions such as what percentage of poststroke depressed patients have recurrent depressions, whether recurrent depressions occur more frequently over time, whether recurrent depressions last as long as initial depressions, or whether there is a relationship between the type or location of brain injury and the frequency or duration of recurrent depressions have not been determined. There are, however, many examples of recurrent depression after brain injury.

The following case history gives an example of a recurrent depressive disorder following stroke.

CASE STUDY

Mrs. A. was a 35-year-old woman who had been the regional director of marketing for a national company. Deadlines, frequent travel, and sales quotas were all part of her high pressured work. She developed hypertension during her first pregnancy but in spite of this kept up her hectic work schedule. While on a business trip during this pregnancy, however, she suffered a stroke which caused mild weakness of her right side as well as an aphasia characterized by difficulty producing speech but intact comprehension (i.e., non-fluent aphasia). These motor and language impairments were relatively mild and cleared up within several months after the stroke.

When I first saw her, she was about 6 months poststroke and was convinced that there was still something wrong with her as a result of the stroke. She had never experienced prolonged depressive symptoms prior to the stroke. Several physicians had told her there was nothing physically wrong with her and all she needed to do was to get back to work. She did not appear depressed when I first met her. She was talkative and her thoughts and speech were not slowed as frequently occurs in depression. She was not tearful or suicidal. She did, however, feel depressed and had loss of interest, concentration, and motivation. She had returned to work for a couple of hours a day but was unable to concentrate well enough to accomplish even the simple tasks. She had lost interest and pleasure in virtually all of her work or social activities. She no longer had the ambition to climb the corporate hierarchy. She also had sleep disturbance with early morning awakening, loss of appetite and weight, decreased sexual interest, and decreased energy. Her response to antidepressant treatment was dramatic. Between 4 and 6 weeks after beginning nortriptyline, her mood had greatly improved, she returned to work, and was able to concentrate and experience interest and pleasure in her work. Over a period of 2 to 3 months, she changed from somebody who was virtually immobilized vocationally and socially by depression to an effective, energetic woman. She also had a return of some of her previous ambition although she still did not have the same drive to reach the top of the corporate hierarchy as she had prior to the stroke.

After 9 months of taking nortriptyline, she wanted to discontinue her medications because she felt that she had fully recovered and did not want to continue taking medication which produced a dry mouth and constipation. The medication was tapered over a period of about 6 weeks and then stopped. She remained well approximately one year but then had a recurrence of the same symptoms that I initially observed. She was uninterested in work, had no feeling of pleasure in any of her usual activities, was unable to concentrate or attend to the demands of work or home, had difficulty sleeping, lost her appetite, and felt depressed. These symptoms again subsided after restarting her antidepressant medication which she continued to take for another year. After that year, she again insisted on stopping her antidepressant medication. Over the next 2 years of follow-up, she remained free of depressive symptoms but it is clear from her previous history that the possibility of another recurrence of depression still exists.

Recurrence of depression is clearly an issue which requires further research. In primary depression, the likelihood of recurrence is dependent upon the number of prior episodes and time since the previous depression. Whether these factors are also important in predicting recurrence of poststroke depression needs to be examined. Questions such as how long patients should prophylactically take antidepressants or whether treatment influences the likelihood of recurrence need to be answered before important patient management decisions can be made.

In summary, several follow-up studies have consistently demonstrated two findings. First, the majority of poststroke major depressions are over by 12 months poststroke. Remissions of depression occur even without treatment. It is noteworthy that a natural course of approximately 9 months has been observed in primary depression (i.e., depression in patients with no brain lesion) (Rennie 1942). The finding by Morris et al. (1990) of 39 weeks mean duration for poststroke major depression suggests a similarity between primary and poststroke major depression. Secondly, there are a group of poststroke depressions which do not remit within a year and become chronic major depressions. This probably reflects the fact that major and minor depressions include a mix of different etiologies. Patients who develop chronic poststroke depression may have a premorbid vulnerability, such as a personality trait or family history of mood disorder that leads to prolonged depression. These prolonged depressions, however, did not correlate significantly with severity of poststroke physical impairment. Other patients may have no such vulnerability and hence depressions of significantly shorter duration.

Whatever the cause of these chronic depressions, identification of the clinical correlates and effective treatment for these disorders are important goals of research into poststroke mood disorders.

REFERENCES

Astrom, M., Adolfsson, R., and Asplund, K. Major depression in stroke patients: a 3-year longitudinal study. *Stroke* (1993a) 24:976–982.

Astrom, M., Olsson, T., and Asplund, K. Different linkage of depression to hypercortisolism early versus late after stroke: A 3-year longitudinal study. *Stroke* (1993b) 24:52–57.

Berg, A., Psych, L., Palomaki, H., *et al.* Poststroke depression – an 18-month follow-up. *Stroke* (2003) 34(1):138–143.

Burvill, P. W., Johnson, G. A., Jamrozik, K. D., *et al.* Prevalence of depression after stroke: the Perth Community Stroke Study. *Br J Psychiatr* (1995) 166:320–327.

House, A., Dennis, M., Mogridge, L., *et al.* Mood disorders in the year after first stroke. *Br J Psychiatr* (1991) 158:83–92.

Morris, P. L. P., Robinson, R. G., and Raphael, B. Prevalence and course of depressive disorders in hospitalized stroke patients. *Int J Psychiatr Med* (1990) 20:349–364.

Pohjasvaara, T., Vataja, R., Leppavuori, A., *et al.* Depression is an independent predictor of poor long-term functional outcome post-stroke. *Eur J Neurol* (2001) 8(4):315–9.

Rennie, T. A. C. Prognosis in manic-depressive psychoses. *Am J Psychiatr* (1942) 98:801–814.

Robinson, R. G., Starr, L. B., Kubos, K. L., *et al.* A two year longitudinal study of post-stroke mood disorders: findings during the initial evaluation. *Stroke* (1983) 14:736–744.

9

Delayed-onset depression

Another issue related to the course of poststroke depression is time of onset of depression. Why do some patients develop depression during the acute poststroke period while other patients develop it several months or even years following stroke. We have recently examined this issue using our group of 142 patients with longitudinal follow-up to determine the frequency of acute- versus delayed-onset major and minor depression during the first 2 years following stroke. The follow-up evaluations were conducted at 3, 6, 12, and 24 months following stroke.

The background characteristics of the patients are shown in Table 9.1. Patients who developed major depression during the acute poststroke period tended to be younger than those who developed delayed-onset major depression, although the age distribution across diagnostic groups was not significantly different. There was no significant difference in the frequency of major versus minor depression among patients with acute- or delayed-onset depression.

There were no significant differences in any of the other background characteristics or previous history of psychiatric disorder. Similarly, there were no significant differences between groups in the use of medications; that is, antihypertensives, steroids, psychotropics, or other drugs. Two of the patients with acute depressions and one with delayed-onset depression were receiving antidepressant medication. There were no significant differences in the neurological findings between the diagnostic groups. Of the 26 patients with acute-onset depression, 7 had aphasia while 4 of the 21 patients with delayed-onset depression had aphasia ($p = $ NS). Furthermore, there were no significant differences between groups in the frequency of right- or left-hemisphere brain injury or in the frequency or existence of bilateral or brain stem lesions. Of the 47 patients with acute depression, 22 had left hemisphere lesions that could be visualized on computed tomography (CT) scan, 12 had right hemisphere lesions, 12 had bilateral lesions. These findings were not significantly different to those relating to the 21 patients with delayed-onset depressions in which six had left hemisphere lesions, two had right hemisphere lesions, and one had bilateral lesions. Moreover, there was no significant difference

Table 9.1. Characteristics of study population

| Characteristic | Major depression | | Minor depression | | No depression |
	Acute ($n = 27$)	Delayed ($n = 27$)	Acute ($n = 20$)	Delayed ($n = 19$)	($n = 49$)
When depression was diagnosed					
At initial hospitalization	27	0	14	0	0
3 or 6 months after discharge	0	12	0	13	0
1 year after discharge	0	3	0	3	0
2 years after discharge	0	12	0	3	0
Age (mean ± SD)	54.0 ± 13.5	59.2 ± 11.1	54.2 ± 15.83	59.4 ± 10.7	61.2 ± 12.0
Race (number of black)	17	17	15	11	33
Sex (number of female)	20	16	5	10	11
Marital status (number of married)	9	14	7	10	25
Socioeconomic status (classes IV–V)	23	19	15	14	33
Handedness (number of right)	23	22	19	16	43
Diagnosis of alcoholism (number of positive)	4	0	1	2	5
Previous psychiatric history (number of positive)	8	3	2	3	3

between the depressed groups in terms of the anterior extent of their lesion; however, there was a significant difference of this type between the depressed and non-depressed groups. Patients with acute- or delayed-onset depression had lesions that were more anterior than those of non-depressed patients. Furthermore, the correlation between the severity of depression and the proximity of the lesion to the frontal pole was significant for patients with acute-onset depression ($r = -0.65$, $p < 0.05$) and for patients with delayed-onset depressions ($r = -0.87$, $p < 0.05$) (i.e., the closer the lesion was to the frontal pole the more severe the depressive symptoms) (see Chapter 10 for a fuller discussion of this phenomenon). Thus, patients with acute-onset depression and those with delayed-onset depression both showed a significant association between the existence of a left anterior lesion and the presence of depression.

During the acute hospitalization, the severity of depressive symptoms as measured by the Hamilton depression (Ham-D) scale, Zung depression scale, or the total score on the present state examination, was significantly higher for patients with acute-onset major depression than for those with late onset major depression or the non-depressed (e.g., Hamilton $p < 0.001$) (Table 9.2). The depression scores

Table 9.2. Scores on measures of mood, cognitive impairment, physical impairment, and social functioning in 142 patients who did or did not become depressed following a stroke

Measure	Major depression Acute (n = 27) Group 4		Delayed (n = 27) Group 3		Minor depression Acute (n = 20) Group 2		Delayed (n = 19) Group 1		No depression (n = 49) Group 0	
	Mean	SD	Mean	SD	Mean	SD	Mean	SD	Mean	SD
Present state examination										
At Initial hospitalization[a]	22.4	7.9	10.2	6.8	12.9	4.8	5.1	3.9	4.4	3.3
At follow-up[b]	16.4	10.1	25.3	8.8	9.9	8.1	9.8	3.9	4.1	4.3
Ham-D scale										
At initial hospitalization[c]	15.9	5.3	6.7	4.7	9.7	3.7	4.8	3.7	4.3	3.4
At follow-up[d]	12.6	6.3	16.9	6.8	9.0	5.3	7.6	3.8	4.1	3.9
Mini-mental score										
At initial hospitalization	21.3	6.3	23.0	5.2	23.2	4.9	25.5	3.5	23.3	5.3
At follow-up	24.0	5.3	22.3	6.1	22.5	6.8	25.4	4.5	25.2	4.9
JHFI										
At initial hospitalization[e]	7.7	6.3	7.1	6.2	5.7	4.6	4.9	4.7	4.0	4.7
At follow-up[f]	5.2	5.1	5.1	5.4	3.6	4.3	1.3	2.4	1.6	2.6
Social functioning examination										
At initial hospitalization[g]	0.25	0.14	0.21	0.14	0.26	0.18	0.16	0.09	0.15	0.11
At follow-up	0.22	0.14	0.27	0.16	0.21	0.13	0.17	0.11	0.17	0.16

[a] Group 4 > 3, 2, 1, 0; 3 > 1, 0; 2 > 1, 0; 1 > 0.
[b] Group 4 > 2, 1, 0; 3 > 4, 2, 1, 0; 2 > 0; 1 > 0.
[c] Group 4 > 3, 2, 1, 0; 2 > 1, 0.
[d] Group 4 > 2, 1, 0; 3 > 4, 2, 1, 0; 2 > 0.
[e] Group 4 > 0.
[f] Group 4 > 1, 0; 3 > 1, 0.
[g] Group 4 > 0; 2 > 0.

for patients with delayed-onset depression and those with no depression, however, were not significantly different at the time of the initial in-hospital evaluation indicating that there were no early signs of incipient or subclinical depression. Furthermore, there were no significant correlations between severity of depressive symptoms and severity of impairment in either the delayed- or the acute-onset depression groups (i.e., correlations between Ham-D score and mini-mental state examination score or activities of daily living (Johns Hopkins functioning inventory or JHFI), score were not significant at the time of diagnosis of depression for both acute- and delayed-onset depressions). There was, however, a significantly greater impairment

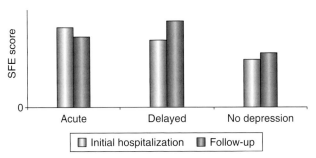

Figure 9.1   Social functioning examination (SFE) scores in patients with major depression diagnosed at the time of acute hospitalization for stroke (acute) or at 6-, 12-, or 24-month follow-up (delayed) or patients who were never depressed. Patients who developed delayed-onset major depression had higher (more impaired) social functioning than the acute-onset and non-depressed patients both at the time of initial evaluation and at follow-up (i.e., follow-up was at 6 months poststroke for acute-onset and non-depressed groups and at the onset of depression for the delayed-onset group). Although both acute- and delayed-onset depressed patients showed deterioration in social functioning over time, the delayed-onset patients had significantly more social impairment at the time they became depressed than either of the other groups. The data for this figure is shown in Table 9.2.

of activities of daily living (JHFI) scores for patients with acute-onset major depression compared to those with no depression (Table 9.2).

In addition to the findings that both acute- and delayed-onset depressions are related to anterior lesion location and acute-onset major depression is related to greater impairment of activities of daily living, probably the major finding of this study is that the quality of social functioning tended to be more impaired in patients with delayed-onset major depression compared to those with acute-onset major depression, acute- or delayed-onset minor depression, or no depression ($p < 0.025$) (Fig. 9.1). It might be suggested that impaired social functioning in patients with delayed-onset major depressions could be related to deterioration of their social functioning after the development of depression but before the follow-up assessment when depression was diagnosed. Thus, impaired social functioning might be hypothesized to be a consequence rather than a cause of depression. It seems unlikely, however, that this is a full explanation since the social functioning examination scores of patients with delayed-onset depression showed that they were more impaired than patients with acute-onset depression at 6 months post-stroke (Table 9.2). If depression had led to deterioration in social functioning, one might expect that the acute-onset depression patients would have deteriorated in social functioning by 6-month follow-up. Since patients with delayed-onset depression had more impaired social functioning than those with acute-onset depression, it seems possible that inadequate social functioning may have contributed to the onset of major depression after hospital discharge (i.e., delayed-onset depressions).

Andersen (1994) and Berg *et al.* (2003) have also examined the frequency of delayed-onset depressions. Andersen found that among 209 patients evaluated for depression within 6 weeks of stroke, 18 cases had onset between 6 weeks and 3-month follow-up, 7 more between 3- and 6-month follow-up and 2 more cases by 1 year. Using a Ham-D of >12, 49% of all depressions began after the initial acute evaluation (28% before 3 months, 14% before 6 months, and 7% before 1 year). Berg *et al.* (2003) reported that 5 of 88 patients (6%) had Beck depression scores >9 for the first time between 6 and 12 months following stroke.

As indicated previously, there are likely to be numerous etiologies for depressive disorders following stroke. The available data support the idea that some acute- and some delayed-onset major depressions are related to lesion location. The differences between acute- and delayed-onset depressions, however, suggest that severity of physical impairment may contribute more to the acute onset of depression than to delayed onset of depression. Thus, some acute-onset depressions may be caused by physiological responses to injury of specific brain structures while other acute-onset depressions may be a psychological response to physical impairment. A delayed onset of depression, on the other hand, may sometimes be related to delayed physiological responses to injury of specific brain structures while at other times they may represent a psychological response to the patient's perception of inadequate social support following their discharge from hospital. The issue of social functioning and its role in depression will be discussed in more detail in Chapter 16 "Relationship of depression to social functioning."

REFERENCES

Andersen, G., Vestergaard, K., Riis, J. O., *et al.* Incidence of post-stroke depression during the first year in a large unselected stroke population determined using a valid standardized rating scale. *Acta Psychiatr Scand* (1994) 90:190–195.

Berg, A., Psych, L., Palomaki, H., *et al.* Poststroke depression – an 18-month follow-up. *Stroke* (2003) 34(1):138–143.

10

Relationship to lesion location

Background

Since the 1860s when Broca described the clinical–pathological correlation between verbal impairment and left hemisphere stroke, neurologists have been searching for the anatomical substrates of mental as well as physical function. Even today, behavioral neurologists study the anatomical substrates of emotion (Damasio and Geschwind 1985). Some clinicians, however, have found it difficult to believe that all poststroke depressions may not be a psychological response to impairment. Thus, a controversy about the relationship between depressive disorder and lesion location has continued since the first publication of this text. In fact, Carson *et al.* (2000) reported a meta-analysis of all studies of poststroke depression that examined the association between depression (as determined by diagnostic criteria or rating scale cut-off scores) and lesion location. They concluded that "this systematic review offered no support for the hypothesis that the risk of depression after stroke is affected by the location of the brain lesion." Moreover, Gainotti *et al.* (1999) stated that our work had been criticized on "factual grounds," because several authors "using verbal and non-verbal measures of depressed mood failed to observe a significant relationship between the severity of poststroke depression and lesion location in the frontal lobe." Gainotti *et al.*, however, failed to cite the numerous studies that did find a significant relationship between depression and frontal lobe lesions. A more balanced systematic literature review by Bhogal *et al.* (2004), however, concluded that the association between left hemisphere lesion location and poststroke depression was dependent upon whether patients were sampled as inpatients or from the community and whether they were examined during the acute as compared to chronic period following stroke. Inpatients during the acute stroke had significant associations between left hemisphere lesions and poststroke depression (odds ratio (OR): 1.36, confidence interval (CI): 1.05–1.76 inpatients; OR: 2.14, CI: 1.50–3.04 acute patients).

As indicated previously, I believe this continuing controversy, reflects the fact that the association between specific clinical symptoms and lesion location does not have a history of success in psychiatry. Based in part on our findings with patients with brain lesions and in part on hypometabolic or hypermetabolic activity in specific brain regions associated with primary (i.e., no known brain lesion) mood disorder, however, neuropsychiatrists are beginning to formulate a neuroanatomy which may mediate mood disorders (Mega and Cummings 1994; George *et al.* 1994–1995; Drevets *et al.* 1997; Mayberg *et al.* 1997). These and other findings led Soares and Mann in 1997 to conclude "decreased prefrontal blood flow and metabolism in depressed unipolar and bipolar patients are the most consistently replicated findings and correlate with the severity of illness. Basal ganglia abnormalities have also been found in depressed unipolar and bipolar patients."

These findings from primary depressive disorder as well as the findings that left frontal atrophy (Jorge *et al.* 2004) or left frontal or left basal ganglia lesions (Fedoroff *et al.* 1992) were associated with depression following traumatic brain injury and that left but not right nigrostriatal dysfunction was associated with major depression in unilateral Parkinson's disease (Starkstein *et al.* 1990) provide considerable evidence that there is a neuroanatomy which mediates depressive disorder across a variety of neuropsychiatric disorders involving dysfunction of the left hemisphere. Given these findings, it would be expected that lesions which disrupt a neuroanatomical circuitry associated with depression could lead to depressive disorder in patients with stroke. This, however, is an empirical question and I will review the world's literature to assess the evidence for and against this hypothesis.

Effects of interhemispheric and intrahemispheric lesion location

We first examined the effect of unilateral ischemic lesions on depression in a series of patients who had no known risk factors for depression and were admitted to hospital after an acute stroke lesion (Robinson *et al.* 1984a). All patients were right-handed and had a single stroke lesion of the right or left hemisphere which was visible on computed tomography (CT) scan. Patients were included only if they had no previous personal or family history of psychiatric disorder.

Major or minor depression was found in 14 of 22 patients with left hemisphere lesions and 2 of 14 patients with right hemisphere lesions ($p < 0.01$) (Robinson *et al.* 1984a). In addition to the increased frequency of depression in patients with left hemisphere lesions, the intrahemispheric lesion location was also an important determinant of the existence of depression. Among 10 patients who had left *anterior* lesions (i.e., the anterior border of the lesion was *rostral* to 40% of the overall anterior–posterior length of the brain on CT scan), 6 had depression as compared to only one of eight patients with left posterior lesions (i.e., the anterior border of the lesion was caudal to 40% of the anterior–posterior distance) ($p < 0.05$). Thus, patients with left anterior hemisphere injuries were found to have a significantly greater frequency of major depression than patients with any other lesion location.

We also looked at this issue in another study of 45 patients with single lesions restricted to either cortical or subcortical structures in the right or left hemisphere (Starkstein *et al.* 1987). The background characteristics of these patients who are grouped according to whether they had a cortical or subcortical lesion location are shown in Table 10.1. Patients with subcortical lesions had infarcts limited to the basal ganglia, thalamus, or white matter of the internal capsule without any involvement of cortical gray matter or subcortical white matter. Patients with cortical lesions had ischemic damage of the cerebral cortical gray matter or underlying white matter.

We found that 44% of patients with left cortical lesions were depressed (i.e., 4 of 16 had major depression) and 39% of patients with left subcortical lesions were similarly depressed (i.e., 4 of 13 with major and 1 of 13 with minor depression). In contrast, only 11% of patients with right cortical lesions (none of nine with major and one of nine with minor depression) and 14% of patients with right subcortical lesions were depressed (one of seven with major, zero of seven with minor

Table 10.1. Characteristics of patients: lesion location

	Left Cortical ($n = 16$)	Right Cortical ($n = 9$)	Left Subcortical ($n = 13$)	Right Subcortical ($n = 7$)
Age (mean $\pm$ SD)	59 ± 12	54 ± 13	63 ± 12	54 ± 8
Sex (% male)	60	88	54	57
Race (% black)	50	33	80	100
Marital status (% married)	87	100	100	86
Mean # children	2	2	3	3
Origin (% rural)	27	11	31	14
Mean # siblings	3	3	4	3
Tobacco use (% >pack/day)	44	22	23	29
Previous medical illness (% life threatening)	25	22	28	29
Time since stroke (mean days $\pm$ SD)	23 ± 25	18 ± 14	19 ± 21	20 ± 19
Education (mean years $\pm$ SD)	9 ± 3	11 ± 4	9 ± 3	8 ± 3
Family history of psychiatric disorder (% positive)	6	23	11	14
Personal history of psychiatric disorder (% positive)				
Alcoholism	19	15	11	28
Other	6	0	11	14

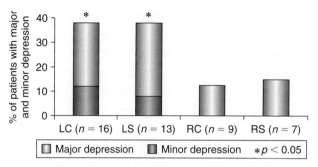

Figure 10.1   The percent of patients with major or minor depression divided by stroke lesion location. LC = left cortical, LS = left subcortical, RC = right cortical, RS = right subcortical. Patients with either left cortical or left subcortical lesions had a significantly higher frequency of major depression during the acute post-stroke period than patients with right hemisphere lesions (data from Starkstein, Brain 1987).

depression) (Fig. 10.1). Patients with lesions of the left hemisphere had significantly higher rates of depression than patients with right hemisphere lesions, regardless of the cortical or subcortical location of the lesion ($p < 0.01$).

The patients were further grouped according to whether they had anterior and posterior lesions using the anatomical criteria that the anterior border of the lesion was located in the frontal lobe. All five patients with left cortical anterior lesions involving the frontal lobe had depression (three major and two minor depression) as compared to only 2 of 11 patients with left cortical posterior lesions whose rostral border involved the temporal, parietal, and/or occipital cortex (one major, one minor depression, $p < 0.01$). Moreover, four of the six patients with left subcortical anterior lesions had major depression (none had minor depression) as compared to one minor depression (none with major depression) among seven patients with left subcortical posterior lesions ($p < 0.01$).

In a subsequent study (Starkstein et al. 1988) which included the 20 patients with subcortical lesions from the previous study as well as five new patients, we compared patients with lesions limited entirely to the basal ganglia/internal capsule with those having thalamic lesions of the right or left hemisphere with no evidence of other brain lesions. Basal ganglia (caudate and/or putamen) lesions produced major depression in seven of eight patients with left hemisphere lesions but in only one of seven patients with right hemisphere lesions. None of the patients with left ($n = 6$) or right ($n = 4$) thalamic lesions had major depression ($p < 0.001$).

The largest study examining clinical–pathological correlations in patients with stroke was reported by Vataja et al. (2001). Twelve to twenty weeks following stroke, 275 patients were examined, using the Structured Interview for Clinical Assessment in Neuropsychiatry (SCAN) and diagnostic and statistical manual (DSM)-IV diagnostic criteria for depressive disorders. The authors did not evaluate the hypotheses that patients with left frontal or left basal ganglia lesions in the first 2 months following stroke would have a greater frequency of major depressive disorder than patients with comparable right hemisphere lesions and that there would be a significant correlation between the proximity of the lesion to the frontal pole and severity of depression. Of the 275 patients, 83 (30%) had prior stroke and 54 (20%) had prior depression. A logistic regression analysis examining independent magnetic resonance imaging (MRI) correlates of the existence of depression was conducted. Depressed patients ($n = 71$) with major depression and ($n = 38$) with minor depression were found to have an increased mean frequency of infarcts in the genu of the internal capsule on the left side (OR: 3.2; 95% CI: 1.0–10.1) and in the pallidum of either side (OR: 1.6; 95% CI and over 1.1–2.3). In addition, the mean volume of infarcts in right occipital lobe was smaller in depressed compared with non-depressed patients (OR: 0.98; CI: 0.96–0.99). These authors have recently published a secondary analysis of this data utilizing the 70 who had a single infarct on magnetic resonance (MR) scan. A logistic regression analysis found that infarct localization in the pallidum of either side was the only correlate of poststroke major or minor depression. When a separate analysis of each hemisphere was done, lesions of the caudate and pallidum on the left hemisphere were significantly associated with depression while lesions of these structures in the right hemisphere were not (Vataja *et al.* 2004).

Studies by other investigators have sometimes shown similar lateralized effects of stroke lesions but sometimes have not. The variable which seemed most likely to account for differences in findings between studies was "time since stroke". For example, in contrast to our studies of acute stroke patients examined 1–2 weeks following stroke, a study of 88 Australian patients seen in a rehabilitation hospital 8.4 weeks (average) following stroke found that 43% of patients with left hemisphere lesions had major or minor depression and 38% of patients with right hemisphere lesions had depression (Morris *et al.* 1990). Similarly, Eastwood *et al.* (1989) examined 87 patients admitted to rehabilitation hospital 12 weeks (average) after stroke. Of 28 patients with left hemisphere lesions, 50% had either major or minor depression while among 45 patients with right hemisphere stroke 62% had major or minor depression. Thus, both of these studies which examined patients in rehabilitation hospitals at approximately 2–3 months poststroke failed to show a lateralized effect of hemispheric brain injury on frequency of depression.

Changes over time in lesion locations associated with depression

We examined the effect of time since stroke on the relationship between lesion location and depression (Shimoda and Robinson 1999). Using the same population of stroke patients with 2-year follow-up (i.e., 142 patients), we identified patients who had a single stroke lesion involving either the right or left middle cerebral artery (MCA) distribution that was visible on CT scan and who had a follow-up evaluation either at 3 or 6 months (short-term follow-up) or at 12 or 24 months (long-term follow-up). Of 60 patients who met these qualifications, 41 were seen at short-term follow-up and 46 were seen at long-term follow-up. There were no statistically significant differences between the short- and long-term follow-up groups in terms of age, gender, race, marital status, education, socioeconomic status, frequency of family or personal psychiatric history or prevalence of major or minor depression (39% of the short-term follow-up patients and 43% of the long-term follow-up patients had in-hospital major or minor depression). The frequency of depression in patients with right and left hemisphere lesions during the initial evaluation and at the short- and long-term follow-up is shown in Fig. 10.2. During the initial evaluation, patients with left hemisphere stroke had a significantly higher prevalence of both major and minor depression (as defined by DSM-IV criteria) than patients with right hemisphere stroke ($p = 0.0006$) (Fig. 10.2). At short- and long-term follow-up, however, there were no significant differences between right and left hemisphere lesion groups in terms of the frequency of major or minor depression. Thus, failure by other investigators to find a lateralized effect of hemispheric lesion location as summarized by Carson *et al.* (2000) was probably the result of including studies that were conducted after the first 2 months following stroke.

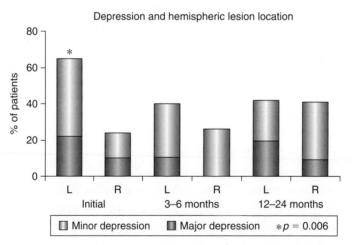

Figure 10.2 The frequency of major and minor depression defined by DSM-IV criteria associated with single lesions of the right or left hemisphere during the acute stroke period and at follow-up. The lateralized effect of left hemisphere lesions on both major and minor depression was found only during the acute stroke period. At 3–6- and 12–24-month follow-up, there were no hemispheric lesion effects on the frequency of depression.

To test the hypothesis that depressive disorders are more frequent in patients with left frontal or left basal ganglia lesions over the first 2 months following stroke, we conducted our own meta-analysis (Robinson 2003). The results of the meta-analysis are shown in Table 10.2. All studies which examined patients within 8 weeks following acute stroke and compared the relative risk of major depression following left anterior versus left posterior stroke or left anterior versus right anterior stroke were included. Meta-analyses utilizing 126 patients, based on the fixed model effect found a relative risk of 2.29 (95% confidence interval, 1.55–3.33) and using the random model, found a relative risk of 2.29 (95% confident interval, 1.55–3.37) (Table 10.2). The random model is a more conservative statistic which assumes that there are random variations in the inter study variance. The fixed model does not make this assumption. When the effect of left anterior versus right anterior lesion location on the risk of major depression was compared, the odds ratio was 2.18 using the fixed model (95% confidence interval 1.44–3.30) and using the random model was 2.16 (95% confidence interval 1.28–3.64). Thus, by defining the parameters of the analysis, the statement by Carson *et al.* at the beginning of this chapter appears to be at least overstated. On the other hand, the Carson *et al.* (2000) analysis helped to define the parameters of the lesion location hypothesis. I stated in the first edition of this text that lesion location and depression were phenomenon of the first few months following stroke. Although we do not know why this phenomenon of asymmetry in association with depression is a temporally related phenomenon, it suggests that pathophysiological changes provoked by the acute stroke are occurring within a 2-month period which initially promotes depressive disorder associated with left anterior hemisphere lesions and then changes in some way to allow both right and left hemisphere lesions to lead to depression. In fact, our data as well as other investigators (Finset *et al.* 1989; Sharpe *et al.* 1994; Shimoda and Robinson 1999) suggest that by 2 or more years poststroke, depressive disorders may be more common following right posterior lesions than any other lesion location.

Correlation between the severity of depression and anterior–posterior lesion location

In addition to the association of depression during the first 2 months following acute stroke with left frontal and left basal ganglia lesion location. A clinical–pathological correlation between the severity of depression, as measured by depression rating scales, and the distance of the lesion from the frontal pole on CT or MRI scan image, as measured by the distance in millimeters between the anterior border of the lesion and the frontal pole, was first reported in 1981 by Robinson and Szetela.

Table 10.2. Meta-analysis of the relationship of depression to lesion location

	N	Left anterior	Left posterior	Relative risk	95% CI	p	N	Left anterior	Right anterior	Relative risk	95% CI	p
Astrom (1993)	21	12/14	2/7	2.62*	1.20–8.63	0.017	25	12/13	2/12	5.54*	1.55–19.82	0.000
Morris (1996)	20	9/10	3/10	3.00*	1.14–7.91	0.006	29	9/14	3/15	3.21*	1.08–9.51	0.016
Robinson (1984)	18	6/7	4/11	2.36*	1.02–5.45	0.040	16	6/6	4/10	2.27*	1.09–4.75	0.028
Robinson (1986)	15	6/7	2/8	2.35*	1.16–9.54	0.019	11	6/6	2/5	2.23	0.85–5.87	0.46
House et al. (1990)	13	1/1	7/12	1.3	0.52–3.28	0.642	15	1/1	7/14	1.50	0.58–3.87	0.506
Herrmann (1995)	17	7/7	3/10	2.95*	1.21–7.13	0.007	NA	NA	NA	NA	NA	NA
Gainotti et al. (1999)	22	1/4	8/18	0.56	0.95–3.32	0.474	16	1/4	8/12	0.38	0.07–2.15	0.146
Fixed combined	128	42/50	29/76	2.29*	1.6–3.4	0.000	112	35/44	26/68	2.18*	1.4–3.3	0.000
Random combined	126	42/50	29/76	2.29*	1.5–3.4	0.000	112	35/44	26/68	2.16*	1.3–3.6	0.004

$*p < 0.05$. Major depression was significantly more frequent following left anterior lesions than right anterior or left posterior lesions. (Reprinted from (Robinson 2003) with permission.)

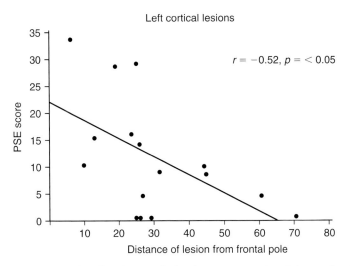

Figure 10.3 Scattergram showing the correlation between severity of depression (as measured by the Present state examination (PSE) scores) and proximity of the anterior border of the lesion from the frontal pole. Patients all had cortical lesions.

In 1984, the study previously described involving a new group of 36 patients with single lesions of the right ($n = 14$) or left ($n = 22$) hemisphere also found a significant inverse correlation between the severity of depressive symptoms as measured by combined score on the Zung depression scale, Hamilton depression scale and total score on the present state examination and the distance from the anterior border of the lesion to the left frontal pole ($r = -0.92$, $p < 0.01$).

In the right hemisphere, however, the correlation was in the opposite direction with more posterior lesions being associated with more severe depressive symptoms ($R = +0.76$, $p < 0.05$). Although the correlation was strongest in patients with left anterior lesions, if patients with left posterior lesions (i.e., anterior border of the lesion was caudal to 40% of the overall anterior–posterior length of the brain) were included (total increased from 11 to 22 patients), the correlation decreased to $r = -0.54$ but remained significant ($p < 0.01$). A similar correlation between the severity of depression and distance of the lesion from the frontal pole was also found in our previously described study of patients with cortical lesions (i.e., lesions restricted to the cortex) of the left hemisphere ($n = 16$) ($r = -0.52$, $p < 0.05$) (Fig. 10.3) or subcortical lesions (i.e., lesions only involving subcortical gray matter) of the left hemisphere ($n = 13$) ($r = -0.68$, $p < 0.01$) (Fig. 10.4) (Starkstein *et al.* 1987). We have also found a similar correlation between proximity of the lesion to the frontal pole and severity of depression in left-handed patients

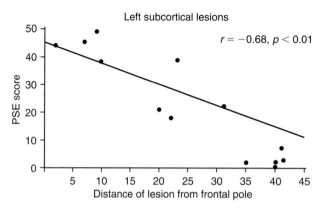

Figure 10.4   Scattergram showing the correlation between severity of depression (as measured by the present state examination (PSE)) and proximity of the anterior border of the lesion from the frontal pole: Only patients who had lesions restricted to the basal ganglia, thalamus or internal capsule of the left hemisphere were included.

with single left hemisphere lesions ($n = 13$) ($r = -0.78, p < 0.01$) (see Chapter 11) (Robinson *et al.* 1985b).

Similar correlations have now been reported by investigators in Canada, UK, Germany, and Australia. Some investigators found that the correlation between the severity of depression and the proximity of the lesion to the frontal pole applied to combined right and left hemisphere lesion groups (Sinyor *et al.* 1986; House *et al.* 1990) while others found this to be the case only among patients with left-sided lesions (Eastwood *et al.* 1989; Morris *et al.* 1992).

We recently examined changes in this correlation over time in 60 patients with single lesion CT scans and follow-up over 2 years (Shimoda and Robinson 1999). Correlations between the severity of depression, as measured by total score on the present state examination, and the proximity of the lesion to the frontal pole are shown in Fig. 10.5. During the initial evaluation, there were significant correlations between severity of depression and both proximity of the lesion to the left frontal pole and lesion volume ($n = 34$). At short-term (i.e., 3–6 months) follow-up, there were significant correlations between the severity of depression and the distance of the anterior border of the lesion from the frontal pole for both left ($n = 26$) and right ($n = 15$) hemisphere lesions. At long-term (i.e., 12–24 months) follow-up, there was no significant correlation between the severity of depression and prox-imity of the lesion to the frontal pole or lesion volume among patients with left hemisphere stroke ($n = 25$). Among patients with right hemisphere stroke ($n = 21$), however, both lesion volume and proximity of the lesion to the occipital pole correlated with the severity of depression (Fig. 10.5).

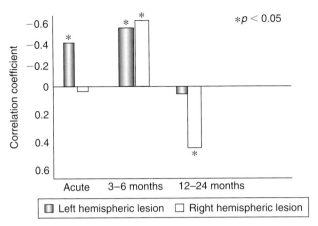

Figure 10.5 Spearman correlation coefficients between severity of depression as measured by Present State examination (PSE) total score and distance of the lesion from the frontal pole as measured on CT scan. A negative correlation indicates that depression increased with proximity of the lesion to the frontal pole and a positive correlation indicates depression increased with proximity of the lesion to the occipital pole. During the acute stroke period, depression severity correlated with proximity of the lesion to the frontal pole but only among patients with left hemisphere lesions. During short-term follow-up, proximity of the lesion to the frontal pole was correlated with more severe depression for both right and left hemisphere lesions. At long-term follow-up, severity of depression was significantly correlated with proximity of the lesion to the occipital pole (i.e., lesions further away from the frontal pole) but only for patients with right hemisphere lesions. These findings demonstrate the dynamic nature of clinical–pathological correlations in poststroke depression.

Based on the finding that there was a significant correlation between the severity of depression and the proximity of the lesion to the left frontal pole during both the acute and 3–6-month follow-up, we recently conducted a meta-analysis of studies which examined patients during the first 6 months following stroke (Tables 10.3 and 10.4) (Narushima *et al.* 2003). A total of 163 patients with left hemisphere lesions had been examined in a total of eight independent studies. Results found a fixed model Z statistic of -7.04 ($p < 0.001$) and a random model Z of -4.68 ($p < 0.001$). The pooled correlation coefficient was -0.53 in the left hemisphere using the fixed model and -0.59 employing the random model (Table 10.3). Correlation coefficients, however, in the right hemisphere between the severity of depression and the proximity of the lesion to the frontal pole during the first 6 months following stroke were non-significant ($n = 150$ in 5 studies) with pooled correlation coefficient, fixed model, $r = -0.20$; random model, $r = -0.23$ ($p = $ NS, Table 10.4). Thus, the correlation between the proximity of the lesion to the frontal pole and severity of depression was significantly stronger for the left hemisphere than the right hemisphere.

Table 10.3. Description of the studies examining the association between severity of depression and the distance of the lesion from the frontal pole in the left hemisphere

Author	Left hemisphere			Population	Scale	Interval	Quality	Remarks
	CC	N	Pooled R					
Eastwood et al. (1989)	R = −0.74	11	−0.74	Rehabilitation	GDS	2.5 months	6	*PH(+) n = 4
Herrmann et al. (1993)	Rho = −0.445	20	−0.445	Acute/rehabilitation	CDS	2 weeks	7	*All left lesion, aphasics, PH(−)
House et al. (1990)	Rho = −0.38	33		Community	PSE	6 months	7	*PH(−)
	Rho = −0.21	28	−0.341		BDI			NS
Lipsey et al. (1983)	R = −0.65	15	−0.645	Acute/rehabilitation	ODS	1.5 months	6	*Bilateral lesions, PH(−)
	R = −0.64	15			HamD			
Morris et al. (1992)	R = −0.872	14	−0.872	Rehabilitation	MARDS	2 weeks	7	*PH(+) removed
Robinson et al. (1985a)	Rho = −0.87	13	−0.87	Acute/rehabilitation	ODS	2.5 months	6	*All left handed, PH(+) removed
Sinyor (1986)	R = −0.28	19	−0.28	Rehabilitation	CDI	2 months	5	NS PH(−)
Overlapped Baltimore studies								
Parikh et al. (1987)	R = −0.41	28		Acute	Mean	6 months	7	*
Robinson et al. (1984a)	R = −0.54	18		Acute	ODS	2 weeks	6	*
Robinson (1984b)	R = −0.65	17		Acute	The PS	2 weeks	6	*
	R = −0.56				HamD			*
	R = −0.70				Zung			*

Study	R	N		Condition	Scale	Weeks		Notes
Shimoda (1999)	R = −0.42	34		Acute	PSE	2 weeks	7	*
	R = −0.28	34			HamD			NS
Starkstein et al. (1987)	R = −0.52	16		Acute/rehabilitation	PSE	3 weeks		*Cortical
	R = −0.39				HamD			NS
	R = −0.50				Zung			*
	R = −0.68	13		Acute/rehabilitation	PSE			*Sub-cortical
	R = −0.64				HamD			*
	R = −0.33				Zurg			NS
	R = −0.46	29		Acute/rehabilitation	PSE	3 weeks	7	*Cortical and sub-cortical
Combined Baltimore group								
	Rho = −0.46	43	−0.441	Acute/rehabilitation	PSE	2 weeks	8	*PH(+) removed
	Rho = −0.36	43			HamD			*
	Total N =	163	−0.53, $p < 0.001$ fixed model −0.59, $p < 0.001$ random model					

The overlapped Baltimore studies are listed but only the combined data with unique patients was used in the analysis. The definition of abbreviations is provided in Table 10.4. (Reprinted from (Narushima et al. 2003) with permission.)

Table 10.4. Description of the studies examining the association between severity of depression and the distance of the anterior border of the lesion from the frontal pole in the right hemisphere

Author	Right hemisphere			Population	Scale	Interval	Quality	Remarks
	CC	N	Pooled R					
Herrmann et al. (1995)	$R = -0.55$	15	−0.55	Acute	CDS	1 month	7	*All PH (−)
House et al. (1990)	$R = -0.34$ $R = -0.23$	28 30	−0.284	Community	BDI PSE	6 months	7	NS All PH (−) NS
Morris et al. (1992)	$R = -0.057$	9	−0.057	Rehabilitation	NARDS	2 weeks	7	NS PH (+) removed
Sinyor et al. (1986)	$R = 0.10$	16	−0.1	Rehabilitation	CDI	2 months	5	NS All PH (−)
Overlapped Baltimore studies								
Parikh et al. (1987)	$R = -0.52$ $R = -0.65$ $R = -0.40$	10		Acute	PSE HamD Zung	3 or 6 months	6	NS ★ NS
Robinson et al. (1984a)	$R = 0.76$	12		Acute	ODS	2 weeks	6	★
Robinson (1984b)	$R = 0.63$ $R = 0.73$ $R = 0.62$	10		Acute	PSE HamD Zung	2 weeks	6	★ ★ ★
Robinson (1985a)	Not stated $Rho = -0.65$	10		Acute	Mean HamD	3 or 6 months	7	NS NS
Shimoda (1999)	$R = -0.02$ $R = 0.17$	26		Acute	PSE HamD	2 weeks	7	NS NS
Starkstein (1987)	$R = -0.65$ $R = -0.22$ $R = -0.43$	9		Acute/rehabilitation	PSE HamD Zung	3 weeks	6	*cortical lesion NS NS

R = −0.08	7	Acute/rehabilitation	PSE	3 weeks	6	NS Sub-cortical lesion
R = −0.18			HamD			NS
R = −0.41			Zung			NS
Not stated	16	Acute/rehabilitation		3 weeks	7	NS Cortical and sub-cortical

Combined Baltimore group

Rho = −0.17	38	Acute/rehabilitation	PSE	2 weeks	8	NS PH(+) removed
Rho = 0.003	38		HamD			NS
Total N =	106					

−0.20, p-NS fixed model − 0.23, p-NS random model

The overlapped Baltimore studies are listed but only the combined data with unique patients was used in the analysis. CC: correlation coefficient; CDI: composite depression index; CDS: Cornell depression scale; GDS: geriatric depression scale; HamD: Hamilton depression scale; Mean: Mean (Zung, HamD, PSE); MARDS: Montgomery and Asberg depression rating scale; N: number of patients; NS: not significant; ODS: overall depression scale; PSE: present state examination; PH = ±patients with/without past psychiatric history; * $p < 0.05$.

Scoring System

	0	1	2
Scale	None	Not standardized	Standardized
Imaging	Not stated	CT/MRI Results unclear	Imagery and psychiatric data done blind
Comprehension deficit	Not stated	Clinical	Operational Criteria
N	$N < 20$	$20 = <N < 30$	$N \geqslant 30$

Reprinted from Narushima *et al.* (2003) with permission.

Relationship between depression and MCA versus posterior circulation

MCA versus posterior circulation infarcts

Although brainstem and cerebellar strokes are less common than cerebral hemisphere strokes, they, nevertheless, constitute an important group of brain infarcts. In contrast to the motor and sensory symptoms that are common in patients with hemispheric infarcts involving the MCA, patients with infarcts of the vertebral-basilar artery have symptoms of cranial nerve dysfunction, such as dysphagia or diplopia or cerebellar dysfunction, such as ataxias or intention tremor (see Chapter 4 for a review of "Vascular anatomy and clinical symptoms").

We compared depression associated with infarcts of the posterior circulation (PC) (i.e., vertebral-basilar arteries supplying the brainstem, cerebellum, thalamus, and posterior hemispheres) and infarcts of the MCA circulation (MCA) (i.e., large areas of frontal, temporal, and parietal cortex and subcortical structures including the basal ganglia) (Starkstein *et al*. 1988). This study included 37 consecutive patients with clinical findings or CT scan evidence indicating a first episode stroke in the PC as well as a consecutive series of 42 patients with single stroke lesions involving the MCA territory. The background characteristics of these groups were not significantly different in age, gender, education or prior psychiatric or medial history. All patients were evaluated during the first 30 days following stroke except for two patients with PC infarcts who were assessed during the second month poststroke.

Cranial nerve abnormalities were found in 41% of the PC group and none of the MCA, while cerebellar signs were found in 24% of the PCA group and none of the MCA group. Based on clinical signs or CT scan imaging, 39% of the patients with PC group lesions had cerebellar involvement, 30% had midbrain lesions, 26% had lesions of the pons, 22% had paramedian infarcts of the tegmentum, and 9% had lateral medullary infarcts. Among patients with MCA group infarcts, 55% had left hemisphere lesions and 45% had right hemisphere lesions.

Among the 37 patients in the PC group, 27% were found to be depressed immediately after the acute lesion (four had DSM-III major and six had DSM-III minor depression). Among the 42 patients with MCA lesions, 48% developed depression immediately after the acute infarct (11 had major depression and nine had minor depression). This higher frequency of depression among the MCA compared with the PC group just failed to reach statistical significance ($p = 0.054$).

At 6-month follow-up, 82% of the patients with MCA lesions who were depressed (major or minor) in hospital remained depressed (Fig. 10.6). Among patients with PC lesions who were depressed (major or minor) at the in-hospital evaluation only 20% remained depressed at the 6-month follow-up ($p < 0.05$). At 1- or 2-year follow-up, the percentage of patients with continued depression was

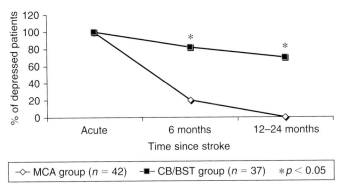

Figure 10.6   The percent of patients depression after an acute stroke who remained depressed at
6 months and 1- or 2-year follow-up. Patients with brainstem or cerebellar infarcts
(CB/BST) recovered from depression (without treatment) significantly more quickly than
patients with left or right MCA (i.e., hemispheric) infarcts (data from Starkstein *et al.*
1988).

68% for the MCA group and zero for the PC group ($p < 0.05$). Although the significantly shorter course of depression in the PC as compared to the MCA group
might be hypothesized to result from the PC group having smaller lesion volumes
than the MCA group, there was no significant correlation between lesion volume
and the severity of depression for the combined group of MCA and PC lesion
patients either in hospital or at 1- or 2-year follow-up.

The relationship between depression and impairment was examined by dividing
MCA and PC lesion patients into those with major depression, minor depression
or no depression. Among patients with PC lesions, neither intergroup comparisons using ANOVA (e.g., mini-mental state examination scores across the three
diagnostic groups) nor dimensional comparisons using correlational analysis (e.g.,
Hamilton depression score correlated with mini-mental state examination score)
demonstrated a significant relationship between depression (diagnosis or severity)
and cognitive impairment (measured by the mini-mental state examination),
activities of daily living (measured by the Johns Hopkins functioning inventory
(JHFI)), or social support (measured by the social functioning examination).
Among the patients with MCA lesions, however, patients with major depression
had significantly higher (i.e., more impaired) JHFI scores (activities of daily living)
than patients with minor depression or no mood disorder ($p < 0.05$).

Right hemisphere lesions

Although the frequency of major depression in the acute poststroke period has
been found in several studies to be greater following left frontal cortical or left
basal ganglia lesions than for any other lesion location, depressions do occur in
many patients with right hemisphere lesions during both the acute and chronic

poststroke periods. We, therefore, examined the clinical correlates of depression associated with right hemisphere lesions to compare them with the clinical correlates of left hemisphere lesion location. This work included a consecutive series of 93 patients who had acute stroke lesions of the right hemisphere. Lesion location was based on CT findings and/or clinical diagnosis and patients were included only if there was no previous history or CT scan evidence of prior brain injury.

The 93 acute stroke patients consisted of both males and females in their late 50s and early 60s, primarily from lower socioeconomic classes (i.e., Hollingshead class IV and class V) examined 2 to 3 weeks poststroke (Table 10.5). There were 46 patients with no mood disturbance, 17 patients with major depression, 11 patients with minor depression, and 19 patients with undue cheerfulness. There were no statistically significant differences in age, gender, education, race, or marital status or time since stroke. The classification of "undue cheerfulness" was based on either a self-report of elevated or expansive mood or clinical observation of inappropriately cheerful affect or disinhibited behavior during the mental status interview.

One of the major findings was that patients with major depression had a significantly higher frequency of psychiatric disorder among their first- or second-degree relatives (i.e., 29% with 55% of these being alcoholism and 45% depression)

Table 10.5. Characteristics of right hemisphere lesion patients

Characteristic	Right hemisphere				Left hemisphere
	No depression ($n = 46$)	Undue cheerfulness ($n = 19$)	Major depression ($n = 17$)	Minor depression ($n = 11$)	Major depression ($n = 27$)
Age, years (mean ± SD)	64 ± 10	60 ± 14	60 ± 11	62 ± 8	56 ± 13
Gender (% females)	35	42	47	36	52
Race (% blacks)	65	74	41	55	59
Socioeconomic status:					
Hollingshead class IV or V	87	74	82	82	89
Marital status (% married)	54	37	42	36	44
Handedness (% right-handed)	87	90	100	100	89
Education (mean years ± SD)	6.5 ± 3.7	8.2 ± 4.3	8.4 ± 3.4	8.8 ± 3.5	9.3 ± 2.8
Familial history of psychiatric disorders (% positive*)	6	5	29	9	4
Personal history of psychiatric disorders (% positive)	15	5	29	36	6
Time since stroke (mean days ± SD)	13 ± 12	11 ± 6	16 ± 9	20 ± 18	14 ± 11

*$p < 00.05$.

compared with other diagnostic groups (i.e., 6% for no diagnosis, 5% undue cheer-fulness, 9% for minor depression, and 5% for major depression following left hemi-sphere stroke) (Fig. 10.7).

In addition, among patients with undue cheerfulness, there was a significantly higher frequency of lesions involving the right frontal operculum compared with depressed (major and minor) and non-depressed patients. Of 12 patients with undue cheerfulness, five had right frontal opercular lesions compared with four of 25 non-depressed and one of 17 depressed patients ($p < 0.05$). On the other hand, patients with depression (both major and minor) showed a significantly higher frequency of lesions involving either the right parietal cortex (i.e., six of nine with major depression and five of eight with minor depression compared to 1 of 12 with undue cheerfulness and 9 of 25 with no depression; $p = 0.02$) or the right lateral frontal cortex (i.e., two of nine with major depression and four of eight with minor depression compared to none of 12 with undue cheerfulness and one of 25 with no depression; $p < 0.01$).

Morris et al. (1990) examined family history in a study of 88 Australian patients in a rehabilitation hospital 8.4 weeks poststroke and found a significantly higher frequency of family history of psychiatric disorder among patients with major depression (i.e., 11 of 16 or 73%) compared to patients with minor depression (i.e., 5 of 18 or 28%) or no depression (i.e., 20 of 54 or 37%) ($p < 0.03$). Patients with major depression following right hemisphere lesions had a positive family

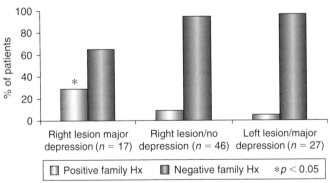

Figure 10.7   The percent of patients with and without a family history of psychiatric disorder (defined by having seen a professional for treatment of an emotional disorder) following an acute right hemisphere infarction. Patients with major depression following a right hemisphere lesion were significantly more likely to have a family history of psychiatric disorder than those without major depression or patients with major depression following a left hemisphere lesion. These data suggest that some poststroke depressions may be related to genetic vulnerability and the factors associated with major depression following right or left hemisphere lesions may be different.

history in 71% of the cases (i.e., five of seven) similar to patients with major depression following left hemisphere lesions (i.e., 67% or six of nine patients).

Patients with right hemisphere lesions have also been studied by Finset *et al.* (1989) who found that among 42 patients with CT-verified single right hemisphere lesions, ischemic damage involving white matter underlying the parietal cortex was associated with a higher frequency of depression (5 of 13 patients) than lesions in any other location in the right hemisphere (7 of 29 patients) ($p < 0.02$). House *et al.* (1990) reported on a group of 21 patients with CT-verified right hemisphere lesions examined 1 month following their first stroke. Of the three patients with major depression following a right hemisphere lesion, all of them had a right posterior lesion (i.e., three major depressions of eight patients with right posterior injury) compared with none of the patients with right anterior ($n = 7$) or right intermediate ($n = 6$) lesion locations ($p < 0.03$). Sinyor *et al.* (1986) examined 16 patients with single CT-verified right hemisphere lesions studied an average of 56 days poststroke. There was a significant quadratic relationship between depression scores and the distance between the anterior border of the lesion and the frontal pole in patients with right hemisphere lesions (i.e., patients with the most anterior and most posterior lesions of the right hemisphere had the highest depression scores, $p < 0.05$). Another study by Stern and Bachman (1991) examined 19 patients with CT-verified single right hemisphere lesions an average of 16 months poststroke. Lesions were classified as dorsal or ventral, frontal or non-frontal. Dysphoric mood was significantly more severe in patients with right ventral non-frontal as compared with right ventral frontal lesions. This suggests that right temporal lesions are associated with depressed mood. Finally, Astrom *et al.* (1993) and Eastwood *et al.* (1989) found no association between lesion location in the right hemisphere and the existence of poststroke depression.

Insular lesions

We have recently examined the relationship between psychopathology and lesions of the insular cortex. The insular cortex is the in-folded cortex surrounding the central fissure beneath the motor and sensory cortex. Seven patients with left insular stroke and six patients with right insular stroke were compared with six patients having left hemisphere non-insular stroke and six patients with right hemisphere non-insular stroke. Patients were studied between 4 and 8 weeks following acute stroke and were examined using the present state examination and DSM-IV diagnoses. Increased frequency of feelings of anergia and under activity (Fisher's exact $p = 0.002$) as well as tiredness (Fisher's exact $p = 0.002$) were found among patients with right insular stroke compared to patients with non-insular lesions or left insular lesions. We hypothesized that feelings of decreased energy or motivation after right insular damage may result from disconnection between the insula and the frontal cortex or anterior cingulate cortex, structures that have been associated with willed action and motor behavior (Manes *et al.* 1999).

Frontal lobe lesions

We have also recently examined the relationship between depression and frontal lobe lesions involving either the lateral frontal cortex ($n = 8$) or the medial frontal cortex ($n = 8$) (Paradiso *et al.* 1999). The groups were composed of three women and five men with traumatic head injuries, and five men with strokes studied within the first 2 months following brain injury. The mean ages of the medial lesion group was 39.5 ± 17 years SD and the lateral lesion group was 44.1 ± 17 years SD. There were no statistically significant differences in group background characteristics.

Six of the eight patients with lateral lesions had depressive disorder (three major and three minor depressions) while the medial lesion group had only two depressions (one major and one minor depression) ($p < 0.05$). Similarly, five of the eight patients in the lateral lesion group had generalized anxiety disorder (GAD) while only one patient in the medial group had this disorder ($p < 0.04$). At 3-month follow-up, there were no significant intergroup differences in the frequency of depressive disorder or GAD. Patients with lateral lesions, however, showed greater severity of depressive symptoms, impairment in activities of daily living, and social functioning compared to the medial lesion group ($p < 0.05$). In addition during the initial evaluation, five patients in the lateral group and one in the medial lesion group showed decreased emotion and motivation ($p < 0.04$) while, at 3 months, five patients in the lateral group and none in the medial lesion group showed these symptoms ($p < 0.003$). There were no significant differences between the groups in the frequency of mania, hypomania, or symptoms of disinhibition.

This study found that patients with single lesions of the lateral prefrontal cortex had significantly greater frequency of depression and anxiety disorders and symptoms of decreased emotion and motivation than patients with medial frontal lesions both during the acute injury and at 3-month follow-up. It was surprising that the medial lesion group did not show significantly higher frequency of symptoms of euphoria, disinhibition, loss of emotion or apathy compared to the lateral lesion group. Although apathy has been associated with damage to the cingulate cortex and mesial frontal regions (Marin 1991; Cummings 1993). Okada *et al.* (1997) found decreased blood flow in the right dorsal lateral frontal and left frontal temporal cortex in 40 patients with apathy after stroke compared with non-apathetic stroke controls. Similarly, Cummings found personality but not mood changes after damage to the frontal cingulate circuit (Cummings 1993). Thus, medial frontal activity may be necessary to experience emotions including depressed mood while lateral prefrontal damage appears to disrupt mood and drive while leaving intact the ability to experience these emotions.

In summary, during the first 2 months following stroke, a meta-analysis of the world's literature found that the frequency of major depression following left frontal or left basal ganglia stroke is more than two times as great as that associated with right anterior lesions or left parietal–occipital lesions. Similarly, over the first 6 months following stroke, a meta-analysis of the world's literature found a significant correlation between the proximity of the lesion to the left frontal pole and severity of depressive symptoms. These studies as well as the large study by Vataja et al. implicate the frontal-basal ganglia-thalamic circuits in the mediation of post-stroke depression. Studies of specific areas of brain injury have found that depressive disorder is more common following basal ganglia as compared with thalamic stroke and with MCA compared with PC strokes. Among patients with right hemisphere stroke, depression was associated with a family history of psychiatric disorder and both anterior and posterior lesion location. Although depression was not associated with lesions of the insular cortex, they were associated with tiredness and amotivational states. Lateral prefrontal lesions were associated with increased frequency of both depression and anxiety disorders compared with medial frontal lesions. There are numerous areas for further research including the mechanism by which these dynamic changes in laterality occur over the first several months following stroke and the mechanism by which lesions of strategic areas of the brain lead to depressive disorder.

REFERENCES

Astrom, M., Adolfsson, R., and Asplund, K. Major depression in stroke patients: a 3-year longitudinal study. *Stroke* (1993) 24:976–982.

Bhogal, S. K., Teasell, R., Foley, N., *et al.* Lesion location and poststroke depression. Systematic review of the methodological limitations in the literature. *Stroke* (2004) 35:794–802.

Carson, A. J., MacHale, S., Allen, K., *et al.* Depression after stroke and lesion location: a systematic review. *Lancet* (2000) 356(9224):122–126.

Cummings, J. Frontal-subcortical lesions and human behavior. *Arch Neurol* (1993) 50:873–880.

Damasio, A. R., and Geschwind, N. *Anatomical Localization in Clinical Neuropsychology*, Vol. 1. Elsevier, 1985.

Drevets, W. C., Price, J. L., Simpson Jr., J. R., *et al.* Subgenual prefrontal cortex abnormalities in mood disorders. *Nature* (1997) 386(6627):824–827.

Eastwood, M. R., Rifat, S. L., Nobbs, H., *et al.* Mood disorder following cerebrovascular accident. *Br J Psychiatr* (1989) 154:195–200.

Fedoroff, J. P., Starkstein, S. E., Forrester, A. W., *et al.* Depression in patients with acute traumatic brain injury. *Am J Psychiatr* (1992) 149:918–923.

Finset, A., Goffeng, L., Landro, N. I., *et al.* Depressed mood and intra-hemispheric location of lesion in right hemisphere stroke patients. *Scand J Rehabil Med* (1989) 21:1–6.

Gainotti, G., Azzoni, A., and Marra, C. Frequency, phenomenology and anatomical-clinical correlates of major post-stroke depression. *Br J Psychiatr* (1999) 175:163–167.

George, M. S., Malloy, L. C., Slate, S. O., *et al.* Pilot MRI study of brain size in nervous pointer dogs. *Anxiety* (1994–1995) 1(3):129–33.

Herrmann, M., Bartles, C., and Wallesch, C.-W. Depression in acute and chronic aphasia: symptoms, pathoanatomical-clinical correlations and functional implications. *J Neurol Neurosurg Psychiatr* (1993) 56:672–678.

Herrmann, M., Bartels, C., Schumacher, M., *et al.* Poststroke depression: is there a pathoanatomic correlate for depression in the postacute stage of stroke? *Stroke* (1995) 26:850–856.

House, A., Dennis, M., Warlow, C., *et al.* Mood disorders after stroke and their relation to lesion location: a CT scan study. *Brain* (1990) 113:1113–1130.

Jorge, R. E., Robinson, R. G., Moser, D., *et al.* Major depression following traumatic brain injury. *Arch Gen Psychiatry* (2004) 61(1):42–50.

Lipsey, J. R., Robinson, R. G., Pearlson, G. D., *et al.* Mood change following bilateral hemisphere brain injury. *Br J Psychiatry* (1983) 143:266–273.

Manes, F., Paradiso, S., and Robinson, R. G. Neuropsychiatric effects of insular stroke. *J Nerv Ment Dis* (1999) 187(12):707–712.

Marin, R. S. Apathy: a neuropsychiatric syndrome. *J Neuropsychiatr Clin Neurosci* (1991) 3:243–254.

Mayberg, H. S., Brannan, S. K., Mahurin, R. K., *et al.* Cingulate function in depression: a potential predictor of treatment response. *Neuroreport* (1997) 8(4):1056–1061.

Mega, M. S., and Cummings, J. L. Frontal-subcortical circuits and neuropsychiatric disorders. *J Neuropsychiatr Clin Neurosci* (1994) 64(4):358–370.

Morris, P. L. P., Robinson, R. G., and Raphael, B. Prevalence and course of depressive disorders in hospitalized stroke patients. *Intl J Psychiatr Med* (1990) 20:349–364.

Morris, P. L. P., Robinson, R. G., and Raphael, B. Lesion location and depression in hospitalized stroke patients: evidence supporting a specific relationship in the left hemisphere. *Neuropsychiatr Neuropsychol Behav Neurol* (1992) 3:75–82.

Morris, P. L. P., Robinson, R. G., Raphael, B., *et al.* Lesion location and post-stroke depression. *J Neuropsychiatry Clin Neurosci* (1996) 8:399–403.

Narushima, K., Kosier, J. T., and Robinson, R. G. A reappraisal of post-stroke depression, intra and inter-hemispheric lesion location using meta-analysis. *J Neuropsychiatr Clin Neurosci* (2003) 15(4):422–430.

Okada, K., Kobayashi, S., Yamagata, S., *et al.* Post stroke apathy and regional cerebral blood flow. *Stroke* (1997) 28:2437–2441.

Paradiso, S., Chemerinski, E., Yazici, K. M., *et al.* Frontal lobe syndrome reassessed: comparison of patients with lateral or medial frontal brain damage. *J Neurol Neurosurg Psychiatry* (1999) 67(5):664–667.

Parikh, R. M., Lipsey, J. R., Robinson, R. G., *et al.* Two-year longitudinal study of post-stroke mood disorders: dynamic changes in correlates of depression at one and two years. *Stroke* (1987) 18:579–584.

Robinson, R. G. The controversy over post-stroke depression and lesion location. *Psychiatric Times* (2003) 20(7):39–40.

Robinson, R. G., and Szetela, B. Mood change following left hemispheric brain injury. *Ann Neurol* (1981) 9:447–453.

Robinson, R. G., Kubos, K. L., Starr, L. B., *et al.* Mood disorders in stroke patients: importance of location of lesion. *Brain* (1984a) 107:81–93.

Robinson, R. G., Starr, L. B., and Price, T. R. A two-year longitudinal study of post-stroke mood disorders: dynamic changes in associated variables over the first six months of follow-up. *Stroke* (1984b) 15:510–517.

Robinson, R. G., Lipsey, J. R., Bolla-Wilson, K., *et al.* Mood disorders in left handed stroke patients. *Am J Psychiatry* (1985a) 142:1424–1429.

Robinson, R. G., Starr, L. B., Lipsey, J. R., *et al.* A two year longitudinal study of post-stroke mood disorders: in-hospital prognostic factors associated with six month outcome. *J Nerv Ment Dis* (1985b) 173:221–226.

Robinson, R. G., Lipsey, J. R., Rao, K., *et al.* Two-year longitudinal study of post-stroke mood disorders: comparison of acute-onset with delayed-onset depression. *Am J Psychiatry* (1986) 143:1238–1244.

Sharpe, M., Hawton, K., Seagroatt, V., *et al.* Depressive disorders in long-term survivors of stroke: associations with demographic and social factors, functional status, and brain lesion volume. *Br J Psychiatr* (1994) 164:380–386.

Shimoda, K., and Robinson, R. G. The relationship between post-stroke depression and lesion location in long-term follow-up. *Biol Psychiatry* (1999) 45:187–192.

Sinyor, D., Jacques, P., Kaloupek, D. G., *et al.* Post-stroke depression and lesion location: an attempted replication. *Brain* (1986) 109:539–546.

Soares, J. C., and Mann, J. J. The functional neuroanatomy of mood disorders. *J Psychiatr Res* (1997) 31(4):393–432.

Starkstein, S. E., Robinson, R. G., and Price, T. R. Comparison of cortical and subcortical lesions in the production of post-stroke mood disorders. *Brain* (1987) 110:1045–1059.

Starkstein, S. E., Robinson, R. G., Berthier, M. L., *et al.* Depressive disorder following posterior circulation compared with middle cerebral artery infarcts. *Brain* (1988) 111:375–387.

Starkstein, S. E., Mayberg, H. S., Berthier, M. L., *et al.* Mania after brain injury: neuroradiological and metabolic findings. *Ann Neurol* (1990) 27:652–659.

Stern, R. A., and Bachman, D. L. Depressive symptoms following stroke. *Am J Psychiatry* (1991) 148(3):351–356.

Vataja, R., Pohjasvaara, T., Leppavuori, A., *et al.* Magnetic resonance imaging correlates of depression after ischemic stroke. *Arch Gen Psychiatr* (2001) 58(10):925–931.

Vataja, R., Leppavuori, A., Pohjasvaara, T., *et al.* Poststroke depression and lesion location revisited. *J Neuropsychiatr Clin Neurosci* (2004) 16(2):156–162.

11

Relationship of depression to cerebral dominance and structural asymmetries

Background

In Chapter 10, I discussed studies demonstrating an association during the acute stroke period between major depressive disorder and lesions of the left dorsolateral frontal cortex or left basal ganglia. Although there is a statistically significant increase in the frequency of major depression among patients with lesions of the left anterior brain region, not all patients with left frontal or left basal ganglia lesions develop depression. We therefore questioned whether patients who had a left anterior brain lesion without depression might have structural differences in their brains compared with those patients who developed depression after left frontal lesions. We have addressed this question in two different studies examining the effect of handedness and structural hemispheric asymmetry on the frequency and clinical correlates of depressive disorder.

Patients with left sided motor dominance

In the first study, a consecutive series of 30 patients who were left handed, without evidence of mixed motor cerebral dominance, was evaluated for depressive disorders (Robinson *et al.* 1985). Patients were included if they reported the predominant use of their left eye for vision, left hand for writing and eating, and left foot for kicking. Patients also had to have a single stroke lesion without a clinical history or computed tomography (CT) scan evidence of prior brain injury. The study included 18 patients with left hemisphere lesions and 12 patients with right hemisphere lesions (Table 11.1). The right and left hemisphere lesion groups were not significantly different in any background characteristics except that the right lesion patients were significantly older than patients with left hemisphere lesions ($p < 0.05$). Of the overall group of 30 patients, eight patients had major depression, three patients had minor depression, and 19 patients were not depressed. Among the 18 patients with left hemisphere lesions, seven had major, and three

Table 11.1. Demographic data on 30 left-handed stroke patients according to hemisphere of lesion

Characteristics	Left hemisphere lesion ($n = 18$)	Right hemisphere lesion ($n = 12$)
Age (mean ± SD)	53 ± 14	63 ± 12
Male (%)	55	75
Married (%)	50	25
Widowed (%)	11	50
Hollingshead socioeconomic class IV or V (%)	83	83
History of alcohol abuse (% positive)	17	8
Personal history of psychiatric disorder (% positive)	11	8
Previous history of stroke (% positive)	28	25
JHFI (mean ± SD)	9.0 ± 7.0	7.1 ± 6.0
Mini-mental (mean ± SD)	20.8 ± 6.9	21.8 ± 4.5
Days since stroke (mean ± SD)	49 ± 64	24 ± 35

JHFI: Johns Hopkins functioning inventory.

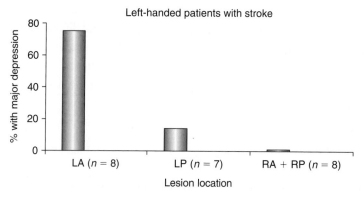

Figure 11.1 The percent of left-handed patients with major depression who had left anterior (LA), left posterior (LP) or right anterior or posterior lesions (RA + RP). There was a significantly greater frequency of major depression among the patients with left anterior lesions than any other location.

had minor depression while eight were not depressed. Among the 12 patients with right hemisphere lesions, one had a major depression while 11 were not depressed ($p = 0.025$ comparing the frequency of depression in patients with right versus left hemisphere lesions). When patients were divided into those with anterior and posterior lesions, patients with left anterior lesions had a significantly higher frequency of depressive disorder than patients with left posterior lesions or patients with right hemisphere anterior or posterior lesions (Fig. 11.1) ($p < 0.001$). In

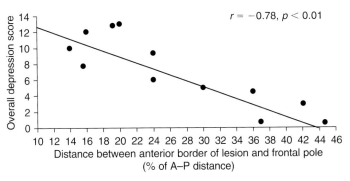

Figure 11.2 Correlation between severity of depression and proximity of the anterior border of the lesion to the frontal pole among 13 patients who were left handed and had a single lesion of the anterior left hemisphere. This is the same kind of correlation in the left anterior hemisphere found in right-handed patients (see Chapter 10). A–P: anterior–posterior.

addition, among 13 patients whose left hemisphere lesion border was anterior to 45% of the anterior–posterior distance, there was a significant correlation between proximity of the lesion to the frontal pole and the severity of depression (Fig. 11.2). This is the same kind of correlation between depression and proximity of the lesion to the frontal pole that was previously found in patients who were right handed (see Fig. 10.5).

The major question that we could not satisfactorily answer in this study is how many of these left-handed patients had right hemisphere dominance for language. It would be expected that approximately 60–70% of left-handed patients (i.e., patients with right hemisphere motor dominance) would show the same left hemisphere dominance for language as patients who were right handed (Rasmussen and Milner 1977). Since we found that left hemisphere (especially left anterior) lesions were associated with major depression, one might hypothesize that damage to the language dominant hemisphere and, therefore, language impairment were the factors that led to depression. Depression, however, was not significantly associated with aphasia (of 11 patients with depression, five had aphasia; of 19 non-depressed patients, four had aphasia, $p = $ NS). Furthermore, we assumed that 60% of left-handers would show left hemisphere dominance for language and, therefore, in these patients left hemisphere lesions would be associated with depression and only 40% would show the reversed pattern of right hemisphere lesions associated with depression. Using this assumption for distribution of language dominance, 5 of the 12 patients with right hemisphere lesions (i.e., 40%) should have the reversed pattern (i.e., right lesions associated with depression). Of these five patients, three would be expected to be depressed (i.e., 60% of left hemisphere lesion patients were depressed) but only one was found. Similarly, in the left lesion group, seven (i.e., 40%) would be expected to have the reversed pattern and no depression while 60% of the remaining 11 patients should be depressed. In fact, 10% or 92% of the left lesion patients who were expected to have left hemisphere language dominance were depressed. This distribution of depressions and hemispheric injury was significantly different than the expected distribution (i.e., distribution based on the assumed pattern of language dominance).

This study indicated that the association of left anterior lesions with depression in left-handers was just like the association previously reported in right-handers. Even when language dominance was taken into account, the number of depressed patients with left hemisphere lesions was higher than expected and the number of depressed patients with right hemisphere lesions was lower than expected if depression vulnerability was linked with language dominance. Thus, the association of left anterior lesions with major depression does not appear to be associated with motor dominance (i.e., handedness) or perhaps language dominance. It should be emphasized, however, that we did not test for language dominance and our conclusions about the lack of association with language are therefore tentative.

Patients with typical and reversed brain asymmetries

The second study was undertaken to assess depression in patients with evidence on CT scan of reversed anatomical organization of the brain (Starkstein *et al.* 1991). LeMay and Kido (1978) first reported normal brain asymmetries on CT scans. They found that 78% of right-handed males had a greater occipital length in the left hemisphere compared with the right hemisphere and 67% had a greater left than right occipital width. On the other hand, the right frontal length was greater than the left in 70% of subjects and the right frontal width was greater than the left in 53% of individuals studied. Although these findings have been extensively replicated (Chui and Damasio 1980; Weinberger *et al.* 1982), the functional significance of these structural brain asymmetries remains uncertain. Some investigators (Bear *et al.* 1986) reported an increased frequency of asymmetries (especially occipital asymmetries) in left-handed patients while other investigators have reported a similar frequency of asymmetries in both right- and left-handers (Chui and Damasio 1980). Chui and Damasio (1980) suggested that the asymmetries were probably related to language dominance rather than handedness. Studies of aphasic patients, however, have shown no association between language dominance and brain asymmetries (Naeser and Borod 1986). Thus, although the functional significance of brain asymmetries remains uncertain, frontal and/or occipital asymmetries are seen in approximately one-third of patients and, they are presumably associated with some hemispheric asymmetry in brain activity or function.

We examined patients with reversed brain asymmetries and compared the frequency of depressive disorders with that in patients with normal brain asymmetries. All patients had a single stroke lesion which involved either the right or left hemisphere and a CT scan which demonstrated a single lesion but no mass effects of the lesion or lateral head tilt, so asymmetries on CT scan could be adequately assessed.

Asymmetries were assessed in the lowest CT cut showing both the frontal horns of the lateral ventricles and the trigone (i.e., the lateral ventricular region where the body, occipital horn and temporal horn join together). An asymmetry index was calculated by subtracting the area in the left occipital pole from the comparable area in the right hemisphere and dividing by the sum of the two areas. Interrater reliability for these measurements was high ($r = 0.99$, $n = 20$). Patients were considered to have reversed asymmetry when the asymmetry index was more than two standard errors above the mean.

The numbers of patients and their background characteristics, based on the type of brain asymmetry (typical or reversed) and side of lesion (left or right hemisphere) are shown in Table 11.2. Patients were mainly in their 50s and early 60s with a slight predominance of black males and lower socioeconomic classes. No significant differences were observed between groups with the exception of education which was lowest in the right lesion group with typical asymmetry. Findings from the neurological examination revealed no significant intergroup differences except for aphasia which was observed only in patients with left hemisphere lesions.

The frequencies of major and minor depression in each of the groups is shown in Fig. 11.3. In patients with typical (i.e., normal) brain asymmetries in the occipital pole, the frequency of depression was significantly higher among patients with left (i.e., 10 of 23 patients had major depression) as compared with right (i.e., 2 of 16 patients had major depression) hemisphere lesions ($p < 0.05$). The association of left hemisphere lesions with major depression in patients with the normal pattern of brain asymmetry was reversed in patients with the opposite pattern of occipital asymmetries. Among patients with reversed occipital asymmetry, major depression was associated with right hemisphere lesions in three out of eight patients compared to none of nine patients with left hemisphere lesions ($p < 0.1$, trend).

When patients with *typical* asymmetries were grouped according to whether they had an anterior or posterior lesion location, the highest frequency of depression was found among patients with left anterior lesions (seven out of eight patients, 88%) compared with 3 of 15 patients with left posterior lesions (20%, $p < 0.05$, Fig. 11.4). Among the patients with *reversed* asymmetries, two of five patients with right anterior lesions and one of three patients with right posterior lesions had major depression. Finally, the frequency of major depression in patients with *typical* asymmetries and left anterior lesions was significantly greater

Table 11.2. Demographic data for patient with typical and reversed occipital asymmetries

Characteristics	Left lesion groups		Right lesion groups	
	Anterior	Posterior	Anterior	Posterior
(A) Patients with typical occipital asymmetries				
Number of patients	8	15	9	7
Age, mean years ± SD	53.8 ± 17	60.4 ± 15	62.4 ± 9.9	57.1 ± 11
Gender (% female)	63	33	44	29
Race (% blacks)	75	53	33	57
Socioeconomic status (% Hollingshead class IV–V)	100	73	78	71
Marital status (% married)	25	53	55	57
Education, mean years ± SD	9.2 ± 2	10.7 ± 3	8.5 ± 3	11.2 ± 5
Alcoholism (% hospitalized because of alcoholism)	12	13	0	29
Familial history of psychiatric disorder (%)	0	13	11	0
Personal history of psychiatric disorders (%)	12	0	0	0
Handedness (% right handed)	88	80	100	100
Time since stroke, mean days ± SD	15.7 ± 11	13.4 ± 10	16.7 ± 10	14.2 ± 7
(B) Patients with reversed occipital asymmetries				
Number of patients	4	5	5	3
Age, mean years ± SD	57.7 ± 18	58.2 ± 10	59.0 ± 7	62.3 ± 11
Gender (% female)	75	20	20	66
Race (% blacks)	50	60	40	100
Socioeconomic status (% Hollingshead class IV–V)	75	40	80	66
Marital status (% married)	25	60	40	33
Education, mean years ± SD	10.5 ± 1	13.4 ± 4	11.8 ± 2	13.3 ± 4
Alcoholism (% hospitalized because of alcoholism)	500	20	60	33
Familial history of psychiatric disorder (%)	0	0	0	0
Personal history of psychiatric disorders (%)	0	0	0	0
Handedness (% right handed)	75	80	80	100
Time since stroke, mean days ± SD	14.2 ± 11	14.2 ± 12	20.4 ± 11	19.3 ± 15

than among patients with left anterior lesions and *reversed* occipital asymmetries (Fisher exact test $p < 0.025$).

In contrast to these strong associations of depression with occipital asymmetry patterns, we did not find the reversal of the association between major depression and left anterior lesion location among patients with frontal brain asymmetries. There were 19 patients with *reversed* frontal asymmetry; in the group with *typical* frontal asymmetry, five of seven patients (71%) with left anterior lesions had major depression compared with three of five patients (60%) with reversed frontal asymmetry and a left anterior lesion (p = NS). Thus, reversal of frontal asymmetry did not produce a significantly different frequency of depression following left anterior

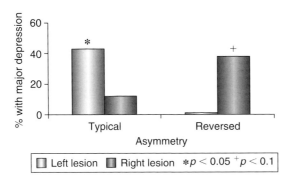

Figure 11.3   The percent of patients who had poststroke depression associated with typical (i.e., normal) occipital brain asymmetry as assessed on axial CT scan. Patients with typical occipital asymmetries had a significantly higher frequency of major depression following left as compared with right hemisphere stroke. Among patients with reversed occipital brain asymmetry, however, there was no association of major depression with left hemisphere lesions. There was a trend for right hemisphere lesions to be associated with depression among patients with reversed brain asymmetry. The frequencies of depression in patients with right or left hemisphere stroke were significantly different in patients with typical as compared to reversed brain asymmetries ($p < 0.025$).

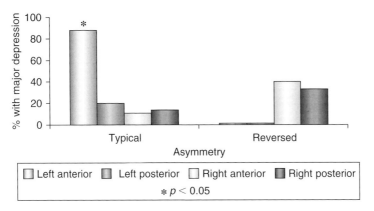

Figure 11.4   The percent of patients with major depression divided into anterior, posterior, right and left lesion location who had typical (i.e., normal) and reversed occipital brain asymmetry. The expected pattern of major depression associated with acute left anterior brain injury was found only in patients with typical occipital asymmetry. There was a trend for patients with reversed occipital asymmetry to an increased frequency of depression associated with right hemisphere rather than left hemisphere stroke.

brain injury. This suggests that posterior asymmetries may be more important than anterior asymmetries in producing the lateralized response to unilateral brain injury.

Findings from this study demonstrated that the association between poststroke major depression and left anterior lesions (i.e., left frontal and left basal ganglia lesions) applied to patients with typical occipital asymmetries and was significantly less frequent among patients with reversed occipital asymmetries. Patients with reversed occipital brain asymmetries appeared to have major depression associated with right hemisphere lesions. The reason that depression and left anterior lesion location were not associated with one another among patients with reversed brain asymmetries may be related to reversal of neurochemical or neuroanatomical pathways which have been hypothesized to mediate depression (see Chapter 21).

Although the functional and anatomical basis of reversed brain asymmetries remains to be established, several studies have found that the presence of either a typical or reversed pattern of brain asymmetry may play a role in the extent of a patient's recovery from stroke related deficits. For example, Schenkman *et al.* (1983) reported that patients with reversed cerebral asymmetries showed *greater* recovery from functional impairments than patients with typical brain asymmetries. They suggested that the inherent flexibility of the cerebral organization of humans (as evidenced by reversed brain asymmetries) may significantly determine outcome following stroke. Pieniadz *et al.* (1986) also reported that recovery may be improved in patients with reversed asymmetries. Patients with global aphasia and reversed occipital asymmetries showed a better recovery in specific language deficits than patients with global aphasia and typical asymmetries.

In summary, although it remains unclear whether a reversed pattern of occipital brain asymmetries seen on CT scan is associated with cerebral dominance for language (the data from the present study showed no cases of aphasia in patients with reversed asymmetries and right hemisphere lesions), the reversed pattern of occipital asymmetry seems to play a role in the association of depression with lesion location following stroke. Patients with typical occipital asymmetries showed the expected increased frequency of major depression associated with left anterior lesions. In patients with reversed occipital asymmetries, however, there was no longer an association between left anterior lesions and major depression (see Fig. 11.4). Further research may elucidate the functional significance or anatomical basis of reversed asymmetries as well as the presumed asymmetry in neural pathways which mediate reversal in hemispheric lesions associated with depression.

REFERENCES

Bear, D., Schiff, D., Saver, J., *et al.* Quantitative analysis of cerebral asymmetries. Fronto-occipital correlation, sexual dimorphism and association with handedness. *Arch Neurol* (1986) 3(6):598–603.

Chui, H. C., and Damasio, A. R. Human cerebral asymmetries evaluated by computed tomography. *J Neurol Neurosurg Psychiatr* (1980) 43:873–878.

LeMay, M., and Kido, D. K. Asymmetries of the cerebral hemispheres on computed tomograms. *J Comput Assist Tomogr* (1978) 2:471–476.

Naeser, M. A., and Borod, J. Aphasia in left handers: lesion site, lesion side, and hemispheric asymmetries on CT. *Neurology* (1986) 36:471–488.

Pieniadz, J. M., and Naeser, M. A. Computed tomographic scan cerebral asymmetries and morphological brain asymmetries: correlation in the same cases post mortem. *Arch Neurol* (1986) 41:403–409.

Rasmussen, T., and Milner, B. The role of early left-brain injury in determining lateralization of cerebral speech functions. *N Y Acad Sci* (1977) 299:355–369.

Robinson, R. G., Lipsey, J. R., Bolla-Wilson, K., *et al.* Mood disorders in left handed stroke patients. *Am J Psychiatr* (1985) 142:1424–1429.

Schenkman, M., Butler, R. B., Naeser, M. A., *et al.* Cerebral hemisphere asymmetry in CT and functional recovery from hemiplegia. *Neurology* (1983) 33(4):473–477.

Starkstein, S. E., Bryer, J. B., Berthier, M. L., *et al.* Depression after stroke: the importance of cerebral hemisphere asymmetries. *J Neuropsychiatr Clin Neurosci* (1991) 3(3):276–285.

Weinberger, D. R., Luchins, D. J., Morihisa, J., *et al.* Asymmetrical volumes of the right and left frontal and occipital regions of the human brain. *Ann Neurol* (1982) 11(1):97–100.

12

Relationship of depression to bilateral hemisphere brain injury

The role of each cerebral hemisphere in emotion regulation has been a topic of speculation and experimental investigation for many years. Flor-Henry (1979), for example, suggested a complex model for the organization of mood. He proposed that the neural substrate for both normal and abnormal mood was predominantly in the non-dominant hemisphere but with bilateral regulation. Thus, according to this hypothesis, euphoria results when the dominant hemisphere no longer receives transcallosal neural inhibition from the non-dominant hemisphere and depression results when the non-dominant hemisphere is released from inhibition by dysfunction in dominant hemisphere. Tucker (1981) has also suggested that the neural substrate for emotion is predominantly in the non-dominant hemisphere. Rather than emphasizing a contralateral release, however, he has suggested ipsilateral release with non-dominant dysfunction leading to positive mood and dominant hemisphere dysfunction manifested as anxious, negative mood. Davidson (1998) suggested that frontal asymmetries recorded by electroencephalography (EEG) in patients with depression (i.e., left frontal inactivation) may reflect deficits in motivation which are independent of current mental state. According to this hypothesis, depressive symptoms emerge based on the cumulative effects of chronic left frontal inactivation and the consequent inability to experience pleasure (Davidson *et al.* 2001). Finally, Kinsbourne and Bemporad (1984) emphasized the integrated functions of the left frontal and right posterior brain areas in mood and suggested that dysfunction in both areas may be involved in depression.

In an effort to examine these hypotheses about the role of hemispheric specialization in depressive disorder, we studied patients with bilateral brain injury (Lipsey *et al.* 1983). Would injury to both hemispheres alter our previous finding of depression being associated with left anterior brain injury? Patients were included in the study if they had computed tomography (CT) scan evidence of bilateral brain injury due to stroke ($n = 13$), or focal traumatic brain injury ($n = 2$). The age of lesions identified on CT scan was categorized by a neuroradiologist (blind to any clinical data) as less than 3 weeks, 3 weeks to 3 months, or greater than 3 months) (depending on relative lucency of the lesion and mass effect).

Patients were grouped according to whether or not they had a left anterior lesion. We hypothesized that there would no longer be an increased frequency of major depression among patients with left anterior lesions and that the existence of bilateral brain injury would be manifested by indifference or apathy rather than depression. In other words, the effect of the right hemisphere lesion could ameliorate the depressive effects of the left frontal lesion. An anterior lesion was defined, as in previous studies, as any lesion whose anterior border was rostral to 40% of the anterior–posterior distance.

Background characteristics such as age (62 $\pm$ 8 SD years left anterior ($n = 8$) versus 59 $\pm$ 20 SD years no left anterior ($n = 6$)), gender distribution (55% male left anterior versus 67% male non-left anterior), social class family or personal prior psychiatric history (none for either left anterior or non-left group), or other background characteristics showed no statistically significant intergroup differences. Of the 15 patients in this study, eight had a single lesion in each hemisphere, five had one lesion of the left hemisphere and two lesions of the right hemisphere, one had two left and one right hemisphere lesions, and one patient had two left and two right hemisphere lesions.

There were no significant differences in neurological findings between patients with and without left anterior brain lesions. Among patients with left anterior lesions, 89% had unilateral motor impairment compared to 100% of patients without left anterior brain lesions. Similarly, 38% of patients with left anterior lesions and 50% of those with no such lesions had aphasia.

Patients with left anterior lesions, however, had significantly more severe symptoms of depression than those without left anterior lesions on the Hamilton depression scale ($p < 0.05$, Fig. 12.1). There were no intergroup differences, however, in terms of the severity of impairment in activities of daily living (Johns Hopkins functioning inventory (JHFI)) or cognitive function (mini-mental state examination) (Fig. 12.1). Furthermore, correlational analysis showed a statistically significant inverse correlation ($r = -0.64, p < 0.05$) between Hamilton depression score and the distance between the anterior border of the lesion and the frontal pole only in the *left* hemisphere (Fig. 12.2). In the two patients who had more than one left hemisphere lesion, the most anterior lesion was chosen for measurement of the distance from the frontal pole. There was no significant correlation, however, between Hamilton depression score and the distance between the lesion and the frontal pole for right-sided lesions. Similarly, there were no significant correlations between Hamilton depression scores and either cognitive impairment (mini-mental state examination) or impairment in activities of daily living (JHFI).

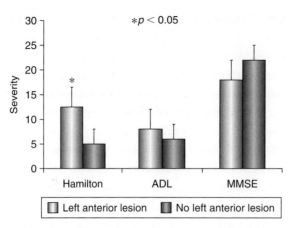

Figure 12.1 Severity of depression (Hamilton), impairment in activities of daily living (ADL) and impairment in cognitive function (mini-mental state examination (MMSE)) in patients with bilateral hemispheric strokes divided into those with one lesion whose anterior border is rostral to 40% of the over anterior–posterior (A–P) diameter of the left hemisphere and those without a left anterior lesion. Patients with left anterior lesions had more severe depressive symptoms than patients without this lesion location but there were no significant differences in the severity of ADL or cognitive impairments.

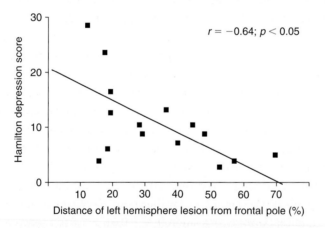

Figure 12.2 Severity of depression as measured by the Hamilton depression scale and proximity of the most anterior left hemisphere lesion to the frontal pole in patients with bilateral strokes. Severity of depression increased with proximity of the lesion to *the left* frontal lobe. Severity of depression, however, was not significantly correlated with right hemisphere lesion location or the age of the most recent stroke.

We next examined whether these findings may have been influenced by the age of the lesions. There was no significant difference between patients with left anterior lesions and those without left anterior lesions in terms of the mean age of their left hemisphere lesions. There was also no significant correlation between the age category (i.e., $<$3 weeks, $>$3 weeks, $>$3 months) of the left hemisphere lesion and the severity of depression. Thus, the increased severity of depression in the left anterior lesion group was not the result of their lesions being more acute than those of the group with no left anterior lesion. Finally, we examined the temporal sequence of the lesions using the lesion age categories. In the group with left anterior lesions, this lesion was more recent in three out of nine patients while the right hemisphere lesion was more recent in the six remaining patients. In the group of patients without a left anterior lesion, the left lesion was the most recent in one of six patients while the right lesion was more recent in the remaining five patients. Thus, a hypothesis of increased frequency of left-sided acute lesions in the left anterior compared with the non-left anterior group was not supported by statistical analysis ($p = $ NS). This finding indicates that the greater severity of depression among patients with left anterior lesions was not explained by the location of the most recent infarct. Most of the patients with left anterior lesions (i.e., the group with significantly higher depression scores) actually had an acute right hemisphere infarct as their most recent lesion.

What are the implications of this study for understanding the mechanisms of depression? Firstly, this study of bilateral lesions indicates the predominance of left frontal pathology over other lesion locations in the mechanism of poststroke depression during the acute period following a second stroke. Secondly, neural mechanisms within the left hemisphere probably played a dominant role in the generation of depression since the existence of a concomitant, frequently acute, right hemisphere lesion did not alter the clinical presentation. The left hemisphere did not appear to be "released" by a right hemisphere lesion and this finding suggests that the mechanism for depression is mediated within the left hemisphere. Thus, the suggestion by Tucker (1981) that contralateral release plays a role in depression is not supported by these findings. These findings are, however, consistent with Davidson's (1998) suggestion that left frontal hemisphere dysfunction may be manifested by the absence of approach motivation and the inability to experience pleasure. The fact that we did not find an augmentation of depression by a combination of left anterior and right hemisphere lesions (i.e., the depression scores were the same as we have previously found in patients with single left anterior lesions) does not lend confirmation (although it also does not disprove) to the suggestion of Kinsbourne and Bemporad (1984) that both right and left hemisphere dysfunction are involved in depression.

In summary, this unusual study of the interaction of the cerebral hemispheres in the etiology of poststroke depression demonstrated that the existence of a left anterior brain lesion was significantly associated with more severe depression independent of the age or temporal sequence of a concomitant right hemisphere lesion. In addition, the proximity of the left anterior lesion to the frontal pole correlated significantly with severity of depression. It should be emphasized, however, that dichotomous distinctions between right and left hemisphere functions in the production of emotion are probably oversimplifications and mediation of emotion using both hemispheres is likely. However, this study of patients with bilateral brain injury is rarely done and does contribute some intriguing findings to our understanding of the role that each cerebral hemisphere plays in the production or maintenance of depression.

REFERENCES

Davidson, J., Pearlstein, T., Londborg, P., *et al.* Efficacy of sertraline in preventing relapse of post-traumatic stress disorder: results of a 28-week double-blind, placebo-controlled study. *Am J Psychiatr* (2001) 158(12):1974–1981.

Davidson, R. J. Affective style and affective disorders: perspectives from affective neuroscience. *Cognition Emotion* (1998) 12(3):307–330.

Flor-Henry, P. Uncertain aspects of the localization of the cerebral symptoms relating and determining emotion. *Biol Psychiatr* (1979) 14:677–698.

Kinsbourne, M., and Bemporad, B. Lateralization of emotion: a model and the evidence. In N. A. Fox and R. J. Davidson, eds., *The Psychobiology of Affective Development*, Hinsdale, N.J.: Lawrence Erlbaum Associates, 1984.

Lipsey, J. R., Robinson, R. G., Pearlson, G. D., *et al.* Mood change following bilateral hemisphere brain injury. *Br J Psychiatr* (1983) 143:266–273.

Tucker, D. M. Lateral brain function, emotion, and conceptualizations. *Psychol Bull* (1981) 89:19–46.

13

Relationship of depression to physical impairment

Background

Apart from studies of the prevalence of poststroke depression, more investigators have examined the relationship between depression and physical impairment than any other association. Perhaps it is an understandable interest because motor impairment represents the most common presenting symptom among patients admitted to hospital with an acute stroke; approximately 70–80% of patients with acute hemispheric stroke present with weakness or paralysis of either the upper and/or lower extremity. Compared with other neurological impairments produced by stroke, such as sensory loss which occurs in about 35% of patients with hemispheric stroke or visual field loss which occurs in about 20%, hemiparesis or monoparesis occurs in the majority of patients admitted to hospital with acute stroke.

Although there is an initial tendency to assume that there is an understandable relationship between poststroke depression and physical impairment, the existing evidence suggests that the relationship is a complex one in which the severity of depressive disorder affects the severity and recovery of physical impairment, and the severity of physical impairment affects the severity and course of depression. In addition, there appear to be dynamic changes over time in the relationship between depression and physical impairment. Using the large database which examined the prevalence of depressive disorders (see Chapter 6), I have summarized the world's literature in Table 13.1 which allows findings from various studies to be compared and readers who are interested in investigating specific studies to identify these studies. The table is divided into three primary areas of investigation. The first area examines the statistical correlation between severity of depression and severity of physical impairment usually measured by activities of daily living (ADL). The second section demonstrates findings concerning the effect of depression on recovery in ADLs while the third section involves studies examining the effect of treatment of depression on recovery in ADLs.

Table 13.1. Relationship of depression and physical impairment

Study	n	Impairment measure	Time since stroke	D versus ND	Univariate analysis D and impairment	Multiple logistic regression	Conclude D and impairment related
I. Relationship of D and physical impairment							
Robinson et al. (1983)	103	JHFI	11 + 14 days		$r = 0.36$	NA	+
Sinyor et al. (1986)	64	PECS	6 week FU		$r = -0.45$, $p < 0.05$	NA	+
Ebrahim et al. (1987)	149	10 items, 0–10-point scale	1 month		$p < 0.01$	NA	+
Eastwood (1989)	87	BI	2–3 months		$r = 0.18$ Ham, $r = -0.33$ GDS	NA	+
Morris (1990)	88	BI	8.4 weeks		$r = 0.11$, $p = $ NS	ADL impairment associated minor D (odds ratio = 0.68, $p = 0.05$)	+ and −
Schubert et al. (1992)	21	BI	1–4 weeks		NS	NA	−
Angeleri et al. (1993)	180	NUDS	37 + 36 months		$r = 0.41$, $p < 0.05$	Beck strongest correlate	+
Astrom et al. (1993)	73	Katz	3 months		$p = 0.020$	NA	+
Schwartz (1993)	91	Crichtondis	90 days		$r = 0.41$, $p < 0.001$	NA	+
Shima (1997)	20	Chart review	1 month to 3 years		No correlation D and ADL	NA	−
Herrmann et al. (1998)	150	FIM	3 months		$r = 0.31$, $p = 0.0001$	NA	+

Study	N	Measure	Time	Finding	Statistic		
Ramasubbu et al. (1998)	626	BI	7–10 days		$r = -0.25$, $p = 0.0001$	NA	+
Paolucci et al. (1999)	470	BI	Approximately 44 days		$p < 0.05$ (odds ratio: 1.99; CI: 1.14–3.46)	NA	+
Kauhanen et al. (2000)	76	Rand physical functioning dimension	12 months		$p < 0.0001$	NA	+
Gainotti et al. (2001)	64	BI	1–4 months		$p < 0.05$	NA	+
House et al. (2001)	448	BI	1 month		$p < 0.004$	NA	+
Berg et al. (2003)	100	Tapping, right	2 weeks		$r = -0.34$, $p < 0.01$	$r = -0.26$, $p < 0.05$	+
Desmond et al. (2003)	421	BI	3 months		$p < 0.05$, odds ratio = 1.815	BI not significant in logistic regression	+
Total				83% of studies found significant association of D with impaired recovery			
II. Effect of D on recovery from physical impairment							
Parikh et al. (1990)	63	JHFI	2 years	D patients showed less functional recovery over 2 years than ND patients	$p < 0.01$	NA	+
Herrmann et al. (1998)	150	FIM, Oxford handicap scale	15 months	D correlates with FIM at 3 months and 1 year	3 months: $r = 0.31$, $p < 0.001$; 1 year: $r = -0.28$, $p < 0.001$	NA	+

Table 13.1. (*Continued*)

Study	n	Impairment measure	Time since stroke	D versus ND	Univariate analysis D and impairment	Multiple logistic regression	Conclude D and impairment related
van de Weg et al. (1999)	85	FIM	6 weeks	No difference in amount change in FIM, D versus ND	14.9 + 9.0 versus 14.2 + 10.2 SD	NA	−
Paolucci et al. (1999, 2000a, b, 2001)	470	BI	83 + 41 SD days	D patients (Ham-D > 18) had greater frequency of BI < 1 compared to ND (odds ratio: 1.99; CI: 1.14–3.46)	$p < 0.05$	NA	+
Pohjasvaara et al. (2001)	256	RS	15 months	Major D versus ND (48% major D had poor outcome versus 27% ND)		D at 3 months and RS at 15 months (odds ratio: 7.5; CI: 1.6–3.8)	+
Sturm et al. (2004)	226	London handicap scale (LHS)	2 years	D at 2 years correlated with LHS at 2 years $p < 0.002$	$r = 0.35$	NA	+

Total   83% of studies found that depression impairs recovery in ADL

III. *Effect of treatment of D on recovery*

Study	n		Treatment		Scale	Design	Results
Lipsey et al. (1984)	34	262 days	Nortriptyline (100 mg/day), $n = 14$, placebo = 20	6 weeks	JHFI	Double blind	Nortriptyline = placebo (at 4 weeks), no ADL difference
Reding et al. (1986)	16	45 days	Trazodone (maximum 200 mg/day), $n = 9$, placebo = 7	32.6 days	BI	Double blind	Trazodone > placebo, mean BI scores improved to 38 for trazodone versus 20 for placebo +
Gonzalez-Torrecillas et al. (1995)	37	4 weeks	Nortriptyline (maximum 75 mg/day) Fluoxetine (maximum 20 mg/day)	6 weeks	BI and KPS	Open study	nortriptyline = fluoxetine > no Rx (at 3–6 weeks) on BI + nortriptyline = fluoxetine > no Rx (at 5 and 6 weeks) on KPS
Dam et al. (1996)	46	1–6 months	16 fluoxetine 14 maprotiline 16 placebo	3 months	BI and HSS	Open label	Good recovery with fluoxetine 75% fluoxetine, 36% maprotiline, 38% + placebo improved after treatment
Palomaki et al. (1999)	100	14.3 days	51 mianserin (maximum 60 mg/day) 49 placebo	12 months	BI and RS	Double blind	Mianserin = placebo (at 2, 6, 12, and 18 mhs)
Paolucci et al. (2000b)	290	36 days	120 fluoxetine 16 maprotiline 9 other	83 days	BI and RMMI	Open label	No difference in ADL recovery comparing 145 D and 145 ND

Table 13.1. (*Continued*)

	n	After stroke (mean days)	Medication	Duration	Results	Design	Significant drug effect
Robinson et al. (2000)	56	10 weeks	16 nortriptyline 23 fluoxetine 17 placebo	12 weeks	FIM and JHFI	Double blind	Nortriptyline > fluoxetine at 9 and 12 weeks; placebo > fluoxetine at 12 weeks on FIM improvement No treatment effect on JHFI improvement
Wiart et al. (2000)	31	47.1 days	16 fluoxetine (20 mg/day) 15 placebo	6 weeks	FIM	Double blind	Fluoxetine = placebo (at 6 weeks)
Chemerinski et al. (2001a)	10	10 weeks	7 nortriptyline	12 weeks	JHFI	Double blind	Responders showed significantly better recovery over + 12 weeks of nortriptyline or fluoxetine compared with non-responders, no significant difference in ADL, between nortriptyline versus placebo groups

Total   44% of studies found treatment improved recovery. Responders to treatment improve more than non-responders

N: number of subjects; D: depression; ND: no depression; GDS: geriatric depression scale; FU: fluoraouracil; PECS: Patient Evaluation Conference System; HSS: hemispheric stroke scale; NUDS: Northwestern University disability scale; SSS: Scandinavian stroke scale.

The relationship between severity of depression and severity of physical impairment

As indicated in Table 13.1, 83% of studies that have examined the relationship between poststroke depression and physical impairment have found that patients with depression are significantly more physically impaired than patients without depression, and furthermore that there is a direct correlation between severity of physical impairment and severity of depressive symptoms (Robinson *et al.* 1983; Eastwood *et al.* 1989; Astrom *et al.* 1993). We have examined our overall acute stroke patient database to examine the relationship between severity of neurological impairment in motor function, sensory deficit, visual impairment, and the severity of depression (Table 13.2). Mean depression scores in patients with upper or lower extremity paresis were not significantly different among patients with mild to moderate motor impairment as compared to those with severe impairment.

Perhaps the most useful way to assess the relationship between physical impairment and poststroke depression is not to look at the severity of motor or sensory

Table 13.2. Severity of neurological impairment and depression

	Weakness			Touch-pain deficit		
	Mild/moderate	Severe	(Significance)	No	Yes	(Significance)
Right arm or leg						
n	220	79		217	22	
Depression	7.9 ± 6.3	8.7 ± 6.2	(NS)	7.5 ± 6.5	6.6 ± 5.9	(NS)
ADL	5.2 ± 4.6	7.9 ± 5.8	(0.0001)	6.1 ± 5.4	4.8 ± 5.9	(NS)
Mini-mental	24.0 ± 5.1	22.6 ± 6.4	(0.0581)	22.5 ± 5.7	25.1 ± 4.1	(0.0394)
Left arm or leg						
n	180	116		213	26	
Depression	7.6 ± 6.4	8.8 ± 6.0	(NS)	7.3 ± 6.4	8.3 ± 6.8	(NS)
ADL	5.6 ± 5.4	6.3 ± 4.6	(NS)	5.9 ± 5.3	6.5 ± 6.5	(NS)
Mini-mental	23.2 ± 5.6	24.2 ± 5.3	(NS)	22.7 ± 5.7	23.5 ± 5.5	(NS)
	Visual field deficit					
	No	Yes				
	278	64				
Depression	7.4 ǀ 6.4	9.3 ǀ 7.0	0.0394			
ADL	5.7 + 5.0	7.5 + 5.6	0.0106			
Mini-mental	23.5 + 5.5	24.05 + 6.0	0.5580			

Depression: Ham-D score. Higher numbers indicate greater severity of depression (values given in mean ± SD).

ADL: JHFI score. Higher numbers indicate greater impairment (values given in mean ± SD).

Mini-mental: lower numbers indicate greater intellectual impairment (values given in mean ± SD).

impairment but to quantitate deficits in performance of daily activities. In our studies, we have used the Johns Hopkins functioning inventory (JHFI) to quantify severity of impairment in ADL. Our more recent studies have utilized the functional independence measure (FIM) as a more widely accepted measurement of ADL impairment. The JHFI assesses the patient's ability to dress themselves, feed themselves, walk, find their way around, express needs, read and write, keep their room in order, and to maintain sphincter control. Although this ADL scale evaluates severity of impairment across a range of activities related to daily care, it is heavily dependent on limitations in physical activity.

As shown in Table 13.1, most studies have found that the severity of impairment in ADL scores is significantly greater in depressed compared with non-depressed patients. Furthermore, some studies have found a statistically significant correlation between severity of impairment in ADL and severity of depressive symptoms. Even when multiple regression or logistic regression analyses have been used to look for independent effects of severity of impairment on depressive disorder, significant relationships have been reported.

Figure 13.1 shows the mean correlation coefficient between the JHFI score and the summed total scores on the Zung, Hamilton, and present state examination (PSE) at 5-time points during 2 years following acute stroke. During the first 6 months following stroke, there was an increase in the mean correlation between severity of impairment and severity of depression. However, at 1- and 2-year poststroke, the strength of the correlation declined.

In addition to this cross sectional look at the relationship between impairment and depression, we have also examined the predictive relationship between ADL and depression scores over the first 2 years following stroke. If severity of physical impairment was causing depression through a psychological response (e.g., grief

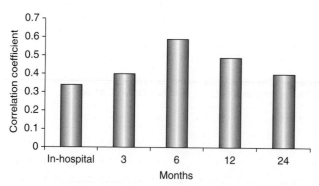

Figure 13.1   Correlation coefficients between ADL (JHFI) scores and depression scores over the first 2 years following stroke. The correlations increased in strength during the first 6-month poststroke and then declined for the next 18 months. The correlation, however, remained statistically significant, throughout the first 2 years following an acute stroke.

secondary to loss of previous lifestyle), one would predict that in-hospital severity of impairment in ADL would predict depression at 3 or 6 months. Similarly, if severity of depression was influencing patients' physical recovery from stroke, one would predict depression in-hospital would be related to ADL impairment at 3 or 6 months. Our data, in fact, supported both explanations as shown in Fig. 13.2. We found that in-hospital measures of depression using either the PSE Hamilton or Zung depression scores correlated significantly with ADL as measured by the JHFI score at 3 months following stroke. Also both the PSE and the Hamilton depression (Ham-D) scores assessed at the time of the in-patient evaluation correlated significantly with measures of ADL at 6-month follow-up. On the other hand, ADL scores (JHFI scores in-hospital were significantly correlated with depression scores at both 3- and 6-month follow-up (Fig. 13.2). These findings suggest that the most physically impaired patients remain the most depressed at follow-up and the most depressed patients remained the most physically impaired at follow-up.

Our finding, however, raises the question of why the relationship between physical impairment and depression may be a dynamic one. It is possible that the strength of the correlation increased for the first 6 months (see Fig. 13.1) because the most severely impaired patients became more depressed over the first 6 months. As shown in our previous analysis, however, part of this increased correlation could

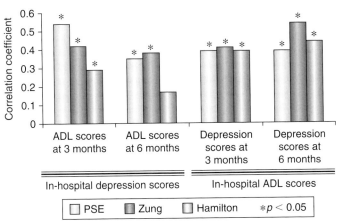

Figure 13.2 Correlation coefficients between depression and ADL impairment over the first 6 months following stroke. There were significant correlations between in-hospital depression or ADL scores and depression or impairment scores at 3- or 6-month follow-up. Note that in-hospital depression appears to weaken in its relationship to follow-up ADL scores over time while in-hospital ADL scores show increasing correspondence with follow-up depression scores. This may suggest that the most physically impaired patients remain the most depressed over the first 6 months following stroke.

represent a failure of depressed patients to recover in their ADL during the initial poststroke period when much of the physical recovery would be expected to take place. A third possible explanation for the increased correspondence between depression and ADL impairment is that both depression and physical impairment are related to another factor. For example, patients who have the greatest degree of cognitive impairment might not be able to participate in stroke rehabilitation and might become the most depressed patients. Although the available data suggest that physical impairment influences depression and vice versa. Multiple regression analyses by Eastwood *et al.* (1989), Morris *et al.* (1990), and ourselves (unpublished data) have shown that the relationship between depression and impairment in ADL is independent of the severity in cognitive impairment, social function, age, education, or other background characteristics.

The effect of depression on recovery in ADL

Examining the effect of depression on recovery in ADL is a complicated task because there are so many variables which have been demonstrated to effect physical recovery from stroke (Table 13.1). The factors which have been shown to influence recovery include baseline neurological deficits, early intervention care, presence of a stroke unit, type of infarct, and the use of physiotherapy (Dove *et al.* 1984). The effect of depression cannot be evaluated unless all of these as well as other factors are either comparable across groups or controlled.

In an effort to control for all of these factors, we studied 25 patients who had either major or minor depression following an acute stroke and some impairment in their ADL score (JHFI score > 0) compared with 38 non-depressed patients who had a comparable degree of physical impairment at the time of their initial evaluation following acute stroke (Parikh *et al.* 1990). Patients were included only if they had survived 2 years since stroke without subsequent stroke or other significant medical illnesses that would have effected their recovery in daily activities. Background characteristics are shown in Table 13.3 including their baseline neurological findings. There were no statistically significant differences in demographic characteristics of the depressed (major and minor depression combined) and non-depressed patients. Similarly there were no significant intergroup differences in neurological findings or in the severity of intellectual impairment or social impairment. Furthermore, all patients received acute care on the same specialized stroke unit and there were no significant differences in the mean time from stroke to receipt of medical care.

Repeated measures analysis of variance (ANOVA) of ADL scores (i.e., Johns Hopkins functioning inventory or JHFI scores) comparing depressed and non-depressed patients in-hospital and at 2-year follow-up showed a significant group-by-time interaction (i.e., change in JHFI scores over time were significantly different

Table 13.3. In-hospital characteristics of the depressed and non-depressed groups[a]

	Depressed[b] ($n = 25$)	Non-depressed ($n = 38$)
Age, year (mean ± SD)	56 ± 12	61 ± 19
Sex (% male)	42	66
Race (% black)	59	56
Marital status (%)		
Married	50	49
Widowed	16	21
Other	34	30
Socioeconomic status (Hollingshead class) (%)		
I–III	13	21
IV–V	87	79
History of CVA (%)	14	16
MMSE (mean ± SD)	21.1 ± 60	22.0 ± 6.0
Social ties checklist (mean ± SD)	4.3 ± 2.0	4.3 ± 1.9
Social functioning examination (mean ± SD)	0.27 ± .20	0.20 ± 0.13
Time from stroke to interview (days ± SD)	11 ± 12	9 ± 6
Stroke type		
Thromboembolism	20	31
Intracerebral hemorrhage	5	7
Neurological examination findings		
Hemiparesis–monoparesis, moderate to severe	10	13
Sensory deficit, moderate to severe	9	14
Visual field deficit, hemianopsia or quadrantanopsia	5	6
Aphasia		
Broca's	2	1
Wernicke's	0	1
Global	2	1
Other	5	3

CVA: cerebrovascular accident.

[a] There were no significant differences in any of the variables between the two groups.

[b] Major and minor depression combined.

for depressed and non-depressed groups, $p < 0.05$ (Fig. 13.3). Repeated measures ANOVA of major versus minor depression, however, did not show any significant differences in the ADL recovery curves for these two kinds of depression. Although the two groups were not significantly different in terms of their JHFI scores in-hospital, *post hoc* analysis revealed statistically significantly lower (i.e., less impairment in ADL) scores for the non-depressed patients compared with the depressed group at 2-year follow-up ($p < 0.01$).

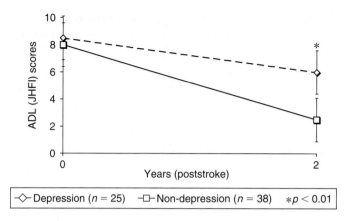

Figure 13.3 JHFI scores among patients with an acute in-hospital diagnosis of poststroke major or minor depression or no mood disorder. Higher scores (mean ± SEM shown) indicate greater impairment. There was a significant group-by-time interaction, demonstrating that depressed patients had less recovery in terms of ADL than non-depressed patients (modified from Parikh *et al. Arch Neurol* 47:785–789, copyright © 1990 American Medical Association. All rights reserved.).

A factor analysis of the 10 items in the JHFI revealed that there were three distinct factors being measured by the JHFI score. Factor 1 included six items related to physical impairment: ability to walk, dress, eat, write, find one's way around and perform routine tasks. Factor 2 included three items related to comprehension and expression of language: comprehension of spoken and written language, and the ability to express one's needs. Factor 3 was one item related to sphincter control. Analysis of each factor independently indicated that there was a significant time-by-group interaction for Factor 1 (i.e., physical impairment) and Factor 2 (i.e., language impairment) but not for Factor 3.

A multiple regression analysis of ADL scores at 2-year follow-up examining the effects of in-hospital depression scores, 2-year depression scores, in-hospital ADL scores, intellectual impairment scores in-hospital and at follow-up, social functioning scores in-hospital and at follow-up, and lesion location (i.e., proximity to the frontal pole) demonstrated that in-hospital depression scores were independently and positively correlated with JHFI scores at 2 years ($r = 0.42, p < 0.05$) (i.e., the lower the in-hospital depression score the less the impairment in ADL 2 years later). The only other significant correlate of ADL scores at 2-year follow-up was the in-hospital JHFI score ($r = 0.40, p < 0.05$). Interestingly, in-hospital ADL scores did not correlate significantly with depression scores at 2 years. This suggests that the most severely impaired patients at the time of the acute stroke were not the most severely depressed patients by 2-year follow-up.

Depressive diagnoses at 2-year follow-up revealed no significant intergroup differences in the frequency or severity of depression. This suggests that the significantly poorer physical recovery in patients with major or minor depression was related to the initial period of depression and not to depressive status at 2-year follow-up.

We also examined other factors which might influence recovery of ADL at 2-year follow-up including lesion location (hemisphere or structure), lesion volume, nature of the ischemic lesion, the existence of aphasia, and the amount of rehabilitation therapy. We also examined the frequency of purely subcortical, purely cortical, and mixed cortical subcortical lesions in the depressed compared with the non-depressed group. There were no significant differences between groups in any of these factors (e.g., total lesion volume for depressed patients was $6.2 \pm 5.25\%$ of total brain volume versus 5.3 ± 3.7 for non-depressed patients, $p = NS$). Similarly, thromboembolic versus hemorrhagic infarcts and lacunar versus non-lacunar infarcts did not explain the differences in recovery between the depressed and non-depressed groups. Finally, the effect of physical, occupational, or speech therapy after hospitalization did not differentiate the depressed and non-depressed groups (e.g., 55% of the depressed and 50% of the non-depressed patients had post-hospital rehabilitation therapy).

Pohjasvaara *et al.* (2001) reported on the relationship between depressive disorder at 3 months following ischemic stroke and outcome 15 months later in a group of 256 patients who were examined for depression among a consecutive group of 486 patients with stroke aged 55–85 years. Diagnostic and Statistical Manual, 2nd ed., revised (DSM-II-R) major depression was diagnosed in 66 (25.8%) and minor depression in 32 (12.5%) of 256 patients 3 months following stroke. Patients with Beck depression inventory scores of 10 or greater or with a diagnosis of major depression had significantly greater frequency of poor functional outcome as measured by the Rankin scale (RS) or the Barthel index (BI) (i.e., depressed patients with RS > II or BI < 17 was 48% compared to non-depressed with RS > II or BI < 17, 27%). A logistic regression analysis demonstrated that the diagnosis of depression as defined by Beck score of 10 or greater was significantly and independently associated with an RS > II (odds ratio: 2.5; 95% confidence interval (CI): 1.6–3.8). However, an RS > II at 3 months was not independently associated with (Beck depression scale 10 or greater at 15 months. Thus depression at 3 months appeared to be a better predictor of functional physical outcome at 15 months than physical outcome was a predictor of depression at 15 months.

Herrmann *et al.* (1998) examined 150 patients at 3 months and 136 patients at 1-year poststroke. Depressive symptoms as measured by the Zung depression scale and the Montgomery Asberg depression rating scale at 3 months following stroke were significantly correlated with ADL as measured by the FIM ($r = -0.31$, $p < 0.0001$) and the Oxford handicap scale ($r = 0.41$, $p < 0.0001$) and at 1 year

($r = -0.28$, $p < 0.001$, FIM; $r = 0.35$, $p < 0.0001$, Oxford handicap scale). Thus, severity of depression at 3 months was significantly associated with greater degree of impairment at 1-year follow-up.

Paolucci et al. (1999) reported that among 470 patients who were a mean of 44 days following stroke, multiple regression analyses failed to show an association between impairment of ADL as measured by the BI or the River mead mobility index (RMMI) and severity of depression as measured by the Ham-D scale. The only significant association with depression was a poor rehabilitation response (i.e., with less change in the BI than no depression) during the course of 83 ± 41-day treatment in a rehabilitation hospital (odds ratio: 1.99; CI: 1.1–4.46). It should be noted, however, that all of the 129 patients with depression with Ham-D scores greater than 18 (i.e., the definition of depression), received either fluoxetine ($n = 118$) or amitriptyline ($n = 11$). Thus, treatment likely influenced the lack of a longitudinal association between depression and impairment in ADLs.

van de Weg et al. (1999) examined 85 patients admitted to a rehabilitation hospital 3–6 weeks following stroke with follow-up 6 months later. Thirty patients (35%) were diagnosed with major depression based on a clinical interview and DSM, 3rd ed., revised (DSM-III-R) criteria. FIM scores at admission were significantly lower (more impaired) in the depressed compared with the non-depressed patients ($n = 55$). At 6 months follow-up, however, there was a 14.9 ± 9.0-point improvement for the depressed patients and 14.4 ± 10.2 for the non-depressed patients ($p = $ NS). Thus, the rate of recovery in ADLs in the depressed patients was equivalent to the rate of recovery in the non-depressed patients. At both admission and at follow-up, however, the depressed patients were more impaired than the non-depressed patients.

Effect of treatment on recovery in physical impairment

The final area of investigation which has generated a surprising number of studies has involved the assessment of antidepressant medications and their effects on recovery from physical impairment or ADL impairment. The first study to demonstrate a positive effect of treatment of depression on recovery in ADLs was reported by Reding et al. (1986). During a 6-week double-blind treatment trial, 16 patients who had a positive dexamethasone suppression test (DST) showed greater improvement in their ADL scores as measured by the BI when they received double-blind treatment with trazodone ($n = 7$) (dose: 50–200 mg/day) as compared with placebo (Table 13.2). Although grouping the patients based on the clinical diagnosis of major or dysthymic depressive disorder did not show a statistically significant effect of trazodone, there was a trend for actively treated depressed patients to improve their BI scores more than depressed patients treated with placebo.

In an open label study, Gonzalez-Torrecillas (1995) compared 26 poststroke depressed patients treated with fluoxetine (20–40 mg/day), 11 poststroke depressed patients treated with nortriptyline (25–100 mg/day), and 11 poststroke depressed patients given no treatment. Patients began treatment 4-week poststroke and the treatment trial lasted 6 weeks. Both neurological function as measured by the Orgogozo scale and ADL as measured by the BI showed significantly greater improvement in patients treated with either nortriptyline or fluoxetine compared with placebo ($p < 0.005$) for both scales (Table 13.1).

Dam *et al.* (1996) reported on 52 severely hemiplegic subjects treated with fluoxetine ($n = 16$), maprotiline ($n = 14$), or placebo ($n = 16$) in an open label design. Patients were in a rehabilitation program between 1 and 6 months following stroke and the duration of treatment was 3 months. There were no significant differences prior to treatment in their BI scores or in their graded neurological scale (HSS) (Adams *et al.* 1987). There were no significant differences between groups in either the BI or HSS score. Based on cluster analysis, patients were divided into those with good recovery and those with poor recovery. The patients treated with fluoxetine had 12 of 16 patients (75%) in the good recovery group at the end of the 3-month protocol compared to 5 of 14 patients (36%) treated with maprotiline and 6 of 16 patients (38%) treated with placebo ($p < 0.05$ fluoxetine versus maprotiline and placebo). In contrast to these positive findings with antidepressant medications, Paolucci *et al.* (2001) performed a case-controlled study in 290 stroke in-patients matched for age ± 1 year and interval between stroke and admission (± 3 days). Of the 145 depressed patients, 120 received fluoxetine (10–20 mg/day), 16 maprotiline (10–20 mg/day), and 9 received other antidepressants (amitriptyline or mianserin). Patients were treated in an open label study and were in a rehabilitation program. The duration of treatment was 83 ± 41 days. The patients with poststroke depression compared to patients without depression showed the same course of recovery with both showing improvement in BI and Rankin scores. The only significant finding was patients with poststroke depression were less likely to have a high response on the Rankin scale compared with non-depressed patients (24.6% versus 15.1%, $p < 0.05$).

In our 12-week treatment study comparing nortriptyline, fluoxetine and placebo, using double-blind methodology, we found no significant difference in ADL as measured by the FIM. The FIM is an 18-item 72-point scale with lower numbers indicating greater impairment. The FIM consists of six domains including self-care, sphincter control, mobility, locomotion, communication, and social cognition. On the FIM, however, there was significantly less recovery in the fluoxetine treated group compared with the nortriptyline or placebo group (Robinson *et al.* 2000).

Other double-blind treatment studies which have measured change in ADL have also failed to show a difference between active and placebo treatment.

Wiart *et al.* (2000) showed a significant time effect but no significant group effect on ADL as measured by the FIM. The study by Fruehwald (2003) found no significant difference in a double-blind-randomized treatment study of 26 patients treated with fluoxetine (20 mg/day) or placebo for 12 weeks. During the 12 weeks of treatment there were no significant differences in improvement in the SSS or Barthel scales, however, at 18-month follow-up the fluoxetine treated group showed a greater degree of recovery than the placebo treated group.

We have conducted three studies which have examined the effect of treatment or remission of depression on recovery in ADL (Chemerinski *et al.* 2001a, b; Narushima *et al.* 2003). Our first study examined 21 patients who had major or minor depression following acute stroke and who had remission of depression defined as >50% reduction in Ham-D score by 3- or 6-month follow-up. Non-remission was a <50% reduction in Ham-D score at the same follow-up interval. The remission group (*n* = 21) had an initial JHFI score of 8.3 ± 5.9 (SD) while the non-remission group (*n* = 34) had an initial JHFI score of 8.0 ± 5.0 (SD) (Fig. 13.4). Repeated measures ANOVA revealed a significant group-by-time interaction with the patients in remission having improved significantly more than the non-remission patients. A factor analysis of the JHFI revealed three distinct factors (Parikh *et al.* 1990): Factor 1 included six motor items, ability to walk, dress, eat, write, find one's way around a familiar setting and ability to perform routine tasks; Factor 2 included three language items, comprehension of spoken and written language and ability to express one's needs; and Factor 3 included only sphincter control. A repeated measures ANOVA for each factor revealed a significant group-by-time interaction for Factor 1

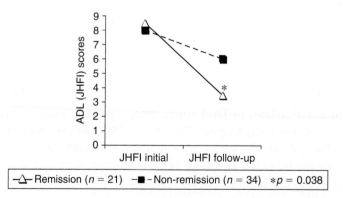

Figure 13.4 ADL scores, as measured by the JHFI, in depressed patients during the acute poststroke evaluation and at 3- or 6-month follow-up. Patients who had remission of their depression sometime between initial evaluation and follow-up showed significantly better recovery in their ADLs than patients who remained depressed (reprinted with permission from Chemerinski *et al. Stroke* (2001b) 32:113–117).

($p = 0.03$) but not Factor 2 ($p = 0.6$) or Factor 3 ($p = 0.5$). There were no significant differences between the remission and non-remission groups in age, race, marital status, years of education, time since stroke or the percent of patients receiving antidepressant therapy (mood improvement 19%, no mood improvement 20%). There were no significant differences between groups in cognitive impairment as measured by the mini-mental state examination (MMSE), lesion volume, cortical or subcortical lesion location, number with motor deficits, sensory deficits, visual field deficits, aphasia, apraxia, neglect or the number who had received physical therapy. There was, however, a significantly higher percentage of women in the non-remission group ($p = 0.01$). When we reanalyzed the data using only male patients, however, there remained a significant group-by-time interaction indicating that the improvement in remitted patients was not due to male/female differences in ADL recovery. There were also no significant differences in the amount of recovery between patients with major versus minor depression. JHFI scores for the remitted major depression patients went from 4.7 ± 3.5 to 3.7 ± 2.9 (SD) while the minor depression patients went from 5.7 ± 5.2 to 2.4 ± 2.4 ($p = $ NS).

Our second study examined the effect of treatment of depression on recovery of ADL comparing 10 patients with a first ever stroke who had major or minor depression who responded to nortriptyline or placebo in a double-blind study and had a score >0 on the JHFI with 10 patients who met the same criteria but who failed to respond to treatment. There were no significant differences between the two groups in age, gender, race, handedness, marital status, years of education, time since stroke, socioeconomic status or personal or family history of mood disorder or history of alcohol abuse. Seven out of 10 patients in the remission group had received active nortriptyline in a double-blind treatment trial while only one of 10 non-remitted patients had received nortriptyline. There were no significant differences between responders and non-responders in hemisphere of injury, volume of lesion, cortical versus subcortical lesion location, initial neurological deficits, or the percent of patients assigned to physical rehabilitation programs.

We then compared trajectories (i.e., the mean slope of the line between 0 and 100 mg of nortriptyline) of JHFI scores among patients whose depression had responded and those who had not. The mean JHFI score trajectory over the 6–9-week study period in the remission group was -0.58 ± 0.35 (SD) while in the non-improvement group, the mean value was -0.08 ± 0.52 (SD) (a negative number indicated continued improvement in JHFI scores) (Fig. 13.5).

The major question which arises from these two studies is what mechanism associated with remission of depression leads to improvement in ADLs and secondly, why have double-blind treatment trials comparing antidepressant treatment with placebo generally failed to show a significant improvement in ADL associated with active antidepressant treatment. I believe the answer to the second

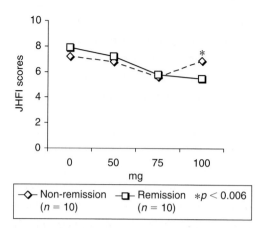

Figure 13.5   ADL as measured by the JHFI during the course of a double-blind treatment trial with
nortriptyline. Data from two studies were merged and patients whose depression
remitted while taking nortriptyline showed significantly better recovery in ADLs at a
nortriptyline dose of 100 mg. Patients received 50 mg at weeks 2–3, 75 mg at weeks
4–6, and 100 mg at weeks 6–9 (reprinted with permission from Chemerinski *et al.*
J Nerv Ment Dis (2001a) 189:421–425).

question is related to the size of the treatment effect. When patients who responded
to active treatment are mixed with those who failed to respond, one would expect
a smaller treatment effect than if only patients who responded to treatment were
compared to patients who failed to respond to treatment. We examined this
hypothesis in our treatment studies and found that the effect size increases from
0.3 to 0.9 when active versus placebo treatment is compared and when responders
versus non-responders are compared (Kimura *et al.* 2000). With an effect size of
0.3, it would take 175 patients to demonstrate a statistically significant difference at
the $p < 0.05$ level between two groups while an effect size of 0.9 would require
treatment groups of only 20 or more to show a statistically significant difference
with an 80% probability.

The second question about why improvement in depression leads to improved
recovery in ADL remains uncertain. It is possible that the improvement in ADL function is mediated by changes in neurochemistry or neurophysiology related to remission of depression (Drevets *et al.* 1992; Mayberg *et al.* 1995). On the other hand,
patients who are no longer depressed may be more motivated to participate in rehabilitation activities and may devote more energy and motivation to their recovery.

Perhaps our most provocative recent study examining physical recovery from
stroke utilized data from our prior treatment study (Robinson *et al.* 2000). We compared 34 patients who received antidepressant treatment during the first month following stroke compared to 28 patients who received antidepressant treatment begun
after the first month following stroke (Narushima and Robinson 2003). Patients

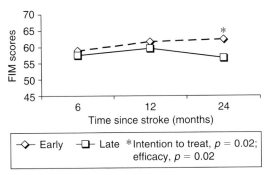

Figure 13.6 Recovery in ADL as measured by the FIM over 2 years of follow-up. All patients were treated for 12 weeks in a double-blind study with fluoxetine or nortriptyline. Patients who received treatment within 1 month after stroke (early) improved significantly more than those who received treatment after the first month poststroke (late). FIM scores were measured at the same times following stroke to control for group differences in time since stroke when the 3-month treatment was given (reprinted with permission from Narushima *et al. J Nerv Ment Dis* (2003) 191(10):645–652).

were treated for 12 weeks and recovery in ADLs was assessed at 12- and 24-month follow-up. The doses of nortriptyline were 25 mg/day for week 1, 50 mg/day for weeks 2–3, 75 mg/day for weeks 4–6, and 100 mg/day for weeks 6–12. Doses of fluoxetine were 10 mg/day for weeks 0–3, 20 mg/day for weeks 4–6, 30 mg/day for weeks 7–9, and 40 mg/day for weeks 10–12. ADLs were assessed using the FIM (Ottenbacher *et al.* 1994). The early treatment group was 19 ± 25 (SD) days poststroke compared to the later treatment patients who were 140 ± 28 (SD) days following stroke. Due to dropouts, death and medical complications, 22 of the 34 early treatment patients and 15 of the 28 late treatment patients completed the 24-month follow-up. There were no significant differences between the early and late treatment patients in their background characteristics, or the total number of therapy hours received.

At the 3-month evaluation, there was a significant group-by-treatment interaction using either intention-to-treat analysis ($p = 0.03$ with the last observation carried forward) or efficacy analysis ($p = 0.03$). The early treatment group improved more quickly than the late treatment group during this first 3 months (Fig. 13.6). During the 3–24-month follow-up, there was a significant group-by-time interaction using either efficacy analysis or intention-to-treat analysis ($p = 0.03$) (Fig. 13.6). The early treatment group continued to show gradual improvement in ADL scores during the 21 months of follow-up while the late treatment group began to show gradual deterioration between 12- and 24-month follow-up. During the 3–24-month follow-up period, there was no significant group-by-treatment effect on the severity of depressive symptoms as measured by the Ham-D score (intention to treat, $p = 0.6$; efficacy, $p = 0.6$). Thus, the late treatment group did not develop more depression than the early treatment group. Since the deterioration in ADL seen in the later treatment group could have been due to time since stroke, we reanalyzed our data to compare the two groups over the same poststroke time period (i.e., 12–24-month poststroke. Using either intention-to-treat or efficacy analysis, there was a significant time-by-treatment interaction on FIM scores between 12 and 24 months after the stroke (efficacy, $p = 0.04$; intention to treat, $p = 0.02$). The early treatment patients improved in their ADLs more than the late treatment patients.

A logistic regression analysis was conducted using intention-to-treat data and examining the effects of initial diagnosis (i.e., depressed or non-depressed), type of treatment (i.e., nortriptyline or fluoxetine), the presence or absence of motor impairment, the presence or absence of past psychiatric history, the presence or absence of continued medication during follow-up, and the time of treatment (i.e., <1 month or >1 month following stroke). Results showed a significant and independent effect of early versus late treatment on FIM scores during 1–2-year follow-up ($p = 0.012$). There was also a near significant effect of continued medication ($p = 0.06$).

Although we do not know why the late treatment patients showed some deterioration in their ADL between 1 and 2 years, we ruled out the development of another physical illness such as recurrent stroke or differences in time since stroke between the two groups. It is possible that anatomical or physiological changes provoked by antidepressants may be more long lasting when they are given closer to the time of injury. Fifteen of the 34 patients in the early treatment group and 17 of 28 patients in the late group had either major or minor depressive disorder ($p = NS$). Thus, although this phenomena will require more research to establish the importance of early treatment on recovery, it suggests that patients should be treated with antidepressants within 1 month following stroke in order to receive the maximum benefit of antidepressant medication on recovery. The early use of antidepressant medication did not appear to work through a greater improvement of depressive symptoms because there were no differences in severity of depression between the early and late treatment group during the 24 months from the beginning to the end of the study.

In summary, this chapter has examined the relationship between physical impairment and depressive disorder following stroke when the two measurements are made at the same time. There was a fairly consistent finding that severity of depression correlates significantly with severity of impairment in ADL. The nature of this relationship was examined in the second part of the chapter. Although there were some studies which failed to find a relationship between depression and recovery in ADL, most of the literature supports the conclusion that the existence of depression in the first few months after stroke is associated with impaired recovery in ADL at 1- or 2-year follow-up. Finally, the third part of this chapter examined the ability of treatment with antidepressant medications to improve recovery in ADL. Although the majority of studies which examined recovery in ADLs between patients receiving active medication and placebo medication have failed to show a significant effect on recovery, when patients who responded to treatment were compared to patients who failed to respond to treatment, a significant effect of treatment response was identified. Perhaps the most provocative finding, however, is a recent one in which patients with or without depression, given antidepressant medication (i.e., nortriptyline or fluoxetine) during the first month poststroke, had significantly better recovery in ADLs over the next 2 years than patients who were given antidepressants >1-month poststroke. These findings suggest that patients' recovery following stroke may benefit from antidepressant therapy and that treatment should be initiated within the first month following stroke in order to obtain optimal treatment results (Narushima and Robinson 2003). This certainly is an observation worthy of further investigation.

REFERENCES

Adams, R. J., Meador, K. J., Sethi, K. D., *et al.* Graded neurologic scale for use in acute hemispheric stroke treatment protocols. *Stroke* (1987) 18(3):665–669.

Angeleri, F., Angeleri, V. A., Foschi, N., *et al.* The influence of depression, social activity, and family stress on functional outcome after stroke. *Stroke* (1993) 24(20):1478–1483.

Astrom, M., Adolfsson, R., and Asplund, K. Major depression in stroke patients: a 3-year longitudinal study. *Stroke* (1993) 24:976–982.

Berg, A., Psych, L., Palomaki, H., *et al.* Poststroke depression – An 18-month follow-up. *Stroke* (2003) 34(1):138–143.

Chemerinski, E., Robinson, R. G., Arndt, S., *et al.* The effect of remission of poststroke depression on activities of daily living in a double-blind randomized treatment study. *J Nerv Ment Dis* (2001a) 189(7):421–425.

Chemerinski, E., Robinson, R. G., and Kosier, J. T. Improved recovery in activities of daily living associated with remission of post-stroke depression. *Stroke* (2001b) 32(1):113–117.

Dam, M., Tonin, P., De Boni, A., *et al.* Effects of fluoxetine and maprotiline on functional recovery in poststroke hemiplegic patients undergoing rehabilitation therapy [comment]. *Stroke* (1996) 27(7):1211–1214.

Desmond, D. W., Remien, R. H., Moroney, J. T., *et al.* Ischemic stroke and depression. *J Int Neuropsychol Soc* (2003) 9(3):429–439.

Dove, H. G., Schneider, K. C., and Wallace, J. D. Evaluating and predicting outcome of acute cerebral vascular accident. *Stroke* (1984) 15:858–864.

Drevets, W. C., Videen, T. O., Price, J. L., *et al.* A functional anatomical study of unipolar depression. *J Neurosci* (1992) 12:3628–3641.

Eastwood, M. R., Rifat, S. L., Nobbs, H., *et al.* Mood disorder following cerebrovascular accident. *Br J Psychiatr* (1989) 154:195–200.

Ebrahim, S., Barer, D., and Nouri, F. Affective illness after stroke. *Br J Psychiatr* (1987) 151:52–56.

Fruehwald, S., Gatterbauer, E., Rehak, P., *et al.* Early fluoxetine treatment of post-stroke depression – a three-month double-blind placebo-controlled study with an open-label long-term follow up. *J Neurol* (2003) 250(3):347–351.

Gainotti, G., Antonucci, G., Marra, C., *et al.* Relation between depression after stroke, antidepressant therapy, and functional recovery. *J Neurol Neurosurg Psychiatr* (2001) 71(2):258–261.

Gonzalez-Torrecillas, J. L., Mendlewicz, J., and Lobo, A. Effects of early treatment of poststroke depression on neuropsychological rehabilitation. *Int Psychogeriatr* (1995) 7(4):547–560.

Herrmann, N., Black, S. E., Lawrence, J., *et al.* The Sunnybrook stroke study. A prospective study of depressive symptoms and functional outcome. *Stroke* (1998) 29:618–624.

House, A., Knapp, P., Bamford, J., *et al.* Mortality at 12 and 24 months after stroke may be associated with depressive symptoms at 1 month. *Stroke* (2001) 32(3):696–701.

Kauhanen, M. L., Korpelainen, J. T., Hiltunen, P., *et al.* Domains and determinants of quality of life after stroke caused by brain infarction. *Arch Phys Med Rehabil* (2000) 81(12):1541–1546.

Kimura, M., Robinson, R. G., and Kosier, T. Treatment of cognitive impairment after poststroke depression. *Stroke* (2000) 31(7):1482–1486.

Lipsey, J. R., Robinson, R. G., Pearlson, G. D., *et al.* Nortriptyline treatment of post-stroke depression: a double-blind study. *Lancet* (1984) i(8372):297–300.

Mayberg, H. S., Liotti, M., Jerabek, P. A., *et al.* Induced sadness: a PET model of depression. *Hum Brain Mapp* (1995) (Suppl 1):396.

Morris, P. L. P., Robinson, R. G., and Raphael, B. Prevalence and course of depressive disorders in hospitalized stroke patients. *Int J Psychiatr Med* (1990) 20:349–364.

Narushima, K., and Robinson, R. G. The effect of early versus late antidepressant treatment on physical impairment associated with poststroke depression. Is there a time-related therapeutic window? *J Nerv Ment Dis* (2003) 191(10):645–652.

Narushima, K., Chan, K. L., Kosier, J. T., *et al.* Does cognitive recovery after treatment of post-stroke depression last? A 2-year follow-up of cognitive function associated with poststroke depression. *Am J Psychiatr* (2003) 160(6):1157–1162.

Ottenbacher, K. J., Mann, W. C., Granger, C. V., *et al.* Inter-rater agreement and stability of functional assessment in the community-based elderly. *Arch Phys Med Rehabil* (1994) 75:1297–1301.

Palomaki, H., Kaste, M., Berg, A., *et al.* Prevention of poststroke depression: 1 year randomised placebo controlled double blind trial of mainserin with 6 month followup after therapy. *J Neurol Neurosurg Psychiatr* (1999) 66:490–494.

Paolucci, S., Antonucci, G., Pratesi, L., *et al.* Poststroke depression and its role in rehabilitation of inpatients. *Arch Phys Med Rehabil* (1999) 80:985–990.

Paolucci, S., Antonucci, G., Grasso, M. G., *et al.* Early versus delayed inpatient stroke rehabilitation: a matched comparison conducted in Italy. *Arch Phys Med Rehabil* (2000a) 81(6):695–700.

Paolucci, S., Grasso, M. G., Antonucci, G., *et al.* One-year follow-up in stroke patients discharged from rehabilitation hospital. *Cerebrovasc Dis* (2000b) 10(1):25–32.

Paolucci, S., Antonucci, G., Grasso, M. G., *et al.* Post-stroke depression, antidepressant treatment and rehabilitation results. A case–control study. *Cerebrovasc Dis* (2001) 12(3):264–271.

Parikh, R. M., Robinson, R. G., Lipsey, J. R., *et al.* The impact of post-stroke depression on recovery in activities of daily living over two year follow-up. *Arch Neurol* (1990) 47:785–789.

Pohjasvaara, T., Vataja, R., Leppavuori, A., *et al.* Depression is an independent predictor of poor long-term functional outcome post-stroke. *Eur J Neurol* (2001) 8(4):315–319.

Ramasubbu, R., Robinson, R. G., Flint, A. J., *et al.* Functional impairment associated with acute poststroke depression: the Stroke Data Bank Study. *J Neuropsychiatr Clin Neurosci* (1998) 10(1):26–33.

Reding, M. J., Orto, L. A., Winter, S. W., *et al.* Antidepressant therapy after stroke: a double-blind trial. *Arch Neurol* (1986) 43:763–765.

Robinson, R. G., Starr, L. B., Kubos, K. L., *et al.* A two year longitudinal study of post-stroke mood disorders: findings during the initial evaluation. *Stroke* (1983) 14:736–744.

Robinson, R. G., Schultz, S. K., Castillo, C., *et al.* Nortriptyline versus fluoxetine in the treatment of depression and in short term recovery after stroke: a placebo controlled, double-blind study. *Am J Psychiatr* (2000) 157:351–359.

Schubert, D. S. P., Taylor, C., Lee, S., *et al.* Physical consequences of depression in the stroke patient. *Gen Hosp Psychiatr* (1992) 14:69–76.

Schwartz, J. A., Speed, N. M., Brunberg, J. A., *et al.* Depression in stroke rehabilitation. *Biol Psychiatr* (1993) 33:694–699.

Shima, S. The efficacy of antidepressants in post-stroke depression. *Keio J Med* (1997) 46(1):25–26.

Sinyor, D., Amato, P., and Kaloupek, P. Post-stroke depression: relationship to functional impairment, coping strategies, and rehabilitation outcome. *Stroke* (1986) 17:112–117.

Sturm, J. W., Donnan, G. A., Dewey, H. M., *et al.* Determinants of handicap after stroke. The North East Melbourne Stroke Incidence Study (NEMESIS). *Stroke* (2004) 35:715–720.

van de Weg, F. B., Kuik, D. J., and Lankhorst, G. J. Post-stroke depression and functional outcome: a cohort study investigating the influence of depression on functional recovery from stroke. *Clin Rehabil* (1999) 13:268–272.

Wiart, L., Petit, H., Joseph, P. A., *et al.* Fluoxetine in early poststroke depression: a double-blind placebo-controlled study. *Stroke* (2000) 31:1829–1832.

14

Relationship to cognitive impairment and treatment

Cognitive impairment and stroke

There are numerous studies which have demonstrated cognitive impairment associated with of specific regions of cerebral infarction (Gazzaniga 2000). Although the focus of this chapter will be on the relationship between depression and cognitive impairment, it is worthwhile to review some of the recent studies which have documented the frequency and severity of cognitive impairment associated with stroke. Perhaps the most well-designed study is the one involving the Framingham cohort (Kase *et al.* 1998). They prospectively studied a group of 74 subjects who had suffered a stroke during a 13-year follow-up and compared them with 74 control subjects who had not suffered a stroke, but were matched for age and sex. The patients who suffered a stroke were noted to have a significantly lower mini-mental state exam (MMSE) score at prestroke baseline (i.e., 27.3 ± 0.3, stroke and 28.1 ± 0.2, control). Following the stroke, however, the mean MMSE in the affected group was 23.6 ± 0.9 compared with a mean mini-mental score of 28.3 ± 0.2 ($p < 0.001$) in the control patients. The decline in cognitive function was correlated with large left-sided strokes as documented on CT scan. The Framingham Study also found that the Center for Epidemiological Studies – depression scale (CES-D) scores indicated significantly more depressive symptoms in the patients with stroke compared with controls. Another study by Censori *et al.* (1996) found that, when 110 hospitalized patients, who had suffered a first ever stroke as documented by CT scan, were examined at 3 months following stroke, 5% showed dementia, as determined by the National Institute of Neurological Disorders and Stroke ARIEN criteria. Considering only patients with supratentorial lesions and with residual deficits of motor or sensory functions, the frequency of dementia was 24.6% (95% confidence interval (CI): 14.5–37.3%). A multivariate analysis identified age, the existence of diabetes, presence of aphasia, large, middle-cerebral artery infarction, and lesions of the frontal lobe, as significant independent correlates of poststroke dementia. Finally, Pohjasvaara *et al.* (1997) found that among 451 patients with acute stroke, cognitive decline was present in 61.7%. In the groups aged 55–64, 65–74, and 75–85, the frequency of cognitive decline was 45.7%, 53.8%, and 74.1%, respectively ($p =$ 0.0008). The frequency of dementia was 18.4% using diagnostic and statistical manual (DSM-IV) criteria. Thus, these studies document the fact that, in the majority of patients suffering a stroke, cognitive impairment is a common consequence of stroke and probably represents the most common mental impairment associated with ischemic lesions.

Cognitive impairment and depression

The nature of the relationship between cognitive impairment and depression appears to involve a complex interaction between depression, the stroke lesion and cognitive impairment. Although one might understandably view cognitive impairment as a cause of depression, their relationship is clearly a more complex one. In 1989, we hypothesized that major depression following left hemisphere lesions produces through some physiological process a greater degree of cognitive impairment than can be explained by the lesions alone and that this represents a post-stroke dementia of depression (Bolla-Wilson *et al.* 1989).

Although some investigators have found that patients with depression were no more cognitively impaired than those without depression (Eastwood *et al.* 1989; Morris *et al.* 1990), most studies have reported that patients with major depression have a greater degree of cognitive impairment than non-depressed patients (Robinson *et al.* 1986; House *et al.* 1991; Kauhanen *et al.* 1999; Spalletta and Caltagirone 2003). In our initial longitudinal study of 103 patients, we found a significant correlation between severity of cognitive impairment, as measured by the MMSE score, and severity of depression, as measured by either the Zung depression rating scale ($r = -0.28$; $p < 0.01$), the Hamilton depression rating scale (HDRS) ($r = -0.22$; $p < 0.02$), or the present state examination (PSE) ($r = -0.38$; $p < 0.02$) (Robinson *et al.* 1983). Furthermore, the MMSE scores of patients with major depression were significantly lower (19.7 ± 4.7 SD) than those of patients with minor depression (22.5 ± 6.3 SD) or no depression (23.4 ± 4.7 SD) ($p < 0.01$).

Subsequently, other investigators have also found that cognitive impairment is significantly greater among patients with major depression compared with non-depressed patients (House *et al.* 1990). Kauhanen *et al.* (1999) examined 106 consecutive patients with acute first ever ischemic stroke. The prevalence of major depression was 9% at 3 months and 16% at 12 months. Patients with major depressive disorder were significantly more impaired than the non-depressed patients (Kauhanen *et al.* 1999). A study by Andersen *et al.* (1996) examined 166 patients 1 year following acute stroke. Depression diagnosis was based on having a Hamilton depression score of 13 or greater. Fifty percent were diagnosed with depression at

Table 14.1. Background characteristics

Baltimore and Iowa stroke patients combined	$n = 357$
Age in years (mean ± SD)	61.3 (13.8)
Education in years (mean ± SD)	10.0 (3.9)
Gender (% male)	57.7
Race (% black)	51.0
Alcohol abuse (% positive)	16.1
Marital status (% married)	46.5
Socio-economic status	
Hollingshead Class I and II	14.9
Hollingshead Class III and IV	85.1
Family history of psychiatric disorder (% with history)	10.8
Personal history of psychiatric disorder (% with history)	10.5

1 month and 79% within 3 months after stroke. Improvement in mood symptoms was correlated with improvement of intellectual function. The Mattis dementia rating scale correlated with the Hamilton depression score in the first year following stroke ($r = -0.22; p = 0.005$). In 53 patients, however, improvement in intellectual performance was absent and the use of antidepressant medication did not lead to a significant improvement in the Mattis dementia rating scale.

Neuropsychological testing showed that major depressed patients had significant impairments in almost all areas of cognitive function in comparison with non-depressed patients. Patients with depression were more impaired at 3 and 6 months in verbal logical thinking, comprehension, non-verbal problem solving, including picture completion and block design, verbal memory, as measured by logical memory and serial learning, visual memory, as measured by visual reproduction, visual recognition and attention, and executive function, as measured by trail making test part A, verbal fluency, and visual constructive functions. These findings held up after patients with aphasias were removed. Thus, detailed neuropsychological testing revealed a significant association between major depression and widespread cognitive impairment (i.e., dementia syndrome).

We have recently examined the relationship between depression diagnosis and cognitive impairment as measured by the mini-mental state in all of the patients which we have examined in our acute stroke depression studies (i.e., 357). This group included our original 103 patients and 254 new patients. The background characteristics of this group are shown in Table 14.1. The mean MMSE scores for these patients are shown in relationship to their depressive diagnosis in Fig. 14.1, study 1. Patients with major depression (i.e., MMSE 19.2 ± 7.4 SD) were significantly more cognitively impaired that those with minor depression or no mood disorder

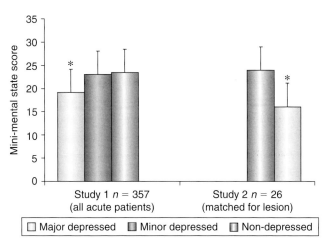

Figure 14.1   Mini-mental scores related to depression diagnoses (i.e., major, minor, or no depression) in two studies. Study 1 included all acute stroke patients with mini-mental exams. Study 2 compared cognitive function in patients with or without major depression who were matched for lesion volume ($\pm$5%) and lesion location. These studies found that major but not minor poststroke depression was associated with greater cognitive impairment than no mood disturbance. $*p < 0.05$ compared with minor or non-depressed.

(MMSE 23.1 + 5.1)($p = 0.0001$). Furthermore, using a score of 23 or less as indicating significant cognitive impairment, in the non-depressed group, 80 of 222 patients (36%) were cognitively impaired, as were 28 of 65 (43%) with minor depression versus 41 of 70 (59%) with major depression ($p = 0.0037$). Thus, in our overall acute stroke population, cognitive impairment as measured by the MMSE was significantly more frequent in patients with major depression compared with minor depression or no depression.

In addition to the effect of depression, we have also found significant associations of cognitive impairment with age, education, and race (Table 14.2). A multiple linear regression analysis found that major depression ($p = 0.0029$), age ($p = 0.0511$), and education ($p = 0.0001$) were all independent factors associated with cognitive impairment following stroke.

In an effort to determine whether there was an interaction between severity of cognitive impairment and severity of major depression, a two-way analysis of variance (ANOVA) of Hamilton depression scores was performed (Factor 1 presence or absence of major depression, Factor 2 presence or absence of cognitive impairment). Results demonstrated the expected effect of depression, that is depressed patients had significantly higher Hamilton depression scores, but no effect of cognitive impairment (i.e., cognitively impaired patients with major depression did not have higher Hamilton scores than non-cognitively impaired patients) and no interaction

Table 14.2. Background characteristics in relationship to depression and cognitive impairment

	In-hospital				
	Not depressed cognitive impairment		Major depression cognitive impairment		
	No	Yes	No	Yes	p
n	179	108	29	41	
Age in years (mean ± SD)	61.1 (14.2)	64.0 (11.6)	57.2 (15.6)	57.9 (14.9)	0.0240[a,b]
Education in years (mean ± SD)	11.1 (3.6)	8.3 (4.1)	11.2 (2.8)	9.0 (3.2)	0.0001[a]
Gender (% male)	57.0	63.9	48.3	51.2	0.3216
Race (% African–American)	40.8	72.2	27.6	56.1	0.0001[a]
Alcohol abuse (% positive)	15.6	11.1	20.7	26.8	0.0644
Marital status (% married)	50.3	40.7	58.6	36.6	0.1217
Socio-economic status (%)					
Hollingshead Class I and II	46.8	18.0	31.0	12.2	
Hollingshead Class III and IV	53.2	82.0	69.0	87.8	0.3623
Family history of psychiatric disorder (% with history)	11.9	6.5	6.9	20.0	0.1017
Personal history of psychiatric disorder (% with history)	9.0	3.7	20.7	26.8	0.0001[b]

[a] Cognitive impaired versus non-cognitive impaired.
[b] Major depression versus not depressed.

between the two. This finding indicates that severity of depression cannot account for the existence of cognitive impairment in those with poststroke major depression.

Effects of depression versus effects of lesion

To separate the effect of stroke from the effect of depression on cognitive impairment, we examined 13 pairs of patients who were matched for lesion size and location, but one patient of the pair had major depression, while the other was non-depressed (Starkstein *et al.* 1988). Patients were matched for lesion location if both of their lesions involved, either totally or partially, the same regions as those defined by Levine and Grek (1984). There were no significant group differences in background characteristics such as age, gender, years of education, or socio-economic status. Depressed patients, however, had significantly lower mini-mental scores than non-depressed patients (Fig. 14.1). Of the 13 pairs of patients, 10 had lower MMSE scores than their respective lesion-matched controls, two had the same scores and only one depressed patient had less cognitive impairment than their non-depressed lesion-matched control ($p = 0.001$).

This study demonstrated that the greater degree of cognitive impairment among patients with major depression compared to non-depressed patients could not be explained by the effect of the ischemic lesion. Our second study which distinguished between the effects of depression and the effects of brain injury administered a battery of neuropsychological tests to assess cognitive function among 53 patients with single stroke lesions of the right or left hemisphere who had no language disturbance except mild anomia (Bolla-Wilson *et al.* 1989).

The neuropsychological examination included orientation, language, remote memory, verbal memory, visual memory, recognition, visual perceptual ability, visual constructional ability, executive motor function, and frontal lobe functions. Patients were grouped according to the hemisphere in which their lesion was located and by the presence or absence of major depression. There were no significant differences between the depressed and non-depressed groups in terms of their background characteristics including age, socio-economic status, years of education, gender, race, handedness, or time since stroke. Similarly, there were no significant differences in neurological findings with 85% of patients being hemiparetic and 50% having a hemisensory deficit. Visual field deficits, hemi-anopsia or quadrant anopsia, were found in one patient with a left hemisphere lesion and five patients with a right hemisphere lesion, none of whom were depressed. In these patients, all testing materials were presented to the non-affected visual field. CT scan analysis found that there were no significant differences between the depressed and non-depressed groups in the frequency of cortical compared with subcortical lesions. The mean lesion volumes for the patients with left hemisphere lesions with major depression ($n = 10$) was 2.0 ± 2.0% of brain volume, and without depression ($n = 16$) was 5.3 ± 1.0%, while in patients with right hemisphere lesions with major depression ($n = 8$) was 3.5 ± 2.0% and without depression ($n = 19$) was (6.8 ± 6.0%). The anterior lesion borders as a percent of the overall anterior posterior distance for the four groups were 30.4 ± 6.0%, 37.9 ± 20.0%, 45.9 ± 17.0%, and 40.5 ± 22.0%, respectively.

In order to compare across various neuropsychological domains, individual scores were converted to standardized Z-scores and are shown in Fig. 14.2. The sum Z-scores demonstrate that there was a significantly greater impairment among patients with left hemisphere lesions and major depression compared to patients with left hemisphere lesions without depression or compared to those with right hemisphere lesions with or without depression ($p < 0.01$). Analysis of individual tests of neuropsychological function indicated that patients with left hemisphere lesions and major depression were more impaired in orientation, language, visual perceptual constructional tasks, executive motor function, and frontal lobe functions compared to patients with left hemisphere lesions but no depression.

Among patients with right hemisphere lesions, however, there were no significant differences between patients with major depression and those who were non-depressed

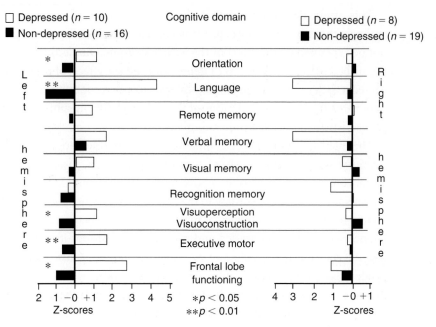

Figure 14.2 The results of neuropsychological testing in patients with major depression (depressed) or no mood disturbance (non-depressed) following a single lesion of the left or right hemisphere. Scores in each cognitive domain were converted to Z-scores so that comparisons could be made across domains. A more positive Z-score indicates a greater degree of impairment. Note that among patients with left hemisphere strokes, patients with major depression were more impaired than the non-depressed in every cognitive domain. Five of these domains reached statistical significance, indicated by asterisks. None of the domains reached significance in the patients with right hemisphere stroke.

in any of the nine cognitive domains. Thus cognitive impairment associated with major depression occurred only among patients with left hemisphere lesions and involved impairments in right hemisphere function and frontal lobe function.

Kauhanen *et al.* (1999) reported similar findings. Patients with first ever stroke and major depression were found to be significantly more impaired than non-depressed patients ($n = 46$ at 3 months and $n = 53$ at 12 months) in verbal and visual memory, non-verbal problem solving, executive function and visuocon-structional tasks at both time points. Although this study did not examine the effect of hemispheric side of injury and they found that both major and minor depression were associated with cognitive impairment, the impairment tended to be more severe in patients with major depression, particularly among patients with dysphasia and major depression ($n = 7$) at 12 months.

Spalleta *et al.* (2002) examined 153 patients with first ever stroke lesions of the right ($n = 87$) or left ($n = 66$) hemisphere who were less than 1 year poststroke. The presence of major depression was based on the structured clinical interview

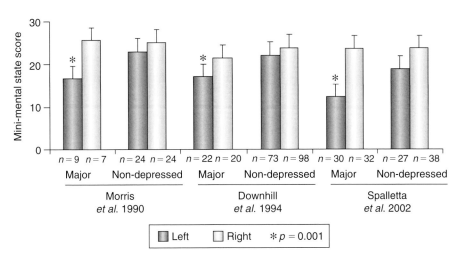

Figure 14.3 MMSE scores following acute stroke in three studies among patients with major or no mood disturbance grouped according to the hemisphere of ischemia. In all three studies, there was a significant difference between patients with major depression following left hemisphere stroke and non-depressed patients with similar lesions (*p = 0.001). Major depression following right hemisphere lesions did not lead to the same phenomenon.

for DSM-IV (SCID) and the severity of cognitive impairment was based on the MMSE. Sixty-two (41%) of the patients had a major depression (32 right lesions, 30 left lesions) while 26 (17%) had a minor depression (17 right, 9 left lesions). Patients with left hemisphere lesion and major depression were found to be significantly more impaired than non-depressed patients with left hemisphere lesions (mini-mental 12.3 ± 9.0 for major depressed versus 18.9 ± 8.5 non-depressed) $p < 0.001$) (Fig. 14.3). Similarly, patients with left hemisphere lesions were significantly more cognitively impaired than patients with right hemisphere lesions even though they both had major depressive disorder (12.3 ± 9.0 SD versus 23.7 ± 7.1 SD) (p = 0.0001). There was no effect of minor depression or side of injury on cognitive function. A series of stepwise multiple regression analyses examining the effects of Hamilton depression score, number of brain regions affected by the stroke, trait anger inventory, age, Hamilton anxiety scale, Barthel Index, diabetes mellitus, and age revealed that among patients with left hemisphere lesions the strongest correlate of mini-mental score was HDRS (r = −0.34) ($p < 0.001$). Numbers of areas of brain injury and the anger trait/anger expression inventory also were independently associated with mini-mental score. Among patients with right hemisphere lesions, only education level was significantly associated with severity of cognitive impairment (r = 0.24) (p = 0.025).

House *et al.* (1990) found that patients with major depression (n = 10), or any other DSM-III axis I diagnosis (n = 27) at 1 month poststroke, were significantly more cognitively impaired as measured by the MMSE than patients with no axis I diagnosis ($n = 52; p < 0.006$). Patients with major depression had the lowest MMSE scores. In addition, for patients with left hemisphere lesions there was a significant correlation between MMSE scores and the severity of depression as measured by the Beck depression inventory (BDI) or the PSE (BDI, $r = -0.55$; PSE $r = -0.43$; $p < 0.003$). For patients with right hemisphere lesions these correlations were weaker or NS (BDI $r = -0.08$; $p = $ NS; PSE $r = -0.39$; $p = 0.04$). At 6-month follow-up, the correlation between BDI score and MMSE was significant for patients with left hemisphere lesions ($r = -0.21$ but NS for patients with right hemisphere lesions $r = -0.06$).

Morris *et al.* (1990) also found a significant association between major depression and cognitive impairment at 2–3 months following acute stroke among patients with left hemisphere lesions. Patients with left hemisphere lesions and major depression ($n = 9$) had a mean MMSE of 16.6 ± 8.6 while non-depressed patients with left hemisphere lesions ($n = 24$) had a mean MMSE of 23.0 ± 7.0 ($p = 0.03$). There were no significant differences in the mental scores between 7 patients with major depression following right hemisphere lesions (25.7 ± 2.3) and 24 non-depressed patients with right hemisphere lesions (25.1 ± 4.0) (Fig. 14.3).

In summary, several studies have demonstrated that during the first year following stroke, major depression is associated with a greater degree of cognitive impairment than could be explained based on the size or location of the stroke lesion. The degree of cognitive impairment among patients with major depression and left hemisphere stroke was also significantly greater than among patients with major depression and right hemisphere strokes or patients with minor depression or no mood disturbance. This phenomenon was also confirmed using detailed neuropsychological testing which showed that a significant number of neuropsychological domains were significantly affected by major depressive disorder following a left hemisphere stroke.

Longitudinal course of cognitive impairment and depression

In our original 2-year longitudinal study of 103 patients (see Table 8.1 for population characteristics), we found that the mean correlation coefficient between the severity of depression and the MMSE score declined from -0.34 ($p < 0.01$) during acute hospitalization to -0.18 at 3 months ($p = $ NS). By 6-month follow-up, however, the correlation had increased to -0.31 ($p < 0.01$). At 1- and 2-year follow-up, however, the correlations were not significant. Thus, in our initial follow-up study, the strength of the relationship between depression and cognitive impairment appeared to decline over time. As mentioned previously, House *et al.* (1990) found a similar phenomenon. The correlation between the BDI and the MMSE score for 76 patients at 1 month poststroke was $r = -0.34$ ($p = 0.001$). At 6 months poststroke, for 107 patients, the correlation was $r = -0.24$ ($p = 0.006$) while at 12 months, for 88 patients, the correlation had fallen to $r = -0.09$ ($p = $ NS). These data suggest that the relationship between depression and cognitive impairment declines with time following stroke.

We examined this phenomenon in all of our acute stroke patients who were seen for at least one follow-up during the first 2 years poststroke ($n = 140$). Longitudinal data obtained at the 3-, 6-, 12-, and 24-month follow-ups were analyzed for the relationship between depression and cognitive impairment (Downhill and Robinson 1994). ANOVA of MMSE scores, comparing major depressed and non-depressed (including or excluding minor depressions) patients in-hospital or at the 3-, 6-, 12-, and 24-month follow-ups demonstrated a significant effect of major depression at the initial in-hospital evaluation (Fig. 14.3) and at 3- and 6-month follow-ups (in-hospital MMSE score 17.3 ± 8.1 for depressed versus 24.1 ± 5.6 for non-depressed patients; $p = 0.01$; 3 months MMSE scores $= 18.5 \pm 9.9$ for depressed versus 24.8 ± 5.0 for non-depressed; $p = 0.01$; 6 months MMSE scores $= 20.2 \pm 9.7$ for depressed versus 24.7 ± 5.7 for non-depressed; $p = 0.1$.

Since the association between depression and cognitive impairment was strongest in patients with left hemisphere lesions, patients were grouped according to the side of their lesion. Patients with a diagnosis of major depression and a left hemisphere lesion were more cognitively impaired than non-depressed patients or patients with major depression and a right hemisphere lesion in-hospital ($p = 0.01$) and at the 3 ($p = 0.006$) and 6 ($p = 0.03$) month follow-ups (Fig. 14.4 bottom panel). The composition of the major depression and non-depressed groups, however, was slightly different at each time point (i.e., at each follow-up, any patient with a diagnosis of major depression was included regardless of whether they had been depressed at a previous evaluation).

This analysis could have "diluted" the effect, if there was something different about patients who had cognitive impairment with major depression in the immediate poststroke period as compared to patients with late-onset major depression. Therefore, we examined the longitudinal course of cognitive impairment in patients with in-hospital major depression regardless of their diagnosis at follow-up (i.e., groups were composed of the same patients at each follow-up time point). There was a significant effect of in-hospital diagnosis of major depression and left hemisphere stroke on cognitive performance at the initial, 6 month ($p = 0.03$), and 12 month ($p = 0.02$) follow-up periods (Fig. 14.4 top panel). There was no significant effect of major depression on cognitive performance at 2 years poststroke and there was no significant effect among patients with right hemisphere stroke at any poststroke time period. These data suggested that in-hospital major depression after a left hemisphere lesion is different than other major depressions and when it

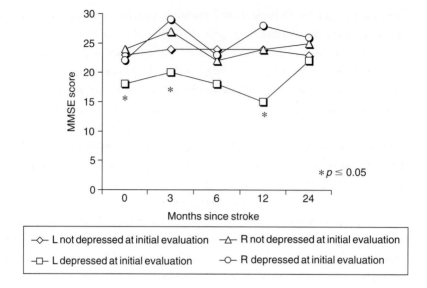

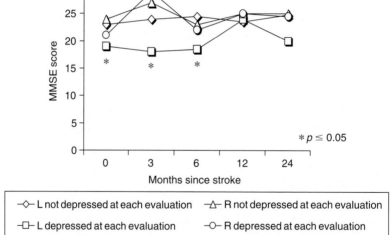

Figure 14.4   MMSE scores of patients grouped according to hemisphere of stroke (Left (L) or Right (R))
with major depression (depressed) or no mood disorder (not depressed) (patients with
minor depression excluded) at the in-hospital evaluation and over 2-year follow-up. The
top panel shows the scores of patients who were depressed at the in-hospital evaluation
and the scores of those same patients (independent of whether they remained
depressed) at each follow-up. The bottom panel shows the scores of all patients with
major depression or no mood disorder at each follow-up (independent of their diagnosis
at prior evaluation). Cognitive function is significantly more impaired in patients with
major depression following left, but not right, hemisphere stroke. The greater cognitive
impairment lasted for about 1 year (data from Downhill and Robinson, 1994).

resolves (within the first year following stroke) major depression is no longer associated with cognitive dysfunction.

Finally, we examined the relationship between in-hospital findings and cognitive function at either 3- or the 6-month follow-up. This study utilized the original group of 103 patients who were evaluated over 2 years following acute stroke. Findings obtained during the initial in-hospital evaluation were correlated with outcome at 3- and 6-month follow-ups (Fig. 14.5). In-hospital depression scores were weakly correlated with MMSE scores at the 3-month follow-up. None of the three measures of depression at the in-hospital evaluation were significantly correlated with MMSE scores at the 6-month follow-up. Thus, depression was only weakly predictive of cognitive impairment at follow-up. Alternatively, MMSE scores at the in-hospital evaluation were not significantly correlated with depression scores at 3-month follow-up. At the 6-month follow-up, however, there were significant correlations between in-hospital MMSE scores and depression scores at follow-up (Fig. 14.5). Thus, cognitive impairment at the time of acute stroke was moderately predictive of depression at 6-month follow-up.

In conclusion, the relationship between cognitive impairment and depression appeared to be as complex as the relationship between physical impairment and

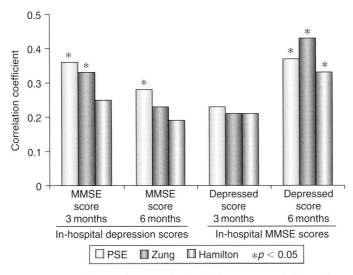

Figure 14.5 Correlation coefficients between in-hospital measures of depression or cognitive impairment and the corresponding measures in the same patients at 3- and 6-month follow-up. Note that in-hospital depression showed declining correlation with cognitive impairment over time while in-hospital mini-mental scores increased in their relationship to depression at follow-up. This may reflect that depressions with cognitive impairment lasted longer than depression without cognitive impairment or that patients with cognitive impairment become more depressed over time.

depression. During the first year poststroke, the most severely cognitively impaired patients remained depressed and the most depressed patients showed the smallest amount of recovery in their cognitive functions.

Effect of antidepressant treatment on cognitive function

Perhaps the most important data which addresses the question about whether cognitive impairment produces depression or depression produces cognitive impairment is treatment outcome. Prior double-blind treatment studies (Lipsey *et al.* 1984; Andersen *et al.* 1994; Robinson *et al.* 2000; Fruehwald *et al.* 2003) have all found that patients treated with active antidepressant medication had no greater improvement in their cognitive function than patients treated with placebo, in spite of the fact that active treatment significantly improved mood. This observation led Andersen to suggest that cognitive impairment may lead to depressive disorder (Andersen *et al.* 1996).

We recently performed a merged analysis of patients from our prior treatment studies to examine whether successful treatment of depression would lead to improved cognitive function (Kimura *et al.* 2000). Patients from the Lipsey *et al.* (1984) treatment study (Baltimore) as well as the Robinson *et al.* study (2000) (Iowa) were included if they had completed the treatment study and had received either nortriptyline ($n = 21$) or placebo ($n = 26$). Background characteristics are shown in Table 14.3. The only significant intergroup difference was a significantly higher frequency of family history of psychiatric disorder in the nortriptyline group than the placebo group ($p = 0.006$). There were no significant differences in stroke type, lesion location, or neurological deficit. Repeated measures ANOVA of the MMSE scores showed no significant group effect or group by time interaction. We next examined treatment effects among patients who did or did not respond to treatment. Responders ($n = 24$), major depression ($n = 15$), minor depression ($n = 9$), had a

Table 14.3. Comparison of Ham-D and MMSE scores for nortriptyline and placebo groups

	Ham-D					MMSE				
Dose	Nortriptyline	(*n*)	Placebo	(*n*)	*p	Nortriptyline	(*n*)	Placebo	(*n*)	*p
0 mg	17.38 ± 4.30	(21)	17.92 ± 3.95	(26)	0.655	23.62 ± 1.24	(21)	24.39 ± 1.02	(26)	0.632
50 mg	12.81 ± 3.86	(21)	13.27 ± 4.79	(26)	0.723	24.95 ± 1.10	(20)	24.76 ± 1.07	(25)	0.903
75 mg	8.38 ± 5.74	(21)	13.12 ± 7.70	(26)	0.024	25.20 ± 1.09	(20)	25.17 ± 1.02	(23)	0.986
100 mg	5.33 ± 6.24	(18)	11.08 ± 7.81	(26)	0.013	26.47 ± 1.14	(17)	25.44 ± 1.14	(25)	0.540

Values are mean ± SD. Total *n* of each group decreased because of missing data.
* Unpaired *t*-test.
Reprinted with permission from Kimura *et al.* (2000).

greater than 50% reduction in Hamilton depression scores and no longer met crite-
rion for major or minor depression and non-responders ($n = 23$), major depression
($n = 18$), minor depression ($n = 5$) had less than 50% reduction in Hamilton rating
scale for depression (Ham-D) scores. The responder group included 16 patients
treated with nortriptyline and 9 with placebo. The non-responder group included
5 patients treated with nortriptyline and 18 with placebo. There were no significant
differences between the responder group and treatment failure group in their baseline Hamilton depression scores (18.3 ± 4.2 responder versus 17.0 ± 3.9 non-
responder). There were also no significant differences between the two groups
in their demographic characteristics, lesion variables or neurological findings.
Repeated measures, ANOVA of mini-mental scores demonstrated a significant
group by dose interaction ($p = 0.005$) (i.e., cognitive function in the responder group
recovered more than the treatment failure group) (Fig. 14.6). Planned comparisons
revealed that the responders had significantly less impaired mini-mental scores than
the non-responders at nortriptyline doses of 75 mg ($p = 0.036$) and 100 mg
($p = 0.024$). Although some placebo patients ($n - 8$) were in the responder group,
there were significantly more nortriptyline-treated patients in this group than in the
non-responder group ($p = 0.0032$). If only nortriptyline-treated patients were used

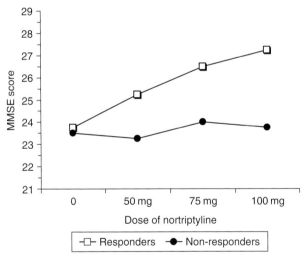

Figure 14.6   Change of MMSE scores in patients with poststroke depression who did or did not
respond to treatment with nortriptyline or placebo in a double-blind study. The data from
two studies was merged based on dose of nortriptyline (i.e., 6-week trial in one and a
9-week trial in the other). Repeated measures ANOVA showed a group by dose interaction
($F3, 108 = 4.45, p = 0.005$) with significantly better MMSE scores in the responder group
at doses of 75 ($p = 0.036$) and 100 mg ($p = 0.024$) (reprinted from Kimura *et al.* (2000)
with permission).

in the treatment response group and only placebo patients in the treatment failure group, there was still a significant group by time interaction ($p = 0.036$). This finding indicates that the failure to demonstrate cognitive improvement in prior studies was not the result of either a nortriptyline drug effect such as sedation or anticholinergic effects or because the cognitive impairment was due entirely to the brain lesion.

As we have previously found that cognitive impairment was associated with major but not minor depression, we examined whether the phenomenon of cognitive improvement with treatment response would occur in patients only with major depression. Among patients with major depression ($n = 33$), responders ($n = 15$) showed significantly greater improvement in cognitive function than non-responders ($n = 18$) ($p = 0.0087$). Among patients with minor depression (nine responders and five non-responders) repeated measures ANOVA of mini-mental scores showed no significant group effect, time effect, or group by time interaction.

This study, using double-blind placebo-controlled methodology, demonstrated for the first time that successful treatment of depression in patients with poststroke major depression produces a significant improvement in cognitive function. The areas of cognitive function on the MMSE that showed significant improvement were attention, concentration and recall. This finding supports our proposal that poststroke major depression with cognitive impairment represents a reversible dementia of depression.

One might logically wonder why improved cognitive function associated with mood improvement was not noted in prior treatment studies. The answer to this question is related to effect size. Nortriptyline treatment of depression as demonstrated in the present study produced a mean change of 12.1 points on the Ham-D or a 69.5% decline compared with a 36.8% (6.8 points) decline in the placebo group. The effect size was 0.71. This effect size is much larger than the effect of nortriptyline on mini-mental scores (i.e., 9.6%, 1.8 points for active treatment and 5.6%, 1.3 points for placebo treatment) with an effect size of 0.16. It would take a group size of 598 patients to demonstrate a significant effect of nortriptyline on cognitive function with an 80% probability. By dividing patients on the basis of response to treatment, the effect on the mini-mental score was 17.2% (3.0 points) for responders and 1.3% (0.14 points) for non-responders for an effect size of 0.96. This allowed a significant difference to be detected with a group size of only 47.

Another significant finding from this study was that improved cognitive function was related to mood improvement and not to the use of nortriptyline itself. Approximately one-third of the patients responding to treatment were taking placebo and showed the same cognitive improvements as those taking nortriptyline. The fact that mood improvement with placebo was associated with the same cognitive

Table 14.4. Demographic characteristics of depressed and non-depressed patients

Characteristic	Depressed ($n = 17$)		Non-depressed ($n = 42$)		Significance
	Mean	SD	Mean	SD	
Age (years)	58.5	15.6	65.3	12.5	NS
Education (years)	10.5	2.8	11.1	3.7	NS
Days since stroke	51.4	77.2	36.1	53.2	NS
	n	%	n	%	
Male sex	13	76.5	28	66.7	NS
Caucasian race	14	82.4	31	73.8	NS
Married	10	58.8	29	69.1	NS
Socio-economic status Hollingshead Class IV or V	12	70.6	20	47.6	NS
Right handedness	15	88.2	39	92.9	NS
Prior psychiatric history	5	31.3	4	9.5	NS
Family psychiatric history	2	11.8	7	16.7	NS
DSM-IV Major depression	10	58.8	0	0	$p < 0.05$
	($n = 6$)		($n = 10$)		
Received antidepressant treatment from primary care physician	35.3		31.3		NS

Reprinted with permission from Narushima *et al.* (2003).

improvement as nortriptyline suggests that reversal of the pathophysiological changes related to depression, not the biochemical effects of nortriptyline, was responsible for the cognitive improvement.

We have also recently examined the longitudinal course of treated depression and cognitive dysfunction among 17 patients treated for poststroke depression ($n = 10$ major depression; $n = 7$ minor depression) compared to 42 patients without treatment who remained non-depressed throughout a 2-year follow-up (Table 14.4) (Narushima *et al.* 2003). The patients were taken from the Iowa treatment study (Robinson *et al.* 2000) ($n = 27$ non-depressed; $n = 12$ depressed) as well as the previously described Baltimore longitudinal and treatment studies ($n = 20$ non-depressed; $n = 5$ depressed). The initial mean score on the Hamilton depression score for the depressed patients was 15.1 ± 1.2 SD, and the non-depressed patients mean was 5.6 ± 4.7 SD ($p = 0.01$). The depressed patients represented all patients who had responded to treatment and remained in remission without other illnesses from 3 months to 2 years following stroke. The non-depressed patients represented all patients who remained non-depressed throughout the 2 years and had no intervening physical illness. Repeated measures ANOVA showed a significant group

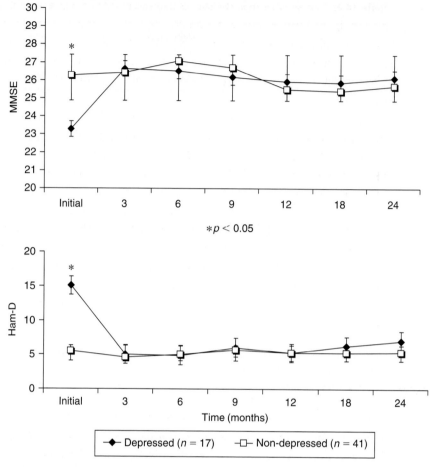

Figure 14.7 Scores over 2 years on the MMSE and the Ham-D for patients whose poststroke
depression responded (i.e., greater than 50% reduction in Ham-D score) and remained
non-depressed for 2 years compared to similar patients who were never depressed
throughout the 2-year follow-up. Note in the top panel that after the improvement over
the first 3 months, MMSE scores remained unchanged through the 2 years of observation
(reprinted with permission from Narishima et al. AJP 2003).

by time interaction with the depressed group improving in Ham-D scores more
than the non-depressed group over the first 3 months ($p = 0.01$) (Fig. 14.7 bottom
panel). The initial mean mini-mental score for the depressed patients was
23.3 ± 4.2 which was significantly more impaired than the initial mean score of
26.3 ± 3.1 SD for the non-depressed group, $p = 0.01$. Mini-mental scores for the
depressed patients improved significantly by the 3-month follow-up to a mean of
26.6 ± 3.5 ($p = 0.04$) and remained unchanged for the next 2 years (final score:
mean = 26.1 ± 23.6 SD) (Fig. 14.7 top panel).

A logistic regression analysis examining the effects of lesion volume, improvement in Ham-D score at 3-month follow-up, and motor deficit on improvement in mini-mental scores (i.e., the variables which were significantly different between the two groups) showed a significant and independent effect of response of depression during the acute phase ($p = 0.04$) and no significant effect of lesion volume ($p = 0.08$) or motor deficit ($p = 0.22$).

This study demonstrated that patients who were effectively treated for poststroke depression sustained the improvement of cognitive function over a 2-year period. The degree of cognitive impairment due to depression was 3.3 points on the MMSE which represented the difference between the initial score and the mean score of 26.6 after remission of depression. This study also found that the cognitive impairment due to ischemic brain injury independent of depression did not improve between 1 and 24 months poststroke. In our earlier study, comparing patients with major depression, with non-depressed patients matched for lesion size and location (Starkstein *et al.* 1988), a difference of 5.8 points in mini-mental score was found (i.e., 16.6 ± 7.8 depressed; 22.4 ± 6.6 non-depressed) ($p = 0.02$). Thus, the improvement shown in the current study probably represents a mean effect of depression when lesion size and location are not strictly controlled.

Longitudinal course

Some studies of elderly populations with dementia of depression have shown long-term cognitive deterioration. Alexopoulos (1993) followed up elderly patients with reversible depressive dementia without stroke and found that 33% developed an irreversible dementia about 33 months later. On the basis of this finding the authors proposed that patients who have late onset depression with reversible dementia may include some who have preexisting early stage dementia. Moroney (1996) followed up on non-demented stroke patients for 53 months and found that hypoxic events after stroke such as seizures resulted in a higher risk for subsequent dementia. The absence of deterioration of cognitive function in our patients over 2 years in the current study may have been due to the fact that they were younger than patients in other studies and the follow-up was shorter. Further cognitive deterioration after initial stroke may be related to age, time since stroke, or subsequent reinjury of the central nervous system such as another stroke or transient hypoxic event which may precipitate the onset of a neurodegenerative disorder. This may have been the case in our study if we had followed our patients for a longer period of time. However, the finding that patients without subsequent illnesses maintain their improved level of cognitive functioning following treatment of depression for at least 2 years is a positive finding and demonstrates the importance of identification and treatment of poststroke depression.

Mechanism of cognitive impairment

The finding that patients with major depression had significantly lower MMSE scores than non-depressed patients only during the first 6–12 months following stroke and that cognitive impairment occurred primarily in patients with major depression associated with left hemisphere lesions suggested that depression itself may not have played a major role in producing cognitive impairment. If depression produced cognitive impairment, all patients with major depression regardless of whether they had a right or left hemisphere lesion should be cognitively impaired. Furthermore, if depression led to cognitive impairment this relationship should be seen at all times following stroke and not be diminished in strength after the first year poststroke. Similarly, the data did not support the contention that cognitive impairment led to depression. Although in-hospital cognitive impairment correlated with depression at 6, but not 3, months follow-up (Fig. 14.5), the improvement in cognitive function associated with treatment or remission of depression would not be expected. A stable cognitive impairment that led to depression would be expected. Furthermore, of 26 patients with MMSE less than 23 in hospital only 2 (8%) developed depression at 3 months and 4 (15%) at 6 months while among 36 patients with MMSE greater than 23, 6 (17%) developed depression at 3 months and 7 at 6 months (18%) ($p =$ NS). Thus, cognitive impairment did not lead to the development of depression.

The third possibility suggested for the association of major depression and cognitive impairment was that depression and cognitive impairment may be produced by a unique physiological state. None of the data would be inconsistent with this suggestion and, in fact, the finding that patients with a particular type of lesion (i.e., left hemisphere) and major depression had the most prominent cognitive impairment suggests that a physiological state produced by left hemisphere stroke may have led to both depression and cognitive impairment. Thus, if poststroke depressions are seen as a group of disorders with multiple etiologies, some major depressions associated with left hemisphere stroke may have a particular mechanism or pathophysiology which produced cognitive impairment. In contrast, depressions produced by other mechanisms (e.g., genetic vulnerability) may lead to major depression based on a different neurophysiological or psychological process which does not cause cognitive impairment.

The laterality finding was a particularly interesting phenomenon. As previously discussed, this finding was also reported by House *et al.* (1990) and Morris *et al.* (1990) (Fig. 14.3). Although the explanation for why left but not right hemisphere strokes produced a dementia of depression is unclear, it parallels the laterality findings in patients with acute stroke in which left anterior lesions were associated with a greater frequency of major depression than right anterior lesions (see Chapter 10).

In an effort to investigate a mechanism for this laterality phenomenon, we studied 26 patients with acute stroke (not included in these longitudinal studies) using positron emission tomography (PET) imaging of cortical serotonin S_2 receptor binding (Morris *et al.* 1993). Among the group of 26 patients, MMSE scores were found to correlate significantly with the amount of S_2 serotonin receptor binding (as measured by [C-11] *N*-methylspiperone (NMSP) uptake) in uninjured areas of frontal and parietal cortex in both the right and left hemisphere (Fig. 14.8). The correlation of MMSE score with serotonin receptor binding, however, was strongest in the left frontal cortex (Fig. 14.8). When the individual items of the MMSE were examined, there were significant correlations between the amount of S_2 receptor binding in the left frontal cortex and performance on serial 7s ($r = 0.42$; $p = 0.03$), writing a sentence ($r = 0.56$; $p = 0.003$), and copying a design ($r = 0.53$; $p = 0.006$). A study in rats confirmed that the NMSP binding in the cortex was predominantly to serotonin S_2 receptors (Mayberg *et al.* 1990). In addition, right hemisphere lesions in rats produced a different effect on serotonin receptors (i.e., a more widespread decrease in receptor number) than identical left hemisphere lesions (Mayberg *et al.* 1990).

The fact that S_2 receptor binding correlated significantly with MMSE score in several brain regions and across several cognitive tasks (Morris *et al.* 1993) suggests that the serotonergic system played some general rather than specific role in

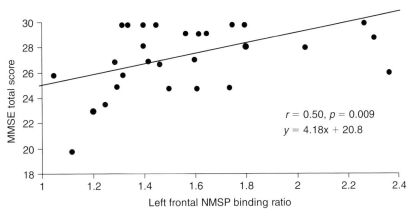

$r = 0.50, p = 0.009$
$y = 4.18x + 20.8$

Figure 14.8 The relationship between mini-mental score and the amount of binding of NMSP in non-injured areas of left frontal cortex in 26 patients with stroke. NMSP binding was measured by PET comparing the number of C11-positron emission counts in a specified region of interest in left frontal cortex to similar counts in a comparable area of cerebellum (i.e., non-specific binding). This gave a binding ratio (i.e., cortical to cerebellar binding) NMSP binding in cortex has been shown to be primarily to serotonin S_2 receptors. The correlation indicates that cognitive function improved with increasing amount of serotonin S_2 receptors in frontal cortex.

cognition. One aspect of cognition which might have influenced a wide range of tasks is attention and concentration. In addition, we have previously found that severity of depression was negatively correlated with S_2 receptor binding in the left but not the right temporal cortex (i.e., as serotonin receptor binding decreased, depression scores increased) (Mayberg *et al.* 1988; Mayberg 1992) (see Chapters 10 and 22). Taken together, these findings suggest the hypothesis that cognitive impairment may be mediated in part by frontal lobe serotonergic mechanisms while depression may be mediated in part by temporal lobe serotonergic mechanisms. Thus, stroke lesions which produce cerebral dysfunction (perhaps as a result of decreased serotonergic receptor stimulation) in both frontal and temporal regions may lead to both major depression and cognitive impairment while lesions which produce decreased temporal serotonergic receptor stimulation (without frontal lobe dysfunction) may lead to depression without dementia.

This hypothesis, that temporal lobe dysfunction subserves depression while frontal lobe dysfunction subserves cognitive impairment might also explain why the association of depression and intellectual impairment was strongest during the acute poststroke period. Acute stroke has been shown to produce a generalized hypometabolism in many non-injured areas of cortex independent of depression (Mayberg 1992). This might produce a decrease in frontal lobe activity which could combine with temporal lobe hypometabolism to produce both dementia and depression. After the acute stroke period was over, there was less general metabolic suppression of frontal lobe function due to stroke and, therefore, a weaker apparent relationship with depression (i.e., the temporal hypometabolism would continue while the frontal hypometabolism would diminish).

In summary, there was substantial evidence that cognitive impairment and major depression were significantly associated with one another in some patients with stroke. Although several factors contributed to poststroke cognitive impairment, including lesion size and location, depression appeared to be associated with an even greater degree of cognitive impairment than could be explained by the lesion alone. This phenomenon occurred primarily following left hemisphere stroke and only with major depression. The available data also suggested that cognitive impairment did not directly produce depression and that only a particular type of depression was associated with cognitive impairment. Although the association of major depression with cognitive impairment could be demonstrated during the first year following stroke, it was strongest during the acute poststroke period. Therefore, it seems possible that both cognitive impairment and depression were the outcome of a third factor, such as serotonergic dysfunction induced by left hemisphere injury. We have hypothesized that decreased serotonin receptor activity in the frontal and temporal lobe led to cognitive impairment and major depression while temporal lobe dysfunction alone led to depression without cognitive impairment. The lateralized effect of stroke on depression and cognitive impairment (i.e., left but not right hemisphere lesions were associated with cognitive impairment and major depression) may have been related to the lateralized effect of stroke on serotonergic receptors (Mayberg *et al.* 1988).

REFERENCES

Alexopoulos, G. S., Meyers, B. S., Young, R. C., *et al.* The course of geriatric depression with "reversible dementia": a controlled study. *Am J Psychiatr* (1993) 150(11):1693–1699.

Andersen, G., Vestergaard, K., and Lauritzen, L. Effective treatment of poststroke depression with the selective serotonin reuptake inhibitor citalopram. *Stroke* (1994) 25:1099–1104.

Andersen, G., Vestergaard, K., Riis, J. O., *et al.* Dementia of depression or depression of dementia in stroke? *Acta Psychiatr Scand* (1996) 94:272–278.

Bolla-Wilson, K., Robinson, R. G., Starkstein, S. E., *et al.* Lateralization of dementia of depression in stroke patients. *Am J Psychiatr* (1989) 146:627–634.

Censori, B., Manara, O., Agostinis, C., *et al.* Dementia after first stroke. *Stroke* (1996) 27(7):1205–1210.

Downhill Jr., J. E., and Robinson, R. G. Longitudinal assessment of depression and cognitive impairment following stroke. *J Nerv Ment Dis* (1994) 182:425–431.

Eastwood, M. R., Rifat, S. L., Nobbs, H., *et al.* Mood disorder following cerebrovascular accident. *Br J Psychiatr* (1989) 154:195–200.

Fruehwald, S., Gatterbauer, E., Rehak, P., *et al.* Early fluoxetine treatment of post-stroke depression – a three-month double-blind placebo-controlled study with an open-label long-term follow up. *J Neurol* (2003) 250(3):347–351.

Gazzaniga, M. S. *Cognitive Neuroscience.* Blackwell Publishing, 2000.

House, A., Dennis, M., Warlow, C., *et al.* The relationship between intellectual impairment and mood disorder in the first year after stroke. *Psychol Med* (1990) 20:805–814.

House, A., Dennis, M., Mogridge, L., *et al.* Mood disorders in the year after first stroke. *Br J Psychiatr* (1991) 158:83–92.

Kase, C. S., Wolf, P. A., Kelly-Hayes, M., *et al.* Intellectual decline after stroke: the Framingham study. *Stroke* (1998) 29(4):805–812.

Kauhanen, M., Korpelainen, J. T., Hiltunen, P., *et al.* Poststroke depression correlates with cognitive impairment and neurological deficits. *Stroke* (1999) 30(9):1875–1880.

Kimura, M., Robinson, R. G., and Kosier, T. Treatment of cognitive impairment after poststroke depression. *Stroke* (2000) 31(7):1482–1486.

Levine, D. N., and Grek, A. The anatomic basis of delusions after right cerebral infarction. *Neurology* (1984) 34:577–582.

Lipsey, J. R., Robinson, R. G., Pearlson, G. D., *et al.* Nortriptyline treatment of post-stroke depression: a double-blind study. *Lancet* (1984) i(8372):297–300.

Mayberg, H. S., Robinson, R. G., Wong, D. F., *et al.* PET imaging of cortical S_2-serotonin receptors after stroke: lateralized changes and relationship to depression. *Am J Psychiatr* (1988) 145:937–943.

Mayberg, H. S., Moran, T. H., and Robinson, R. G. Remote lateralized changes in cortical ^{3}H-spiperone binding following focal frontal cortex lesions in the rat. *Brain Res* (1990) 516:127–131.

Mayberg, H. S. Neuroimaging studies of depression in neurologic disease. In S. E. Starkstein and R. G. Robinson, eds., *Depression in Neurologic Disease*. The Johns Hopkins University Press, 1992.

Moroney, J. T., Bagiella, E., Desmond, D. W., *et al.* Risk factors for incident dementia after stroke: role of hypoxic and ischemic disorders. *Stroke* (1996) 27:1283–1289.

Morris, P. L. P., Robinson, R. G., and Raphael, B. Prevalence and course of depressive disorders in hospitalized stroke patients. *Int J Psychiatr Med* (1990) 20:349–364.

Morris, P. L. P., Mayberg, H., Bolla, K., *et al.* A preliminary study of cortical S_2 serotonin receptors and cognitive performance following stroke. *J Neuropsychiatr Clin Neurosci* (1993) 5:395–400.

Narushima, K., Chan, K. L., Kosier, J. T., *et al.* Does cognitive recovery after treatment of poststroke depression last? A 2-year follow-up of cognitive function associated with poststroke depression. *Am J Psychiatr* (2003) 160(6):1157–1162.

Pohjasvaara, T., Erkinjuntti, T., Vataja, R., *et al.* Dementia three months after stroke: baseline frequency and effect of different definitions of dementia in the Helsinki stroke aging memory study (SAM) cohort. *Stroke* (1997) 28:785–792.

Robinson, R. G., Starr, L. B., Kubos, K. L., *et al.* A two year longitudinal study of post-stroke mood disorders: findings during the initial evaluation. *Stroke* (1983) 14:736–744.

Robinson, R. G., Bolla-Wilson, K., Kaplan, E., *et al.* Depression influences intellectual impairment in stroke patients. *Br J Psychiatr* (1986) 148:541–547.

Robinson, R. G., Schultz, S. K., Castillo, C., *et al.* Nortriptyline versus fluoxetine in the treatment of depression and in short term recovery after stroke: a placebo controlled, double-blind study. *Am J Psychiatr* (2000) 157:351–359.

Spalletta, G., Guida, G., De Angelis, D., *et al.* Predictors of cognitive level and depression severity are different in patients with left and right hemispheric stroke within the first year of illness. *J Neurol* (2002) 249(11):1541–1551.

Spalletta, G., and Caltagirone, C. Sertraline treatment of post-stroke major depression: an open study in patients with moderate to severe symptoms. *Funct Neurol* (2003) 18(4):227–232.

Starkstein, S. E., Robinson, R. G., and Price, T. R. Comparison of patients with and without poststroke major depression matched for size and location of lesion. *Arch Gen Psychiatr* (1988) 45:247–252.

15

Relationship of aphasia to depression

Aphasia remains one of the most perplexing problems for investigators of neuropsychiatric disorders following stroke. Since the diagnoses of all neuropsychiatric disorders requires subjective responses by the patient to verbal or written questions, the existence of even a moderate degree of comprehension deficit may represent a severe obstacle to the diagnoses of numerous neuropsychiatric disorders. This conundrum has led almost all investigators of poststroke neuropsychiatric disorders to exclude patients with moderate or severe comprehension deficits from their studies (Robinson *et al.* 1983; House *et al.* 1990; Astrom *et al.* 1993).

In spite of the fact that almost all investigations of poststroke depression have excluded patients with comprehension aphasia, the hypothesized cause of many poststroke depressive disorders has been aphasia (Gainotti 1972; Benson 1979). Gainotti (1972) hypothesized that the depressive-catastrophic reaction associated with left hemisphere lesions represented an understandable response of depression and angry outbursts to the loss of language because language represents one of the most important elements of the patient's life. Similarly, Benson (1979) hypothesized that depression sometimes represents a secondary psychological reaction to the loss of language. As a result of the exclusion of patients with comprehensive aphasia (e.g., fluent aphasias and global aphasias) two major questions arise. First, what is the true prevalence of depression among patients with aphasia. Does the exclusion of these patients significantly alter our estimates of prevalence rates, as well as clinical and pathological correlates of depression. The second question arising from the exclusion of patients with comprehension impairment is whether alternative means can be devised to diagnose depression in this population of patients that will withstand tests of reliability and validity? Although patients with moderate to severe comprehension deficits have been excluded from our studies, we have included patients with at least mild forms of fluent, non-fluent and global aphasia in most of our studies.

In our initial studies, the existence of moderate to severe comprehension deficit was determined by requiring the patient to score within 10 points following verbal readministration of the Zung depression scale approximately 10 min apart. For the past 20 years, however, we have utilized the Token test which is specifically designed to assess comprehension. The Token test examines the patient's ability to comprehend and carry out verbal instructions related to the shape and color of plastic tokens. For example, in Part 1, patients are asked to point to the red square or the blue triangle. Patients who are unable to pass Part 1 of the Token test which involves only these simple tasks are excluded from our studies. Our studies, therefore, have included patients with mild fluent (i.e., Wernicke's) aphasia, global aphasia, and transcortical sensory aphasia as well as patients with any severity of non-fluent (Broca's) aphasia. Patients with Broca's aphasia are asked the standard questions in the psychiatric interview but their responses may include such non-verbal behaviors as pointing appropriately to yes or no responses or communicating using non-verbal gestures or limited verbal responses.

In our study of 103 patients with acute stroke, 42% of the patients who met study inclusion criteria and had left hemisphere lesions were diagnosed as having fluent, non-fluent, transcortical, or global aphasia, or severe anomia (this does not include the patients who were excluded from the study due to comprehension deficits). Our latest data on the relationship between aphasia and depression is shown in Table 15.1 (Part A). These findings indicate that among patients without significant comprehension deficits, neither major nor minor depression was more common among aphasic as compared to non-aphasic patients.

We also examined the relationship between depression and aphasia in another group of 25 patients who were examined approximately 3 months following stroke. Based on findings from the Boston aphasia examination, patients were grouped according to whether they had non-fluent ($n = 7$), fluent ($n = 8$), or global ($n = 9$) aphasia (Robinson and Benson 1981). Although the groups were not significantly different with respect to their background characteristics, patients with non-fluent aphasia had significantly higher Zung, Hamilton, and Nurses' depression rating scale scores than the other two groups (Fig. 15.1). There were, however, no differences in mean depression scores between patients with fluent aphasia and patients with global aphasia. There were no statistically significant differences between fluent, non-fluent, and global aphasic patients in terms of their severity of impairment in activities of daily living (ADL) (i.e., Johns Hopkins functioning inventory or JHFI score) or severity of cognitive impairment (i.e., mini-mental state exam score). Thus, this study demonstrated that non-fluent aphasic patients had significantly greater severity of depression than fluent or global aphasic patients in the absence of significant differences in their physical or cognitive deficits.

Based on these findings, one might wonder why there is a greater severity of depression in patients with non-fluent as compared to fluent or global aphasia. It might be proposed, for example, that patients with non-fluent aphasia were most

Table 15.1. The relationship between the existence of aphasia and depression

	No of patients with		
	Major depression	Minor depression	No mood disorder
A. Patients with acute stroke ($n = 265$)	($n = 44$)	($n = 51$)	($n = 170$)
Aphasia	8	7	13
No aphasia	36	44	157
(depressed versus non-depressed, NS, $p = 0.1079$)			
B. Patients given Western aphasia			
($n = 25$)			
Anomia ($n = 7$)	2	2	3
Broca's ($n = 6$)	3	1	2
Wernicke ($n = 6$)	0	3	3
Global ($n = 4$)	2	0	2
TCS ($n = 2$)	2	0	0
(depressed versus non-depressed, $p = $ NS)			
C. Patients with subcortical lesions ($n = 25$)			
Basal ganglia			
Aphasia	3	0	0
No aphasia	5	2	5
Thalamus			
Aphasia	0	1	1
No aphasia	0	1	7
(depressed versus non-depressed, $p = $ NS)			

TCS = transcortical sensory aphasia.

depressed because of their greater awareness of their impairments. Another possible explanation, however, is based on lesion location. Patients with fluent and nonfluent aphasias generally have different lesion locations and the lesion locations which are frequently involved in non-fluent aphasia might explain the increased association of this type of aphasia with depression. In an effort to answer this question, we conducted another study of 25 consecutive patients with aphasia evaluated using the Western aphasia battery (Kertesz 1982; Starkstein and Robinson 1988). Seven patients had anomia, six had Wernicke's aphasia, six had Broca's aphasia, four had global aphasia, and two had transcortical sensory aphasia. The depressive diagnoses are shown in Part B of Table 15.1. There was no significant difference in the frequency of depression among patients with milder forms of aphasia (i.e., anomia or transcortical sensory aphasia) compared with more severe forms of aphasia (i.e., Broca's, Wernicke's, or global aphasia). On the other hand, when we examined the relationship with lesion location, there was a consistent

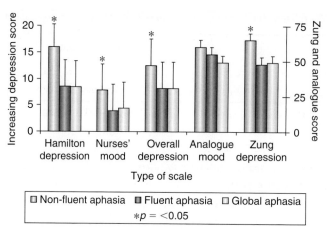

Figure 15.1   Mean ± SEM depression scores using four different measurement scales and an overall scale factoring together the four instruments grouped by type of aphasia. Patients with Broca's (i.e., non-fluent) aphasia ($n = 7$) had the highest depression scores on all scales (significant on four of the five measures) compared to Wernicke's (i.e., fluent) aphasia ($n = 8$) or global aphasia ($n = 9$) (reprinted from Robinson and Benson 1981 with permission from Elsevier).

association between depression and left frontal or left basal ganglia injury. Of the seven patients with major depression and positive computed tomography (CT) scans, all had lesions involving the left anterior brain region (i.e., the left frontal cortex in five cases, and the left basal ganglia in two cases). On the other hand, only one of the 10 non-depressed patients had a left anterior brain injury ($p < 0.01$).

These findings suggest that lesion location rather than type of aphasia may be the most relevant variable in poststroke major depression. The association between Broca's aphasia and the severity of depression reported in the Robinson and Benson study (1981) may be explained by the fact that Broca's area is located in the posterior-inferior aspect of the left frontal lobe (see Fig. 2.1). As discussed in Chapter 10 on the relationship of depression to lesion location during the first two months following stroke, left frontal and left basal ganglia lesions are significantly more frequent among patients with major depression than any other lesion location.

We have also examined the role of subcortical structures in depression and aphasia. The role of subcortical structures in the production and comprehension of language has been the subject of numerous studies [e.g. (Crosson 1985)]. In an effort to clarify the relationship between aphasia and depression, we examined patients with lesions restricted to the subcortical grey nuclei with or without involvement of the white matter of the internal capsule (Starkstein and Robinson 1988). If aphasia led to the development of depression, one would expect that, whether the aphasia was produced by a subcortical lesion or a cortical lesion, depression should follow. Included in this study were eight patients with lesions of the left basal ganglia and seven with lesions of the right basal ganglia. In addition, there were six patients with lesions restricted to the left thalamus and four with right thalamic lesions. Aphasia occurred only in patients with left hemisphere lesions. The frequency of depression in patients with non-fluent, fluent or global aphasia and lesions of the basal ganglia or thalamus is shown in Part C of Table 15.1. There was a significant association between major depression and basal ganglia lesions as compared to thalamic lesions ($p < 0.01$). On the other hand, there was no significant increase in the frequency of depression among patients with basal ganglia or thalamic lesions based on the presence or absence of aphasia. Thus, these findings suggest that, as with cortical lesions, the location of the lesion appears to be a more important factor in determining the frequency of depression than the existence of aphasia.

Herrmann *et al.* (1993) reported on the results of a study of 21 acute and 21 chronic aphasic patients with single stroke lesions of the left hemisphere. The acute stroke patients had significantly higher depression scores (i.e., Cornell depression scale) compared to the chronic stroke patients with non-fluent aphasias (i.e., Broca's or global aphasia) who also had a greater frequency of major depression compared to patients with fluent aphasias (i.e., Wernicke's or anomic aphasia) ($p = 0.0014$). These authors also found a significant linear correlation between the severity of depression and the proximity of the lesion to the frontal pole. These findings are in agreement with our previously described studies of aphasia and are consistent with the hypothesis that non-fluent aphasia does not cause depression but frequently coexists with it because lesion sites associated with depression and non-fluent aphasia are anatomically close.

Astrom *et al.* (1993) also reported a significant association between major depression and aphasia in seven patients with language impairment who could be assessed for depression. Dysphasic patients were significantly more likely to be depressed than non-dysphasic patients both during the acute hospitalization period ($p = 0.001$) and at 3 months follow-up ($p = 0.001$) but not at 1, 2, or 3 years follow-up. Patients, however, were not grouped according to whether they had fluent or non-fluent aphasia, and the relationship between depression and anterior left hemisphere lesions, independent of aphasia, was not examined.

Dam *et al.* (1989) examined 92 patients between 8 and 1280 days since their stroke. Aphasia severity was rated on a 4-point scale ranging from none to severe. These investigators found no significant correlation between Hamilton depression (Ham-D) score and the severity of aphasia.

Damecour and Caplan (1991) examined 54 patients with fluent or non-fluent ($n = 32$) aphasia, who were less than ($n = 23$) or more than ($n = 31$) 6 months poststroke. Zung depression rating scales from significant others and speech pathologists were obtained. Depression was determined using a cutoff score on the Zung. Overall 15% of the population was depressed, but using mean rating scores or frequency of depression, no significant differences were found among the groups either in the acute or chronic stroke period. They concluded that patients with Wernicke's aphasia do not experience depression more frequently than patients with Broca's aphasia and that depression is not frequent in this population. Of the fluent aphasics, 84% were interviewed but the reliability of responses was not reported.

Kauhanen *et al.* (2000) examined a consecutive series of 106 patients (46 women and 60 men, mean age 65.8 years) with first ever ischemic stroke. Patients were evaluated for aphasia during the first week after stoke and for aphasia plus psychiatric and neuropsychological impairment at 3 and 12 months poststroke. Aphasia was diagnosed in 34% of the patients during the acute phase and two-thirds of these patients remained aphasic 12 months later. Seventy percent of the aphasic patients fulfilled DSM-III-R criteria for depression at 3 months and 62% at 12 months poststroke. During this time, the prevalence of major depression in the overall population increased from 11% at 3 months to 33% at 12 months. They concluded that aphasia represented a significant risk factor for poststroke depression. Furthermore, although the overall prevalence of depression decreased from 3–12 months poststroke, patients who continued to have aphasia are increasingly likely to have major depressive disorder. The difficulty in evaluating this study is that the diagnosis of depression was based on observation by relatives or hospital staff without showing the reliability or validity of these assessments.

In an attempt to establish an instrument to assess depression in aphasic patients with stroke, Sutcliffe and Lincoln (1998) developed an observer based depression rating scale called the stroke aphasic depression questionnaire (SADQ). Seventy patients who were discharged to home following acute stroke were evaluated using the SADQ, the hospital anxiety and depression scale (HADS) and the Wakefield depression inventory. The correlation between the aphasia questionnaire score and the HADS was 0.32 using a shortened 10-item version of the scale and 0.67 with the Wakefield depression inventory. Seventeen aphasic patients examined at 4-week intervals demonstrated a test-retest reliability of 0.72.

Although Sutcliffe and Lincoln (Sutcliffe and Lincoln 1998) found a relationship between the SADQ and severity of depression, Leeds *et al.* (2004) examined 65 stroke patients without significant aphasia using the shortened version of the SADQ. The Geriatric depression scale correlated with the SADQ score with a correlation coefficient of 0.40. This relatively weak correlation between patient's self report of depression and relatives scores on the SADQ led the authors to conclude that the SADQ-10 did not appear to be a valid measure of depression. The fact that both the Sutcliffe and Lincoln (1998) and the Leeds (2004) studies found only weak to moderate correlations between self reported depression severity and observer rated depressive symptoms indicates that the problem of assessment of depression in patients with comprehension impairment remains a significant obstacle to the investigation of depressive disorders in these patients.

It has been suggested that the exclusion of aphasic patients with severe comprehension deficits following parietal-temporal lesions may have skewed the association between depression and lesion location to more anterior (i.e., frontal) brain regions (Ross *et al.* 1986). If one assumes that the correlation between depression and anterior-posterior lesion location was an artifact produced by excluding depressed patients with posterior lesions (i.e., fluent aphasics), there would have to be a very high frequency of depression in these excluded aphasic patients to negate the correlation of depression with proximity of the lesion to the frontal pole. Since the frequency of major depression among patients with acute left anterior lesions was found to be approximately 60%, the rate of major depression among patients with comprehension disorders would have to be equally high. If findings in studies of patients with mild forms of fluent and global aphasia are extrapolated, however, the frequency of depression in these groups of patients is significantly lower than that among patients with non-fluent aphasia (Robinson and Benson 1981; Herrmann *et al.* 1993). This conclusion, however, is based on the assumption that patients with mild non-fluent aphasias had the same rate of depression as patients with severe non-fluent aphasia (Robinson and Benson 1981). However, in the Damecour and Caplan study there was a modest correlation between depression severity and fluent aphasia severity ($r = 0.3$–0.6 depending on the scale). The affective appearance and behavior of patients with severe fluent aphasias have been described by Benson (1973) as cheerful or even euphoric and in rare instances as fearful or paranoid, but not depressed. Thus, although it is possible that these patients who cannot be examined could have a very different frequency of depression compared with patients with mild fluent aphasias, the available data suggest that this is not the case.

Although aphasia does not appear to be a cause of depression, depression and aphasia may interact significantly throughout the course of poststroke recovery. In Chapter 14, I discussed in detail our finding concerning the effect of depression on recovery from impairment in ADL (Parikh *et al.* 1990). One of the factors derived from the activities of daily living scale (ADLs) JHFI was language. We found that patients who were depressed (major or minor depression, $n = 25$) immediately after stroke had not recovered in language function to the same extent as patients who were not depressed ($n = 38$) even when other relevant factors were controlled. Thus, although further research, including treatment studies, are needed, there is some evidence to support the hypothesis that there are important effects of depression on recovery from aphasia.

In summary, aphasia is a common sequelae of dominant hemisphere brain injury. Although the loss of language might understandably lead to depression, the available evidence suggests that non-fluent (Broca's) aphasia appears to be associated with the highest frequency of depression. The true prevalence, however, of depression in patients with aphasia and comprehension deficits remains uncertain. The association between non-fluent (Broca's) aphasia and depression may be due to the fact that both depression and non-fluent aphasia result from lesions of the left frontal lobe. The development of alternative diagnostic instruments based on relatives' observations has not led to valid measures of depression in patients with comprehension deficits. Although much of the emphasis has been placed on the effect of aphasia in producing depression, it seems likely that poststroke depression may have a significant impact on patients' recovery from aphasia. Future studies should examine the effect of antidepressant treatment on the clinical manifestations and longitudinal recovery from aphasic disorders.

REFERENCES

Astrom, M., Adolfsson, R., and Asplund, K. Major depression in stroke patients: a 3-year longitudinal study. *Stroke* (1993) 24:976–982.

Benson, D. F. Psychiatric aspects of aphasia. *Br J Psychiatr* (1973) 123:555–566.

Benson, D. F. *Aphasia, Alexia, and Agraphia*. Churchill Livingstone, New York, 1979.

Crosson, B. Subcortical functions in language: a working model. *Brain and Language* (1985) 25:257–292.

Dam, H., Pedersen, H. E., and Ahlgren, P. Depression among patients with stroke. *Acta Psychiatr Scand* (1989) 80:118–124.

Damecour, C. L., and Caplan, D. The relationship of depression to symptomatology and lesion site in aphasic patients. *Cortex* (1991) 27:385–401.

Gainotti, G. Emotional behavior and hemispheric side of the brain. *Cortex* (1972) 8:41–55.

Herrmann, M., Bartles, C., and Wallesch, C.-W. Depression in acute and chronic aphasia: symptoms, pathoanatomical-clinical correlations and functional implications. *J Neurol Neurosurg Psychiatr* (1993) 56:672–678.

House, A., Dennis, M., Warlow, C., et al. The relationship between intellectual impairment and mood disorder in the first year after stroke. *Psychol Med* (1990) 20:805–814.

Kauhanen, M. L., Korpelainen, J. T., Hiltunen, P., et al. Domains and determinants of quality of life after stroke caused by brain infarction. *Arch Phys Med Rehabil* (2000) 81(12):1541–1546.

Kertesz, A. *Western Aphasia Battery*. Grune and Stratton, New York, 1982.

Leeds, L., Meara, R. J., and Hobson, J. P. The utility of the stroke aphasia depression questionnaire (SADQ) in a stroke rehabilitation unit. *Clin Rehabil* (2004) 18(2):228–231.

Parikh, R. M., Robinson, R. G., Lipsey, J. R., et al. The impact of post-stroke depression on recovery in activities of daily living over two year follow-up. *Arch Neurol* (1990) 47:785–789.

Robinson, R. G., and Benson, D. F. Depression in aphasic patients: frequency, severity and clinical-pathological correlations. *Brain Lang* (1981) 14:282–291.

Robinson, R. G., Starr, L. B., Kubos, K. L., et al. A two year longitudinal study of post-stroke mood disorders: findings during the initial evaluation. *Stroke* (1983) 14:736–744.

Ross, E. D., Gordon, W. A., Hibbard, M., et al. The dexamethasone suppression test, post-stroke depression, and the validity of DSM-III-based diagnostic criteria. *Am J Psychiatr* (1986) 143:1200–1201.

Starkstein, S. E., and Robinson, R. G. Aphasia and depression. *Aphasiology* (1988) 2:1–20.

Sutcliffe, L. M., and Lincoln, N. B. The assessment of depression in aphasic stroke patients: the development of the stroke aphasic depression questionnaire. *Clin Rehabil* (1998) 12(6):506–513.

Relationship of depression to social functioning

Social functioning has been recognized for many years to play an important role in development of depression associated with stress or negative life events (Brown *et al.* 1986; Henderson 1990). Furthermore, the effect of social support on psychological distress depends upon the nature of the supportive attachment. Among women in a community sample, for example, inadequate social support from a spouse was found to have a greater emotional impact than lack of support from a non-spousal relationship (Andrews and Brown 1988). Although an acute physical illness, such as stroke, can serve to mobilize social support from friends and family, patients who perceive their support to be inadequate may be more vulnerable to poststroke depression than patients who do not.

We have examined the relationship between poststroke depression and social functioning as measured by the social functioning exam (SFE) (Robinson *et al.* 1985a) and the social ties checklist (STC) (Robinson *et al.* 1985a) in several studies. The SFE was developed to quantify patient satisfaction with their social functioning both before and following a stroke. The SFE is shown in Table 16.1. It is a semi-structured interview in which the examiner, after asking one or several probing questions, rates each item on a 3-point scale: 0, indicates no difficulties, 1, indicates moderate difficulties, and 2, indicates severe impairment. The total score is the raw score divided by the maximum possible score (i.e., 00–1.00) with higher scores indicating greater impairment. The inter-rater agreement for each of these items ranged from 57% to 100% (mean 87%) for 31 patients involved in an inter-rater reliability study (Robinson *et al.* 1985a). The inter-rater reliability correlation coefficient (r) for total score on the SFE was 0.92 ($p < 0.01$) for two observers rating the 31 same interviews. Test-retest reliability for the total score on the SFE for eight acute stroke patients re-examined 1 day after their initial evaluation was $r = 0.90$ ($p < 0.01$). Validity was determined by examining the correlation coefficient between the SFE score and independent clinical severity ratings made by a social worker using standard clinical assessment. In 22 patients, the correlation between clinical ratings (1, indicating no impairment to 4, indicating severe impairment) and SFE score was $r = 0.50$ ($p < 0.05$).

Table 16.1. SFE

_____		Exam No.
_____		Interviewer Number
_____		Informant

1 = *Patient*
2 = *Closest other*
3 = *Closest other person – not spouse*
4 = *Other relative*
5 = *Other friend or acquaintance (Specify)*_____

_____   I.   Relationship with significant other
Whom are you closest to: _____
How close are you?
Is _____ affectionate?
Is _____ considerate of your feelings?

_____   1.   Rate closeness of relationship
Do you and _____ have separate interests or activities?
What kind of interests and activities?
Do you or _____ depend on others to help with everyday activities?

_____   2.   Rate independence
What do you and _____ usually disagree about?
How often?
Resolution

_____   3.   Rate compatibility
(If applicable)
Are there difficulties in your sexual relationship?
Satisfaction
Extra-marital relationship

_____   4.   Rate sexual adjustment
How happy have you been with _____?
Has _____ been the end of _____ that you wanted?

_____   5.   Rate satisfaction with relationship

_____   II.   Relationship with spouse or other partner in the household (Ask question below only if spouse, common-law, or boyfriend/girlfriend of opposite sex and living in the household is not named in I.)
Do you have a close relationship with _____?
Is person affectionate?
Is person considerate of *your* feelings?

_____   6.   Rate closeness
Do you and _____ have separate interests and activities?
What kind of activities?
Are you or _____ dependent on others for routine daily activities?

Table 16.1. (*Continued*)

_____	7.	Rate independence
		What do you and _____ usually disagree about?
		How often?
		Resolution
_____	8.	Rate compatibility
		Are there difficulties in your sexual relationship?
_____	9.	Rate sexual adjustment
		How satisfied are you with this relationship?
_____	10.	Rate satisfaction
_____	III.	Relationship with children – for patients who have living children (and/or stepchildren)
		Do you have a close relationship with any of your children (and/or stepchildren)?
		Are you and they affectionate?
		How often do you see them or talk with them?
_____	11.	Rate closeness of parent-child relationship
_____	IV.	Family relationships
		Do your family pull together in good times and bad?
		Give an example
		Do you have family reunions?
		Has someone been a major source of strength and support for the family over the years? Is that person available now? Has someone taken over that role?
_____	12.	Rate family solidarity
_____	V.	Other persons in household (if person lives with others in a household arrangement)
		Are you and others in the household close?
		Do you spend much time together?
		Do they help with household chores?
_____	13.	Rate relationship with household others
_____	VI.	Rate performance of home and family responsibilities
_____	14.	Is there anybody in your family who is now sick or disabled or needs a lot of care?
		Who? _____ Who takes care of this person? _____
_____	15.	Rate family energy devoted to other ill or dependent members
_____	VII.	Work experience
		Do you (did you) enjoy your job?
_____	16.	Rate satisfaction with work experience
_____	17.	Rate presumed loss of job satisfaction due to present illness
_____	VIII.	Social activities
		What are your social and leisure activities?
		Do you belong to any groups, organizations, church?
		How often do you attend?

Table 16.1. (*Continued*)

		How important are these groups to you?
		What kinds of things do you do there?
		What do you and your friends do together?
		How often?
_____	18.	Rate formal groups in patient's life
_____	19.	Rate informal groups in patient's life
_____	IX.	Spiritual beliefs
		Have your religious beliefs helped you through difficult times?
		In what way?
_____	20.	Rate religious beliefs in coping with difficulties
_____	X.	Economic practices
		How financially comfortable are you?
_____	21.	Rate usual financial security
_____	22.	Rate stability of family income in light of present illness
_____	XI.	Living environment
		What is it like where you live?
		What would you most like to change about where you live?
_____	23.	Rate (physical) adequacy of the residence
		What is your neighborhood like?
		What would you most like to change about your neighborhood?
_____	24.	Rate adequacy of neighborhood
_____	XII.	Use of community resources
		What social agencies do you have dealings with?
		What is the nature of your contact with those agencies?
_____	25.	Rate use of social agency services
_____	XIII.	Health and illness experiences
		How is the health of your family members?
		Where do you go for checkups?
_____	26.	Rate general health of the family
		When family members become ill, to whom do they go for medical care?
		What problems arise in following a medical care plan?
_____	27.	Rate health practices
		Has anybody in your family been sick for a long time or needed a lot of care?
		Who? _____ Who took care of that person? How was the family affected by all this?
_____	28.	Rate family coping with prolonged illness/disability

_____ Number of points scored – social functioning.
_____ Number of applicable questions – social functioning.
_____ Score functioning examination.

The STC is a 10-item questionnaire, which determines the number of social connections available to the patient, such as frequency of seeing friends, membership of clubs, churches or other organizations. Scores range from 0 to 10 with higher numbers indicating fewer social connections. The correlation between SFE and STC scores was $r = 0.65$ $(p < 0.01)$ for the 31 patients with acute stroke involved in our reliability study and the correlation between the SFE score and the Hollingshead social class was $r = 0.41$ $(p < 0.05)$. We have also examined the agreement between ratings based on patient information as compared to information provided by significant others. The percentage agreement between patient ratings and other derived ratings on individual items of the SFE ranged from 50 to 100%. The correlation coefficient between SFE total scores based on information from the patient and information obtained from significant others for 30 cases was $r = 0.60$ $(p < 0.001)$. This agreement was maintained even when we included data from patients who were depressed or had cognitive impairment. Thus, given relatively simple questions about their social situation, patients who were able to participate in these studies gave reliable and accurate information about their social functioning.

The correlation coefficients between SFE scores and Hamilton depression (Ham-D) scores over the course of the 2 years following acute stroke are shown in Fig. 16.1. These correlations were based on findings from our 2-year longitudinal

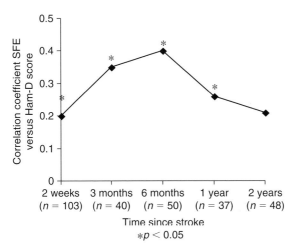

Figure 16.1   Correlation coefficient between HDS and Social Function Exam (SFE) scores over the first 2 years following stroke in 103 patients with acute stroke. Although the strength of the correlation varied over time (the number of patients at each follow-up was 40 at 3 months, 50 at 6 months, 37 at 1 year, and 48 at 2 years). The finding suggests that social functioning is related to depression over the first 2 years following stroke. The strength of the correlation suggests that about 10 to 20% of the variance in depression severity may be related to social functioning.

study of 143 patients with acute stroke. Impairment in social functioning was significantly correlated with severity of depression at the acute in-hospital evaluation and at 6 and 24 months following stroke. In addition, the strength of the correlation between social functioning and depression increased from 0.26 to 0.47 between the in-hospital evaluation and the 6 months follow-up. We also examined SFE scores at each follow-up time point that were compared between patients with major depression and those who were not depressed. Patients with poststroke major depression had significantly higher SFE scores than non-depressed patients in hospital, at 3 months, 6 months, and 12 months poststroke but not at 2 years.

As with physical and cognitive impairment, the relationship between depression and social functioning appears to be both time dependent and complex. For example, it is possible that inadequate social support might lead to depression. On the other hand, depression might lead to deterioration of social relationships and impaired social functioning. Alternatively, depression and social functioning might be related to a third factor, such as cognitive impairment.

In an effort to try to determine the way in which impairment in social functioning influences depression, and vice versa, we examined the relationship between in-hospital measures and outcome 6 months later (Robinson *et al.* 1985b). In-hospital depression scores were not significantly correlated with SFE scores at 3 months, but at 6 months poststroke, the mean correlation between in-hospital depression and follow-up SFE was 0.37 ($p < 0.01$). On the other hand, in-hospital SFE (reflecting prestroke social adjustment) did not predict depression scores at either 3 months or 6 months follow-up. Since in-hospital depression was significantly (although weakly) related to social functioning 6 months later, patients with depression following stroke may undergo social deterioration during the poststroke period. Finding that social withdrawal and deterioration of social function could be a consequence of depression is certainly not surprising. The fact that in-hospital depression did not predict social function at the 3 months follow-up suggests that this process may take several months to occur and the impact of depression on social functioning may not be evident until after the patient is finished with several months of rehabilitation and tries to resume their usual family and social relationships. Limitations in patient's emotional or intellectual capacity to resume these relationships may lead to social withdrawal and deterioration of social functioning.

The other in-hospital factors which significantly correlated with social functioning scores at follow-up were the mini-mental state examination score ($r = -0.43$, $p < 0.01$) and the activities of daily living (Johns Hopkins functioning inventory or JHFI) score ($r = 0.35$, $p < 0.01$). Thus, depression during the acute poststroke period was not the only factor, which contributed to impaired social functioning 6 months later. Again, it is not surprising that limitations of physical and intellectual capacity could lead to social withdrawal and dissatisfaction with social relationships.

We have more recently examined the relationship of depression to individual items of the SFE using a consecutive series of 50 patients selected from our overall group of 215 patients studied at the University of Maryland who had assessment of social functioning at the initial hospitalization and at both short term follow-up (i.e., 3 or 6-months) and at long-term follow-up (i.e., 1 or 2 years). At the time of initial evaluation, seven patients fulfilled DSM-IV criteria for major depression. Fifteen met DSM-IV research criteria for minor depression and 28 were non-depressed. At short-term follow-up, 10 patients had major depression, 10 had minor depression and 30 were non-depressed and at long-term follow-up, 10 patients had major depression, 11 had minor depression and 29 were non-depressed. Using a multiple linear regression analysis, we looked for independent effects of specific items of the SFE on Ham-D score after controlling for age, gender, family psychiatric history, and stroke severity. The individual items at the initial evaluation which were significantly associated with severity of Ham-D scores, were social activities prior to the stroke ($p = 0.04$) and an impaired relationship with the patient's closest other prior to the stroke ($p = 0.05$). At short-term follow-up (i.e., 3–6 months), fear of economic loss due to the stroke ($p = 0.03$) was significantly correlated with Ham-D score and impairment in social activities was nearly a significant predictor of Ham-D score ($p = 0.06$). At long-term follow-up (i.e., 1–2 years) limitations in work experience (e.g., absence of skilled work experience or training) ($p = 0.01$) was a significant predictor of Ham-D ($p = 0.05$) (Robinson *et al.* 1999).

Using logistic regression, controlling for age, gender, family psychiatric history and stroke severity, we also examined whether the patient's diagnosis at the initial evaluation or at short- or long-term follow-up would be predicted by social functioning items prior to the stroke onset (i.e., social functioning evaluation during the initial hospitalization) (Robinson *et al.* 1999). Although none of the social dimensions predicted patients diagnosis at short-term follow-up, relationship with closest other ($p = 0.048$), spiritual beliefs ($p = 0.049$) and social activities ($p = 0.027$) prior to the stroke were all significantly associated with depression diagnosis at 1–2 years following stroke. Thus, this study found that an impaired relationship with the patient's closest other prior to the stroke and limited social activities were associated with depression immediately after the stroke as well as depression 1–2 years later. Within 3–6 months, fears of economic stability and limited social activity were associated with depression while loss of job or job satisfaction was associated with depression at 1–2 years following stroke (Robinson *et al.* 1999).

We have also examined the relationship between social impairment and recovery from stroke (Shimoda and Robinson 1998). In this study we utilized all of the

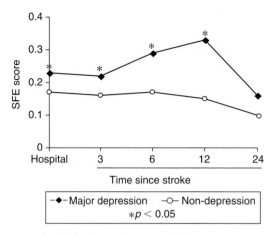

Figure 16.2 SFE scores for patients with major depression and no mood disturbance follow acute stroke and at various follow-up evaluations. Patients with DSM-IV diagnosed major depression ($n = 27$) were significantly more socially impaired (i.e., higher SFE scores) than non-depressed patients ($n = 79$) for the first year following stroke. The initial evaluation reflected pre-stroke social functioning while the follow-up exams reflected post-stroke adjustment. Higher scores indicate greater impairment in social functioning. Note that while non-depressed patients improved in their perception of social functioning over time, patients with major depression showed greater impairment over the first year following stroke. Patients with minor depression ($n = 36$) are not shown but their SFE scores fell between major depression and non-depressed patients.

142 patients admitted for acute poststroke evaluation to the University of Maryland Hospital who received either short-term (3 or 6 months) or long-term (12 or 24 months) follow-up. Of the 142 patients included in the study, 27 had major depression, 35 had minor depression and 79 were non-depressed at the initial evaluation. SFE scores were significantly more impaired in patients with major or minor depression compared with the non-depressed patients (major versus non-depressed, $p = 0.01$) (Fig. 16.2) minor versus non-depressed ($p = 0.04$).

Patients were divided into those with social impairment and those without social impairment based on a score of ≥ 0.2 impaired or < 0.2; non-impaired on the SFE. Patients were also grouped by depression diagnosis (major or minor) or non-depressed. Comparison of background characteristics among the four groups are shown in Table 16.2 (Shimoda and Robinson 1998b). Comparison of characteristics among the four groups revealed significant differences in age, sex, race, socioeconomic status, family, and personal psychiatric history. There were no between group differences in the frequency of motor sensory deficits or other neurological impairments. Because our outcome measures included activities of daily living and cognitive function, patients were matched for initial impairment severity (i.e., JHFI score ± 1

Table 16.2. Demographic information

	Not depressed		Depressed	
	Without social impairment ($n = 58$)	With social impairment ($n = 21$)	Without social impairment ($n = 29$)	With social impairment ($n = 34$)
Age (years + SD)[a]	60.4 ± 12.1	61.8 ± 11.1	57.6 ± 12.3	52.8 ± 13.9
Education (years + SD)	9.8 ± 4.6	7.3 ± 2.5	10.0 ± 3.9	8.7 ± 3.6
Sex, male (%)[b]	63.8	62.0	31.0	61.8
Race, African–American (%)[c]	56.1	90.5	75.9	58.8
Marital status, married (%)	60.0	35.0	39.3	47.8
Socioeconomic status, class IV–V (%)[d]	64.3	100	65.5	75.9
Alcohol abuse, positive (%)	6.9	14.3	3.5	11.8
Family history of psychiatric disorder, positive (%)[e]	10.5	0	0	8.8
Personal history of psychiatric disorder, positive (%)[f]	12.3	0	10.7	26.5
Major depression (%)			37.9	47.1

[a]Significant intergroup differences ($F = 3.3$, $df = 3, 138$, $p = 0.02$).
[b]Significant intergroup differences ($\chi^2 = 9.6$, $df = 3$, $p = 0.02$).
[c]Significant intergroup differences ($\chi^2 = 12.6$, $df = 3$, $p = 0.02$).
[d]Significant intergroup differences ($\chi^2 = 20.8$, $df = 3$, $p = 0.0001$).
[e]Significant intergroup differences ($\chi^2 = 8.0$, $df = 3$, $p = 0.05$).
[f]Significant intergroup differences ($\chi^2 = 10.1$, $df = 3$, $p = 0.02$).
Reprinted with permission from Shimoda and Robinson (1998b).

and mini-mental status examination score ±2). Depressed patients with and without social impairment had a significantly higher frequency of left hemisphere lesions compared with the non-depressed patients (25 of 35 versus 13 of 32, $p = 0.011$).

At short-term follow-up repeated measures ANOVA of JHFI scores (factor 1 presence or absence of in-hospital depression; factor 2 presence or absence of pre-stroke social impairment; factor 3 time) showed significant interactions of depression with time as well as social impairment with time but no significant interaction of social impairment by depression by time (Figs 16.3a and b) (Shimoda and Robinson 1998b). Thus, patients with social impairment or depression did not recover as well in activities of daily living as patients without social impairment or patients without depression at short-term follow-up. At long-term follow-up, repeated measures ANOVA showed a significant effect of depression by time ($p = 0.002$) but no significant effect for social impairment.

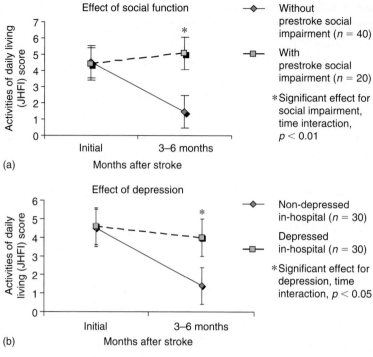

Figure 16.3 (a) The effect of high or low social support on recovery in activities of daily living (JHFI) over short-term (i.e., 3–6 months) follow-up. There was a significant group by time interaction (*F* = 11.0, *f* = 1.56, *p* = 0.002) with the high social support group improving more than the low social support group (reprinted with permission from Shimoda and Robinson (1998b); (b) The effect of presence or absence of depression on recovery in activities of daily living over short-term (i.e., 3–6 months) follow-up. There was a significant group by time interaction (*F* = 4.6, df = 1,56, *p* = 0.04) with the non-depressed group improving more than the depressed group [reprinted with permission from Shimoda and Robinson (1998b)].

Thus, our findings demonstrated for the first time that either depression during the acute stroke period or impairment in social functioning prior to the stroke independently influenced the course of recovery in activities of daily living during the first 3–6 months following stroke.

At short-term follow-up repeated measures ANOVA of mini-mental state examination scores showed a significant interaction of social impairment with time ($p = 0.04$) but no significant effect of depression by time. Thus, patients with social impairment showed significantly less short-term recovery in cognitive examination scores than patients without social impairment. The fact that there was no significant interaction between depression, social functioning and time suggests that both depression and social functioning independently influence physical and/or cognitive recovery following stroke.

We also examined the relationship between recovery from stroke and specific aspects of social functioning (Shimoda and Robinson 1998b). Using multiple regression analysis to control age, sex, family history of psychiatric disorder and stroke severity, we found that health and illness experience in the family prior to the stroke (e.g., prior experience in the family with long-term chronic care) was significantly correlated with recovery in activities of daily living at short-term follow-up ($p = 0.004$). None of the prestroke social dimensions, however, predicted cognitive function at short-term follow-up. At long-term follow-up, prestroke measures of financial security ($p = 0.018$) adequacy of home and neighborhood ($p = 0.038$), and quality of the relationship with the patient's closest other ($p = 0.048$) were all related to the degree of recovery in activities of daily living. In addition, cognitive impairment at long-term follow-up was significantly related to all the same preinjury variables as recovery in activities of daily living that is financial security, $p = 0.007$, adequacy of home and neighborhood $p = 0.041$, quality of relationship with the closest significant other, $p = 0.002$, and quality of social activities ($p = 0.046$).

Many studies have demonstrated that patients have the greatest amount of recovery during the first 3–6 months after their stroke and little change occurs after 6 months (Kelly-Hayes *et al.* 1988; Ernst 1990). Therefore, the effect of social functioning within the most important period for recovery (i.e., the first 3–6 months) makes this a particularly important variable in the recovery of patients following stroke. Treatment of social dysfunction or improvement of social relationships may improve recovery from stroke. Although the mechanism of delayed recovery in activities of daily living and cognitive function associated with impaired social functioning is unclear, one possibility is that lack of social support might prevent patients from regularly attending rehabilitation therapy or decrease motivation during therapy. Although other explanations might also be proposed, these findings do support the need for evaluation of social support at the time of acute stroke and, if needed, intervention to improve social functioning of patients following stroke.

Feibel and Springer (1982), in a study of 91 patients at 6 months following stroke, reported that depressed patients lost 67% of premorbid social activities compared to a 43% loss by non-depressed stroke patients ($p < 0.01$). Astrom *et al.* (1993a) also reported, at 3 months follow-up, only five of 23 patients with major depression (22%) had met a friend or relative, other than their spouse or children, during the week prior to evaluation. In contrast, 27 of 50 non-depressed patients (54%) had met a friend or relative during the same time period ($p = 0.012$). This finding also held true at the 1 year ($p = 0.017$), 2 years ($p = 0.016$), and 3 years follow-ups when only one of 14 depressed patients as compared to 23 of 35 non-depressed patients at 3 years following stroke met a friend or relative outside their immediate family during the week prior to

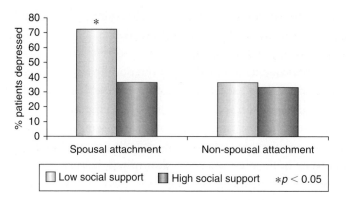

Figure 16.4 The relationship between frequency of depression (major or minor) and patient's perception of spousal and non-spousal social support among 76 Australian patients in a stroke rehabilitation hospital. Patients who identified a spouse as their closest social support but felt their support was low had the highest rate of depression.

evaluation (7% versus 66%, $p < 0.001$). These findings, however, do not address the issue of whether these restricted social contacts following stroke are a cause of depression or whether they reflect the consequences of depression (i.e., social withdrawal, low energy, decreased interest), or whether they may be related to another factor.

Morris *et al.* (1991) examined 96 Australian patients hospitalized for rehabilitation following stroke. Among 96 patients, 76 were examined for perceived adequacy of social support using a modified version of the "interview schedule for social interaction" (ISSI) (Henderson *et al.* 1981). Patients who perceived their social support as low had significantly higher scores on the Montgomery–Asberg depression rating scale (MADRS) (14.9 ± 7.9) than patients with a high degree of support (8.9 ± 6.1) ($p = 0.002$). There were no significant differences, however, between groups with low and high levels of social support in their background characteristics. There were 38 patients who identified a spouse as their closest social support and 38 patients who identified a non-spousal relationship. There were no significant differences between the two groups in terms of the frequency of major or minor depression. Among patients who had a spousal attachment figure, however, low social support was associated with a significantly higher frequency of depression (major plus minor) compared to patients with high level of spousal social support (Fig. 16.4). This relationship between depression and level of social support did not hold for non-spousal attachment figures (i.e., siblings, children, friends).

There were 20 patients in the Morris study who were depressed (major or minor) at the time of the initial interview and were followed up at 15 months after the initial evaluation. The duration of depression was determined by longitudinal assessment using the "composite international diagnostic interview" (CIDI).

The duration of depression in patients who perceived their social support as high was significantly shorter (i.e., 14.3 ± 21.8 SD weeks) than that among patients who perceived their level of social support as low (i.e., 40.8 ± 30.4 weeks) ($p = 0.036$).

The Morris (1991) study also examined the relationship between inadequate social support and the development of depression during the 15 months of follow-up. Of the 21 patients who were non-depressed at the initial in-hospital evaluation and were reevaluated at 15 months, three of four patients with low social support developed depression during the follow-up period compared with only three of 17 patients who had a high level of support ($p = 0.09$, NS). Although this result only indicates a trend, it is consistent with our previously reported finding that patients with delayed-onset-depression (see Chapter 9) had significantly more impaired social functioning scores than patients who never developed depression (Robinson *et al.* 1986).

The interaction between depression and the type of attachment figure providing social support was an unexpected finding. A spousal attachment figure who provides inadequate social support was associated with a significantly increased frequency of depression while a non-spousal attachment figure supplying a low level of support was not. Why patients who perceived inadequate social support from their spouse as opposed to other attachment figures, developed depression is probably a complex issue that may relate to the increased expectations and demands of support in a spousal relationship. It might also reflect personality attributes of the patient that could lead to higher or unrealistic expectations of support. Inadequate support from a spouse may also reflect marital or family dysfunction that preceded the stroke but was intensified by it. Whatever the explanation for this perceived inadequacy of spousal support, it had a marked influence on the frequency of depression in this study and demonstrates that social factors as well as biological (i.e., lesion location) and impairment (i.e., physical and cognitive) variables all probably contribute to depressive disorders.

Inadequate social support also predicted a longer duration of depression. Although the mechanism of this effect is unclear, it could be that feelings of social isolation or loneliness might have perpetuated the depressive state. Although social services are frequently provided for patients suffering from stroke, the intervention tends to be focused on physical limitations and environmental constraints rather than on the perception of adequacy of social or psychological support. These studies underline the fact that perception of social support may play an important role in the development and maintenance of poststroke depression and might provide an avenue for prevention or early treatment of these depressive disorders.

In summary, the relationship between social support and depression in patients with stroke appears to be an interactive relationship that changes over time. Patients with poor social support appear to be more likely to develop depression and patients who are depressed are more likely to deteriorate in their social functioning. We found that specific aspects of prestroke social functioning were associated with the existence and severity of depression at 1–2 years following stroke. At the time of the acute stroke, impaired relationship with a patient's closest other and limited social activities prior to the stroke were associated with depression while at 3–6 months poststroke depression was related to fears of economic stability and limited social activities. Finally, prestroke fears of loss of job satisfaction were predictive of depression at 1–2 years follow-up. This suggests that the focus of patients' social concerns and the areas in which patients may benefit from social intervention may vary over time. The relationship of social functioning to recovery was a surprising finding to us. At 3–6 months follow-up, prestroke impairment in social functioning had a significant effect on the rate of recovery in activities of daily living as well as rate of recovery in cognitive function. At 1–2 years follow-up, financial security, adequacy of home and neighborhood, quality of relationship with a closest other and quality of social activities were all associated with physical and cognitive recovery. These findings as well as similar findings of other investigators provides strong evidence of the importance of social functioning in patients with stroke and the need for further research, particularly into the benefits of social interventions.

REFERENCES

Adams, R. D., and Victor, M. *Principles of Neurology*. McGraw-Hill, New York, 1985.

Andrews, B., and Brown, G. W. Social support, onset of depression, and personality. *Soc Psychiatr Psychiatr Epidemiol* (1988) 23:99–108.

Astrom, M., Adolfsson, R., and Asplund, K. Major depression in stroke patients: a 3-year longitudinal study. *Stroke* (1993) 24:976–982.

Brown, G. W., Andrews, B., Harris, T., *et al.* Social support, self-esteem, and depression. *Psychol Med* (1986) 16:813–832.

Ernst, E. A review of stroke rehabilitation of physiotherapy. *Stroke* (1990) 21:1081–1085.

Feibel, J. H., and Springer, C. J. Depression and failure to resume social activities after stroke. *Arch Phys Med Rehabil* (1982) 63:276–278.

Henderson, S. A. The social psychiatry of later life. *Br J Psychiat* (1990) 156:645–653.

Henderson, S. A., Bryne, D. G., and Duncan-Jones, P. *Neurosis in the social environment*. Academic Press, Sydney, 1981.

Kelly-Hayes, M., Worf, P. A., and Kannel, W. B. Factors influencing survival and need for institutionalization following stroke: the Framingham Study. *Arch Phys Med Rehabil* (1988) 69:415–418.

Morris, P. L. P., Robinson, R. G., Raphael, B., *et al.* The relationship between the perception of social support and post-stroke depression in hospitalized patients. *Psychiatr* (1991) 54:306–316.

Robinson, R. G., Bolduc, P. L., Kubos, K. L., *et al.* Social functioning assessment in stroke patients. *Arch Phys Med Rehabil* (1985a) 66:496–500.

Robinson, R. G., Starr, L. B., Lipsey, J. R., *et al.* A two year longitudinal study of post-stroke mood disorders: in-hospital prognostic factors associated with six month outcome. *J Nerv Ment Dis* (1985b) 173:221–226.

Robinson, R. G., Lipsey, J. R., Rao, K., *et al.* Two-year longitudinal study of post-stroke mood disorders: comparison of acute-onset with delayed-onset depression. *Am J Psychiatr* (1986) 143:1238–1244.

Robinson, R. G., Murata, Y., and Shimoda, K. Dimensions of social impairment and their effect on depression and recovery following stroke. *Int Psychogeriat* (1999) 11(4):375–384.

Shimoda, K., and Robinson, R. G. The relationship between social impairment and recovery from stroke. *Psychiatry* (1998) 61(2):101–111.

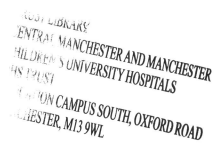

17

Relationship to premorbid risk factors

In previous chapters we have demonstrated the relationship between poststroke depression and stroke-related factors, such as lesion location, severity of physical, or cognitive impairment and social support. Although social support might be argued to be a premorbid risk factor for depression, the dynamic relationship between depression and social functioning makes this an interactive variable with poststroke depression which has already been covered in Chapter 16. In the present chapter, we will focus on both physical and psychological factors that appear to be in existence before the acute stroke event.

It is clear from the discussion in the prior chapters, that stroke-related consequences may play a significant role in poststroke depression but do not explain all of the variants. For example, the meta-analysis of relationship between distances of anterior border of the lesion from the frontal pole and the left hemisphere and severity of depression (Chapter 10, Table 10.3) found a pooled correlation coefficient of -0.53 on the fixed model and -0.59 on the random model. Based on the sample size of 163, these are highly significant correlations. They would explain, however, only about 25–30% of the variance in severity of depression. Similarly, the correlation between depression and severity of impairment in activities of daily living showed a pooled mean correlation coefficient of 0.32. Although this represents a highly significant correlation, it would explain only about 10% of the variance in severity of depression.

The current chapter, therefore, is meant to explore the risk factors existing prior to the onset of stroke which are related to the existence of depression. One of our earliest studies which examined this issue examined 13 patients with poststroke major depression and 13 patients without depression who were matched for the size and location of their lesion (Starkstein *et al.* 1988). Of these patients, 11 pairs had left hemisphere lesions and two pairs had right hemisphere lesions (Fig. 17.1). Patients were matched for size and location of their lesion as follows: using the computed tomography (CT) scan, ratios of lesion area to overall brain area on the axial slice including the body of the lateral ventricle were calculated. Three classes

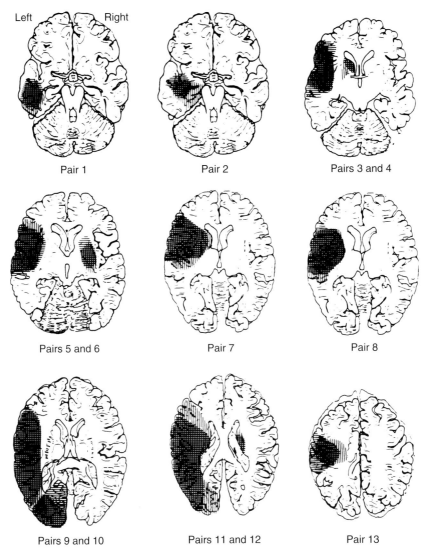

Figure 17.1   Schematic templates of CT scan slices showing the largest cross-sectional area of ischemia for 13 matched pairs of patients – where one of the pair has major depression (vertical lines), the other no mood disturbance (horizontal lines). Although lesions were not precisely identical, lesions were matched for both location and size within the parameters described in the text (from Starkstein *et al. Arch Gen Psychiatry* 45:247–252. Copyright © 1988. American Medical Association. All rights reserved).

of lesion volumes were used; that is, small (1–5%), medium (6–15%), or large (>15%) and patients were matched for these classes of lesion volume. Second, the brain structures involved in the lesion were mapped using the brain regions described by Levine and Grek (1984). Each brain region was classified as being

Table 17.1. Demographic data

	Depressed group ($n = 13$)	Non-depressed group ($n = 13$)
Age (mean ± SD in years)	58 ± 16	58 ± 12
Gender (% female)	23	31
Race (% white)	62	69
Socioeconomic status (% Hollingshead class IV or V)	15	15
Marital status (% married)	54	69
Children (mean number)	3	2
Origin (% urban)	46	46
Siblings (mean number)	3	3
Education (mean number of years ± SD)	10 ± 3	9 ± 2
Tobacco use (% >1 pack/day)	38	69
Time since stroke to depression onset (time to follow-up for non-depressed group) (%)		
<3 months	62	38
3–6 months	8	23
6–12 months	8	8
1–2 years	22	31
Family history of psychiatric disorders (%)	0	0
History of alcohol abuse (hospitalized or had withdrawal symptoms %)	15	15
Time since stroke to CT scan, weeks (mean ± SD)	5.7 ± 14	9.6 ± 21

totally, partially or not involved in the lesion. Patients were then matched according to the site and degree of involvement of the brain region affected by the lesion. Patient pairs were only included if the time elapsed between the stroke and the evaluation for each non-depressed patient was at least as long as that for the matched depressed patient. In addition, all patients were required to have a single stroke lesion of either the right or the left hemisphere visible on CT scan with no previous history of stroke or other brain lesion.

The background characteristics of the study groups are shown in Table 17.1. The patient groups were not significantly different in any of their background characteristics. Patients were predominantly white males in their late 50s. Similarly, there were no significant differences in the frequencies of motor, sensory, or visual deficits, or aphasia (this would be expected based on the fact that patients were matched for lesion size and location).

Evaluations of CT scans included ventricular size and sulcal width, as well as lesion size and location. This was done to determine whether atrophy or degeneration of

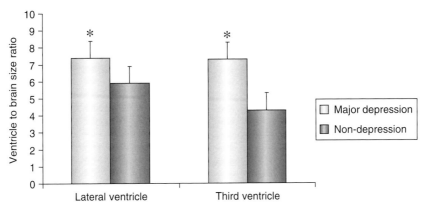

Figure 17.2 Ventricle size to brain size ratios (mean + SEM) for 13 pairs of patients matched for lesion size and location, where one patient of the pair has major depression and the other is non-depressed. Increased ratios reflect greater subcortical atrophy in the depressed compared to non-depressed patients, *$p < 0.05$.

either subcortical or cortical areas of the brain had occurred and whether it was associated with the existence of depression. The ratio of the size of the third ventricle to the overall area of the brain was determined by multiplying the maximal anterior–posterior length of the ventricle by its width and dividing by the overall brain area (i.e., transpineal width multiplied by midsagittal anterior to posterior brain length). The ratio of the size of the lateral ventricle to the overall area of the brain was calculated by dividing the area of the lateral ventricle at the level of the ventricular body by the overall brain area at the same level. Patients with depression were found to have significantly larger third ventricle to brain size ratios ($p = 0.037$) and lateral ventricle to brain size ratios ($p = 0.046$) compared with their lesion-matched controls (Fig. 17.2). Using the lateral to ventricular brain ratio, 10 depressed patients had values that were greater than those of their respective matched controls, while only three patients had lower values ($p = 0.006$). These findings indicate that the depressed patients had a greater amount of subcortical (i.e., basal ganglia, hypothalamic, thalamic, periventricular regions) atrophy on the non-lesion of their brain than their lesion-matched controls. No differences were found between the depressed and non-depressed groups in terms of CT scan measurements of frontal fissure or four cortical sulci ratio (i.e., the sum of the widths of the four widest sulci divided by the transpineal coronal inner table diameter). These findings indicate that, among patients with poststroke major depression, there was evidence of subcortical but not cortical atrophy. This subcortical atrophy probably occurred years before the stroke because it was present within a few days after stroke and on the opposite side of the brain from the lesion (Nasrallah *et al.* 1982). This atrophy may have made the patient more prone to developing depression after the lesion.

In addition to subcortical atrophy, the 13 patients with major depression also had significantly lower mini-mental state examination (MMSE) scores than their lesion-matched controls (depressed 16.6 ± 7.8 versus non-depressed 22.4 ± 6.6, $t = 3.2$, $p = 0.015$). This finding was discussed in detail in Chapter 14 (see Fig. 14.1). In addition, however, there were no significant correlations between the MMSE score and the lateral ventricle to brain ratio or the third ventricle to brain size ratio, suggesting that the degree of subcortical atrophy was not an explanation for the greater severity of intellectual impairment found to occur in patients with major depression as compared with that in non-depressed patients having similar lesions.

In Chapter 10, I described our study of 91 patients with single stroke lesions of the right hemisphere (Starkstein et al. 1989). Of the 17 patients with major depression following right hemisphere stroke, five (30%) had a positive family history of psychiatric disorder (Fig. 10.13). This 30% frequency of family history of psychiatric disorder was significantly greater than that found among 46 non-depressed patients with a right hemisphere stroke lesion or 27 patients with major depression following a left hemisphere lesion ($p < 0.05$). This finding suggests that a genetic predisposition may contribute to the development of depression in some patients with poststroke depression.

Morris et al. (1990) reported similar findings in a study of 99 patients with subacute stroke hospitalized in an Australian rehabilitation hospital. In the Morris study, 11 of 16 patients (69%) with major depression following either right or left hemisphere stroke had a family history of affective or anxiety disorders compared with 5 of 18 patients (28%) with minor depression and 20 of 54 (37%) who were not depressed ($p = 0.04$) (Fig. 17.3). These findings suggest that a genetic predisposition for depression may be a premorbid risk factor brought out by a stroke lesion.

Previous personal history of psychiatric disorder, usually mood disorder, has also been associated with poststroke depression. Of 87 patients in a rehabilitation hospital Eastwood et al. (1989) found a significantly higher frequency of previous psychiatric history among patients with poststroke major or minor depression (12 of 47 patients, 25%) compared to control patients (3 of 32 patients, 9%) ($p < 0.05$). Similar findings were reported by Morris et al. (1990) in which 8 of 16 (50%) patients with major depression had a past personal history of affective or anxiety disorders compared with 5 of 18 patients (28%) with minor depression and 13 of 54 patients (24%) who were not depressed ($p = 0.17$) (Fig. 17.3). Burvill et al. (1995) reported that, at 4 weeks, 4 of 27 males (15%) and 9 of 18 females (50%) with poststroke major depression (difference, $p < 0.001$) had been depressed at the time of the stroke compared to only 6 of 102 men (6%) and two of 77 women (3%) without poststroke depression ($p < 0.01$).

The largest study examining poststroke depression (Desmond et al. 2003) found that among 421 patients examined 3 months after ischemic stroke, compared with

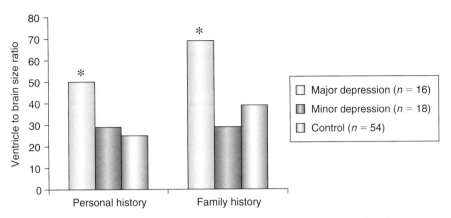

Figure 17.3   Frequency of a previous personal history or family history of psychiatric disorder among patients with major depression, minor depression, or no mood disorder who were hospitalized in a rehabilitation hospital following stroke. Both prior personal history and family history of psychiatric disorder were significantly associated with major depression but not minor depression (data taken from Morris et al. 1990, *$p < 0.05$).

249 stroke-free control subjects, that logistic regression analysis showed that poststroke depression (i.e., structured interview Hamilton depression (Ham-D) score >11) was significantly associated with female sex (i.e., 66% of depressed were female versus 50% of non-depressed, $p = 0.042$) as well as other stroke-related variables such as dementia but no association with prior history of psychiatric disorder (i.e., four of 47 depressed versus 20 of 374 non-depressed). Pohjasvaara et al. (1998) examined 277 patients with ischemic stroke. Multiple logistic regression demonstrated that a history of previous depressive episodes was correlated with a diagnosis of poststroke major depression (odds ratio: 2.9; 95% confidence interval (CI): 1.6–5.5). Astrom et al. (1993), however, found no association between previous personal history of psychiatric disorder (16% had such a history) and the development of major depression among her 80 stroke patients at any time during the 3-year follow-up.

Morris et al. (1992) also examined the mean number of negative life events in patients with poststroke depression. Negative life events occurring during the 6 months prior to stroke were tabulated using the 12-item, list of threatening, negative experiences (Brugha et al. 1985). The negative life events were primarily factual losses which were verified by other family members. The number of negative life events was significantly greater in patients with major depression than in patients with minor depression or no depression. Bush (1999) also examined the relationship of major life events to the development of poststroke depression in 111 patients following acute stroke. Patients were administered the Center for Epidemiological

Studies-Depression (CES-D) at four time periods during the first year following stroke and asked if they had experienced a major life event in the prior 6 months (other than the stroke). Of 25 patients who reported a significant life event during the past 6 months, 28% were in the depressed range on the CES-D compared with only 10% with CES-D scores in the depressed range among 86 patients who did not have a life event. For patients who were 6 months poststroke, the odds ratio of having a depression with a significant life event was 3.33 (95% CI: 1.09–10.13).

Morris et al. (1992) also examined the effect of a personality trait of neuroticism using the brief 8-point form of the neuroticism inventory of Eysenck and Eysenck (1964). The patient and the patient's closest other were asked to respond to the neuroticism questionnaire relative to the patient's personality prior to stroke. Patients with major depression were found to have a significantly higher neuroticism score than non-depressed patients ($p < 0.05$). There were no statistically significant differences between patients with major or minor depression or between those with minor or no depression, indicating that patients with minor depression had a premorbid level of neuroticism that was between those of patients with major and no depression. Aben et al. (2002) also examined the effect of personality vulnerability on poststroke depression. One hundred fifty four patients at 1 month following a first ever stroke filled out a personality inventory, the neo-5-factor inventory (Kosta and McCrae 1985). Depressive symptoms were assessed at 1, 3, 6, 9, and 12 months after stroke. Depression was diagnosed based on the structured clinical interview for Diagnostic and Statistical Manual, 3rd ed. (DSM-III) (SCID-1-R). Multivariate regression analysis of the five personality traits, controlling for age, sex, personal history of depression and level of handicap, demonstrated that the independent correlates of poststroke major or minor depression were neuroticism (hazard ratio: 1.08; 95% CI: 1.04–1.12) and level of handicap (hazard ratio: 1.36; 95% CI: 1.08–1.72). Throughout the 1-year period of follow-up, the cumulative incidence of poststroke depression was significantly higher among the patients scoring in the highest one/third of neuroticism compared with those with low and intermediate scores on neuroticism.

Morris et al. (1992) examined the relationship between the frequency of depression and the number of risk factors including family history of psychiatric disorder, high neuroticism personality trait and one or more negative life events in the past 6 months. The results are shown in Fig. 17.4. The frequency of depression rose from 23% when there were no risk factors to 62.5% when all three risk factors were present.

For many years it has been known that primary depression (i.e., depression with no brain lesion) is more common in women than men (Weissman and Olfson 1995). The effect of gender on poststroke depression has recently been examined in a number of studies.

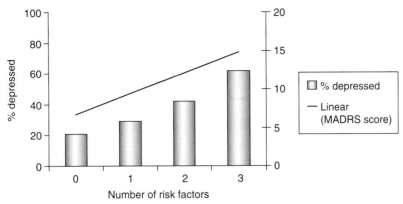

Figure 17.4 Frequency of depression among 99 patients examined in an Australian rehabilitation hospital based on their number of premorbid risk factors (i.e., family history of psychiatric disorder, high neuroticism personality trait, or one or more negative life events in the past 6 months). MADRS = Montgomery–Asberg depression rating scale. The risk of poststroke major or minor depression increased with an increasing number of premorbid risk factors (from Morris *et al.* 1992, reprinted with permission).

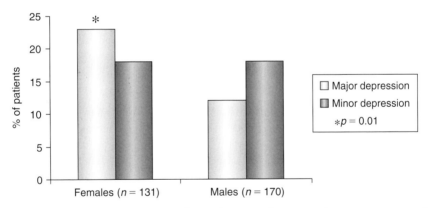

Figure 17.5 The frequency of major and minor depression according to gender among our overall group of 301 patients with acute stroke. The frequency of major depression was significantly higher in females than males. The frequency of minor depression, however, did not differ between genders.

Our examination of gender-related effects on poststroke depression utilized our overall population of 301 patients with acute stroke (Paradiso and Robinson 1998). Among the 170 males, 12.3% had major depression compared with 23.6% of 131 females ($p = 0.01$) (Fig. 17.5). In this analysis, patients with minor depression were included in the non-depressed group because there was no gender-related effect on minor depression. The mean Hamilton scores of male and female patients with major depression, however, were not significantly different (males: 16.5 ± 5.9 versus females: 16.2 ± 5.3), which indicates that the severity of major depression was the same in both sexes. A logistic regression analysis of background characteristics examining the effects of the presence or absence of depression and male and female gender revealed that major depression was associated with younger age ($p = 0.008$), lower socioeconomic status ($p = 0.02$), and a prior history of psychiatric disorder ($p = 0.004$) but no significant effects of gender. When male and female patients were examined separately for background characteristics associated with depression, younger age was associated with depression only in males, and prior psychiatric history was associated with depression only in females.

Analysis of depression, gender, and impairment in activities of daily living (Johns Hopkins functioning inventory, JHFI) revealed significant interactions of gender and JHFI score ($p = 0.04$) on the existence of major depression (Paradiso and Robinson 1998). There were no significant effects of impairment in social functioning and cognitive impairment on gender-related frequencies of depression. Thus, this analysis found that males with the greatest physical impairment were the most depressed.

Analysis of the relationship between depression and lesion location in males and females demonstrated that females with left hemisphere lesions had a significantly greater frequency of major depression than males with left hemisphere lesions. A logistic regression analysis examining the effects of left or right hemisphere lesions and male or female gender on the frequency of major depression demonstrated a significant interaction (Wald $\chi^2 = 4.63$, df = 1, $p = 0.03$) (Fig. 17.6); that is, female patients with major depression were significantly more likely to have a left hemisphere lesion than males with major depression or female patients without major depression.

This study found an interesting but surprising difference between males and females in terms of their correlates with major depression. Females were significantly more likely to have major depression and their depressions were associated with previous personal history of psychiatric disorder and left hemisphere lesion. Major depression in males, on the other hand, was associated with younger age and greater impairment in activities of daily living.

There is a lack of consistency, however, in gender-related differences among studies of poststroke depression (Table 17.2). Andersen et al. (1994) and Angeleri et al. (1993) both found significantly greater frequencies of depression in females compared with males, however, most studies have not found this to be the case. Pohjasvaara et al. (1998), for example, found among 277 patients with acute stroke that there was no significant difference between the depressed and non-depressed patients with regard to gender. In the largest study conducted, however, Desmond et al. (2003) found that 16% of women and only 9% of men developed poststroke

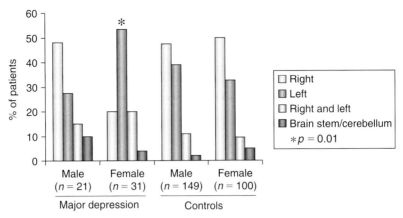

Figure 17.6 The frequency of various lesion locations (i.e., right hemisphere, left hemisphere, bilateral hemisphere, or brain stem/cerebellar) among males and females with and without major depression following acute stroke. Females with major depression were significantly more likely to have a left hemisphere lesion than females without major depression or males with major depression (from Paradiso 1998, reprinted with permission).

depression. A logistic regression found that female sex was an independent risk factor for poststroke depression (odds ratio: 1.70; 95% CI: 0.75–3.84). A merged data analysis of all studies found that depression occurred in 25% of women and 18% of men ($p = 0.0002$) (Table 17.2).

Given the number of factors which have been associated with poststroke depression, a number of hypotheses might be proposed why gender-related differences have not been consistently reported in the literature. Time since stroke, socio-economic status, age, previous personal and family history of psychiatric disorder, premorbid personality, life events, and subcortical atrophy are all factors which have been shown to play a role in the likelihood of developing poststroke major depression. Any of these differences may have masked gender-related differences in the prevalence of major depression. Based on the greater frequency of primary unipolar depression in females compared to males, it seems likely that females suffering a first stroke may be more likely to develop depression than males.

In summary, studies have demonstrated that there are a number of premorbid factors associated with the development of depression following stroke. The fact that a multiple logistical regression analysis found that several factors were independently correlated with the existence of major depression suggests that these risk factors are independent variables which contribute to an increased risk of depression following stroke. Most risk factors for poststroke depression, however, are probably additive. The dose–response gradient shown in Fig. 17.4 between the increasing number of risk factors and the frequency of depression supports this additive concept of risk

Table 17.2. Studies reporting gender based differences in poststroke depression

Study	Gender effect[a]	Time after stroke	Country of study	Depression assessment	p value
Andersen et al. 1994 (n = 285)	F = 40%; M = 21%	1 year incidence	Denmark	HDRS (>12)	<0.001
Angeleri et al. 1993 (n = 180)	F = 19[b]; M = 14	>1 year	Central Italy	BDI	<0.001
Astrom et al. 1993 (n = 98)	Values not reported	≈2 weeks	Sweden	DSM-III	NS
Burvill et al. 1995 (n = 248)	F = 13%; M = 9%	Time of stroke	Perth, Australia	PSE (DSM-III)	>0.3
Dam et al. 1989 (n = 92)	F = 4[c]; M = 2	8–1280 days	Denmark	HDRS	NS
Desmond et al. 2003 (n = 421)	F = 16%; M = 9%		USA	Ham-D scale	0.042
Eastwood et al. 1989 (n = 87)	F = 43%; M = 57%	82 ± 58 days	Canada	RDC	NS
Morris et al. 1990 (n = 88)	F = 44%; M = 56%	60 days	New South Wales, Australia	CIDI DSM-III	<0.008
Pohjasvaara et al. 1998 (n = 277)	Values not reported			PSE and DSM-III	
Sharpe et al. 1994 (n = 60)	F = 30%[d]; M = 10%	31–64 months	Oxfordshire, England	DSM-III-R	<0.09
Sinyor et al. 1986 (n = 64)	F = 56%; M = 41%	Several weeks	Quebec, Canada	SDS (≥ 60)	>0.20
Wade et al. 1987 (n = 379)	F = 26%; M = 19%	3 weeks	Bristol, England	WADI	<0.09
Total (merged data)	F = 25%; M = 18%				p = 0.0002

Note: [a]Percentages (number of depressed/non-depressed females and number of depressed/non-depressed males) are reported, unless noted. In parentheses total patient number. [b]Overall depression severity mean scores. [c]Median HDRS scores for females and males. Frequency of depression noted reported. [d]Fisher's exact test, combined major depression and dysthymia. BDI: Beck depression inventory; HDRS: Hamilton depression rating scale, PSE: present state examination; CIDI: Composite International Diagnostic Interview; SDS: Zung self-rating depression scale; WADI: wakefield assessment depression inventory.

factors and depression. Differences in distribution of risk factors across various stroke populations may explain, in part, why clinical correlates of depression have sometimes varied across studies.

REFERENCES

Aben, I., Verhey, F., Lousberg, R., *et al*. Validity of the Beck depression inventory, hospital anxiety and depression scale, SCL-90, and Hamilton depression rating scale as screening instruments for depression in stroke patients. *Psychosomatics* (2002) 43(5):386–393.

Andersen, G., Vestergaard, K., Riis, J. O., *et al*. Incidence of post-stroke depression during the first year in a large unselected stroke population determined using a valid standardized rating scale. *Acta Psychiatr Scand* (1994) 90:190–195.

Angeleri, F., Angeleri, V. A., Foschi, N., *et al*. The influence of depression, social activity, and family stress on functional outcome after stroke. *Stroke* (1993) 24(20):1478–1483.

Astrom, M., Adolfsson, R., and Asplund, K. Major depression in stroke patients: a 3-year longitudinal study. *Stroke* (1993) 24:976–982.

Brugha, T., Bebbington, P., Tennant, C., *et al*. The list of threatening experiences: a subset of 12 life event categories with considerable long-term contextual threat. *Psychol Med* (1985) 15:189–194.

Burvill, P. W., Johnson, G. A., Jamrozik, K. D., *et al*. Prevalence of depression after stroke: the Perth Community Stroke Study. *Br J Psychiatr* (1995) 166:320–327.

Bush, B. A. Major life events as risk factors for post-stroke depression. *Brain Inj* (1999) 13(2):131–137.

Desmond, D. W., Remien, R. H., Moroney, J. T., *et al*. Ischemic stroke and depression. *J Int Neuropsychol Soc* (2003) 9(3):429–439.

Eastwood, M. R., Rifat, S. L., Nobbs, H., *et al*. Mood disorder following cerebrovascular accident. *Br J Psychiatr* (1989) 154:195–200.

Eysenck, H. J., and Eysenck, S. B. G. *Manual of the Eysenck Personality Inventory*. London University Press, London, 1964.

Kosta P. T., Jr., and McCrae, R. R. *The Neo Personality Inventory Manual*. Psychological Assessment Resources Inc, Odessa FL, 1985.

Levine, D. N., and Grek, A. The anatomic basis of delusions after right cerebral infarction. *Neurology* (1984) 34:577–582.

Morris, P. L. P., Robinson, R. G., and Raphael, B. Prevalence and course of depressive disorders in hospitalized stroke patients. *Int J Psychiatr Med* (1990) 20:349–364.

Morris, P. L. P., Robinson, R. G., Raphael, B., *et al*. The relationship between risk factors for affective disorder and post-stroke depression in hospitalized stroke patients. *Aust N Z J Psychiatr* (1992) 26:208–217.

Nasrallah, H. A., Whitters, M., and Jacoby, C. G. Cerebral ventricular enlargement in bipolar affective disorder. *J Affect Disord* (1982) 4:15–19.

Paradiso, S., and Robinson, R. G. Gender differences in post-stroke depression. *J Neuropsychiatr Clin Neurosci* (1998) 10:41–47.

Pohjasvaara, T., Leppavuori, A., Siira, I., *et al*. Frequency and clinical determinants of poststroke depression. *Stroke* (1998) 29:2311–2317.

Starkstein, S. E., Robinson, R. G., and Price, T. R. Comparison of patients with and without post-stroke major depression matched for size and location of lesion. *Arch Gen Psychiatr* (1988) 45:247–252.

Starkstein, S. E., Robinson, R. G., Honig, M. A., *et al.* Mood changes after right hemisphere lesion. *Br J Psychiatr* (1989) 155:79–85.

Weissman, M. M., and Olfson, M. Depression in women: implications for health care research. *Science* (1995) 269(5225):799–801.

18

Mortality and treatment

Background

The relationship between depression and increased mortality due to physical illness has been a focus of interest among psychiatrists for many years. Maltzberg (1937) reported that the cardiac death rate among melancholic patients was eight times the rate found in the general population. Avery and Winokur (1976) reported that among 519 depressed patients treated with antidepressants or electroconvulsive therapy, there was a significantly increased death rate among patients who had been inadequately treated for depression. Some of the newest studies using large groups of patients have continued to show an association between depressive disorder or depressive symptoms and increased death rate. Unutzer *et al.* (2002) reported on a 7-year follow-up of 2558 Medicare recipients age 65 and older. Subjects with mild to moderate depressive symptoms at baseline did not have an increased risk of mortality compared to those without depressive symptoms. The 3% of older adults with the most severe depressive symptoms, however, had significantly increased mortality even after adjusting for demographics, health risk behaviors, and chronic medical disorders. Similarly, Ensinck *et al.* 2002 in a study in the Netherlands in 2002 reported on 68,965 patients followed for an average of 15 years. Among 1362 depressed patients, 132 had died compared to 4256 deaths among 67,603 non-depressed patients. The adjusted hazard ratio (HR) for depressed versus non-depressed patients was 1.39 (95% confidence interval (CI): 1.16–1.65) indicating a moderate positive association between depression and subsequent mortality. Finally, Gump *et al.* (2005) examined 11,216 men who had participated in a multiple risk factor coronary heart disease intervention trial at 18-year follow-up. Patients who had scored in the highest quartile on the Center for Epidemiological Studies Depression Scale (CES-D) at the end of the treatment trial had an HR of 1.21 for cardiovascular mortality (95% CI: 1.03–1.41, $p < 0.06$) and an HR of 2.03 (95% CI: 1.20–3.44, $p < 0.01$) for stroke mortality at 18-year follow-up. These studies have controlled for many of the short-comings of previous studies in which factors such as age, year of birth, cohort, gender, social class, smoking, systolic blood pressure, alcohol consumption, fasting cholesterol, and medical comorbid illness were not adequately controlled. In spite of controlling for these factors, an association between depression and mortality has held up through many years of study. Murphy (1989) began investigating patients with physical illness and depression and found that the effect of depression on mortality can be seen more strongly among patients with physical illness compared to depressed patients without physical illness.

Mortality and poststroke depression

Increased mortality is perhaps the ultimate validation of the importance of depression in the prognosis of physical illness. Several studies have been conducted among patients with stroke which have documented increased mortality rates among those with depression or depressive symptoms. Our first study was a 10-year follow-up of survival obtained for 91 of original series of 103 acute stroke patients (Morris *et al.* 1993a). Data was obtained by contacting patients' living relatives or searching hospital records. Background characteristics of survivors and non-survivors obtained at the time of the initial evaluation (10 years before follow-up) revealed no significant differences including age, comorbid physical illness, and stroke type or location. At 10-year follow-up, 48 (53%) of the 91 patients had died. In the small portion of cases in which death certificates were available ($n = 18$), the ascribed causes of death were as follows: 28% subsequent stroke, 44% cardiopulmonary arrest, 16% respiratory failure, and 11% other conditions. Impairment scores on the activities of daily living, mini-mental state examination (MMSE), social functioning examination (SFE), and social ties checklist (STC) did not reveal any significant differences between the patients who had survived and the patients who had died, with the exception of social ties, in which patients who had died had significantly fewer social ties than patients who were still alive ($p = 0.03$) (Fig. 18.1). The frequency of death among patients with a diagnosis of major or minor depression was almost identical (Fig. 18.2) and therefore the depressed groups were combined in a single depressed group for subsequent analysis. Depressed patients were more than three times as likely to have died as non-depressed patients (odds ratio (OR): 3.4; 95% CI: 1.4–8.4; $p = 0.007$).

Survival curves for the depressed and non-depressed patients over the 10 years of follow-up are shown in Fig. 18.3. A difference in the probability of survival between depressed and non-depressed patients was evident as early as the first year after stroke. This divergence between the depressed and non-depressed patients in survival continued over the first 5–7 years before the curves began to parallel each other. Since there are many factors which have been associated with mortality following stroke, a multiple logistic regression was carried out examining the

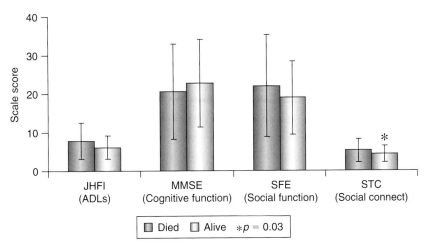

Figure 18.1 Mean ± SD impairment scores at the time of initial in-hospital assessment for 91 patients with stroke who were followed up 10 years later for survival status. Patients who died during the 10-year follow-up had significantly fewer STC than patients who survived. Although differences were not significant, patients who died had greater impairment than survivors on the Johns Hopkins functioning inventory (JHFI), MMSE, and SFE.

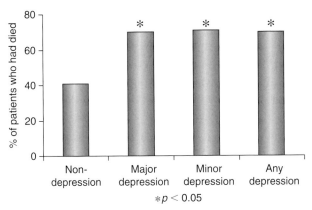

Figure 18.2 Percent of patients with stroke who died during 10 years following stroke. Patients are grouped according to their depression diagnosis at the time of the initial poststroke evaluation. Both major and minor depression were associated with significantly more deaths compared with no depression even though, by 2-year follow-up, patients with in-hospital major depression and non-depressed patients were not significantly different in their Ham-D scores.

factors of age, marital status, gender, social class, social ties, social functioning, mini-mental state score, activities of daily living, alcohol use, medical comorbidity, type of stroke, hemispheric and cortical subcortical lesion location, volume of lesion, impairment, and severity of depression (Hamilton depression (Ham-D) rating

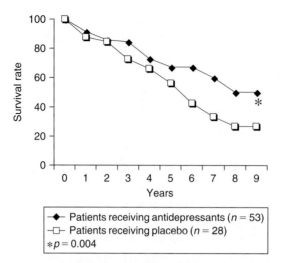

Figure 18.3   Survival rates over 9-year follow-up for stroke patients who received a 12-week course of antidepressants or placebo during the first 6 months following stroke. Probability of survival was significantly greater in the patients receiving antidepressants ($\chi^2 = 8.2$, d.f. $= 1$, $p = 0.004$, Kaplan–Meier survival analysis, and log-rank test) [reprinted with permission from Jorge *et al.* (2003)].

scale) on the likelihood of survival over 10 years. After controlling for all these variables, depression severity was independently associated with mortality outcome (adjusted OR: 3.7; 95% CI: 1.1–12.2; $p = 0.03$). Furthermore, depression and fewer social ties had additive effects on mortality. Patients who were both depressed and had fewer social ties (i.e., impairment scores on the STC above the median) had the highest mortality (12 of 13, 92%). Patients who had either depression or few social ties had intermediate mortality rates (14 of 24, 58%) with depression only and 7 of 15 (47%) with few social ties only. Patients who were non-depressed and had more than the average number of social ties had the lowest mortality (15 of 39, 38%).

The other independent factors associated with mortality were a history of alcohol abuse (OR: 9.1; 95% CI: 2.3–35.9; $p = 0.002$), among 41 patients who had focal lesions which were visualized on Computerized tomography (CT) scan, lesion volume was strongly associated with both mortality and depression status. Patients who died had over twice the lesion volume compared with patients who survived (10.3 ± 9.0 SD% of brain volume, dead versus 4.3 ± 4.5 SD% of brain volume, survived). After matching 11 depressed and 11 non-depressed patients for lesion volume (within ±5%), depressed patients still had a five-fold higher mortality rate than non-depressed patients (OR: 5.4, $p = 0.09$).

Morris *et al.* (1993b) also examined the mortality rate among 99 patients in an Australian rehabilitation hospital. Among the 84 patients in whom mortality data was available at 15-month follow-up, the death rate among patients with an in-hospital diagnosis of major depression was 23% compared with 11% for those with minor depression and 2% for those with no mood disorder ($p = 0.04$). Consistent with our findings from the 10-year follow-up study, patients (mean MMSE 17.1 ± 7.4 dead versus 23.1 ± 6.1 SD alive, $p = 0.02$) who subsequently died were more cognitively impaired, tended to have more severe impairment in activities of daily living ($p = $ NS), however, patients who died tended to have smaller lesions (i.e., 5.0 ± 2.5, 4% dead versus 11.6 ± 8.4% SD alive, $p = $ NS). Combining patients with major and minor depression, depressed patients had a seven-fold higher risk of death than non-depressed patients (OR: 8.1; 95% CI: 0.9–72.9; $p = 0.06$). Death rate among patients with major or minor depression was significantly higher than among non-depressed patients ($p = 0.015$). Morris *et al.* (1993b) also found an interesting association of depression and mortality with premorbid personality traits. Patients who died had higher introversion scores on the Eysenck Personality Inventory as reported by themselves and relatives than patients who died ($p = 0.004$). Multiple logistic regression analysis which examined for independent effects of cognitive impairment, depression, and introversion score, found that both depression ($p = 0.05$) and introversion ($p = 0.02$) were independently associated with mortality while cognitive impairment was not. Thus, both long- and short-term follow-up studies have found in two very different patient populations, that depression, both major and minor, was associated with increased mortality.

Interestingly, Astrom *et al.* (1993) did not find an association between depression and mortality following stroke. Among 21 patients who died during a 3-year study, mortality was associated with older age, being disoriented in hospital, greater impairment in activities of daily living, and more cortical atrophy. However, Burvill *et al.* (1995) at 12-month follow-up found that 5 of 69 patients (7.2%) with major or minor depression had died, 4 of 33 (12.1%) with anxiety disorder had died, but only 5 of 179 (2.8%) without a psychiatric diagnosis had died.

House *et al.* (2001) examined 448 hospitalized patients at 1 month following acute stroke with follow-up at 12 and 24 months. Mood symptoms were assessed using the semi-structured present state examination and the general health questionnaire (GHQ-28). Of the 448 patients, 100 had major depression while 348 did not. At 12-month follow-up, two patients could not be located, but 45 of the 446 patients had died. Causes of death included recurrent stroke, 17 (37.8%), cardiovascular disease, 10 (22.2%), and other causes, 18 (40.0%). The GHQ-D (depression subscale) severe depression and the highest GHQ quartile were significantly associated with mortality. The OR for mortality was 3.1 between the lowest and highest scoring quartiles of the GHQ with a mortality rate of 5% in the lowest quartile and 14% in the highest quartile. Those scoring greater than one on the depression subscale of the GHQ had an OR of mortality of 2.4 compared to those scoring zero. A multiple logistic regression showed that higher GHQ-D score, greater age, lower mini-mental scores, and lower poststroke Barthel scores were all independently associated with increased risk of dying within 12 months.

At 24-month follow-up, a total of 65 patients had died (14.6%) from 446 participating. A similar multiple logistic regression analysis found that GHQ-D subscale score of one or greater remained statistically significant as did older age, and mini-mental scores less than 24. The diagnosis of major depression was not statistically significant (OR: 1.3; 95% CI: 0.65–2.7 at 12 months; OR: 1.7; 95% CI: 0.95–3.0 at 24 months ratio $p = 0.07$). This was probably the result of not including both major and minor depression in the analysis.

Pohjasvaara *et al.* (2002) reported that the only independent correlate of death between 3 and 15 months poststroke was dependent living at 3 months (OR: 2.6; 95% CI: 1.2–5.8) while increasing severity of depression or cognitive impairment were independently associated with dependent living at 15 months poststroke.

The largest study was conducted by Williams *et al.* (Williams *et al.* 2004) in which the records of 151, 119 veterans hospitalized for ischemic stroke who survived more than 30 days were reviewed. Within 3 years following stroke, 2405 had a diagnosis of depression and 2257 had other diagnoses (primarily substance abuse or anxiety disorder). Of the depressed patients, 59.0% were alive at 6 years while 58.7% of the substance abuse and anxiety disorder and 63.6% of the patients with no depression or substance abuse (Hazard ratio 1.13 95% CI: 1.06–1.21, $p < 0.01$ for depression and 1.13, CI: 1.07–1.22, $p < 0.01$ for substance abuse/anxiety disorder). Other factors associated with morality were younger age, white race, and heart disease such as myocardial infarction (HR: 1.59; CI: 1.38–1.62, $p < 0.01$) congestive heart failure (HR: 1.59; CI: 1.52–1.66, $p < 0.01$) and atrial fibrillation (HR: 1.25; CI: 1.19–1.30, $p < 0.01$). The obvious shortcoming of this retrospective review is the low rate of depression (5%) which suggests that many depressions were missed. Furthermore, comorbidity of substance abuse and anxiety disorder with depression was not considered and the protective effect of treatment was not considered. Thus, the risk of depression for mortality was probably underestimated.

Mechanism of mortality following poststroke depression

Based on the fact that our studies found an association between both major and minor depression with mortality, it appears likely that severity of depression is not as important as the existence of some level of depression. Subsyndromal forms of major depression appear to place patients at risk for mortality just as much as major depression (House *et al.* 2001).

The mechanism by which depression following stroke leads to increased mortality over many years remains a topic of debate. Although there are many explanations which could be proposed to explain the association of poststroke depression with mortality, there is a developing literature on the association of mortality with heart rate variability. Tokgozoglu *et al.* (1999) reported that patients with decreased sympathetic and parasympathetically controlled heart rate variability resulting from insular lesions had increased frequency of sudden death. It has also been demonstrated that depression itself influences heart rate variability which can in turn lead to fatal arrhythmias (Carney *et al.* 1988). Depression alters the sympathetic–parasympathetic balance leading to decreased heart rate variability (Dalack and Roose 1990).

Another possible explanation for the increased mortality rate associated with poststroke depression is enhanced platelet aggregation stimulated by serotonergic dysfunction related to depression (Kusumi *et al.* 1991). Increased platelet aggregation could easily lead to myocardial infarction, recurrent stroke, or other mechanisms causing mortality. These mechanisms could extend beyond the period of depression and lead to a long period of increased mortality. Our 10-year follow-up indicated that patients were at increased risk for at least 7 years following stroke. The fact that both syndromal and subsyndromal depression increased the risk of death, suggests that a general mechanism induced by depression, rather than the mechanism which is more specific to the etiology of major depression (presumably the mechanisms of major and minor depression are distinct), is responsible for the increased mortality.

Finding that fewer social ties was also associated with increased death is consistent with reports of increased mortality in patients with cardiovascular disease and poor social support (Case *et al.* 1992; Williams *et al.* 1992). In addition, similar to our findings, Lesperance and Frasure-Smith (1996, 2000) found that both major depression and minor depression following myocardial infarction were associated with a significantly increased death rate. Furthermore, the Glassman *et al.* (2002) "Sadheart study" demonstrated a decrease in adverse events among patients who were treated with sertraline for major depression following myocardial infarction, compared to similar patients who received placebo. All of these findings are consistent with the hypothesis that cerebrovascular and cardiovascular disease combine with physiological changes induced by depressive disorder to lead to increased morbidity and mortality. This leads to the obvious question can morbidity and mortality be decreased by treatment of poststroke depression.

Treatment of morbidity and mortality related to poststroke depression

Our study, described in Chapter 22, Treatment of poststroke depression, included 56 patients with DSM-IV defined major or minor depressive disorder. In addition, this study included 48 patients who were not depressed (i.e., no depressive diagnosis and Ham-D score < 12) at the time of enrollment in the treatment trial (Table 18.1).

Table 18.1. Background characteristics of patients (intention to treat analysis)

	Depressed			Non-depressed		
	Fluox	Nortrip	Placebo	Fluox	Nortrip	Placebo
N	23	16	17	17	15	16
Age (year $\pm$ SD)	65 $\pm$ 14	64 $\pm$ 10	73 $\pm$ 8	66 $\pm$ 13	65 $\pm$ 13	67 $\pm$ 9
Sex (% female)	26*	69	47	12**	53	25
Race (% Caucasian)	83	69	94	94	87	87
Education (year $\pm$ SD)	12 $\pm$ 3	12 $\pm$ 3	11 $\pm$ 3	13 $\pm$ 3	13 $\pm$ 2	11 $\pm$ 4
Married (%)	74	75	59	76	67	63
Hollingshead						
(%I–III)	70	60	65	47	73	69
(%IV–V)	30	40	35	53	27	31
Prior psychiatric history (%)	9	12	18	12	6	0
Family psychiatric history (%)	13	31	12	18	13	6
Since stroke (week $\pm$ SD)	16 $\pm$ 35	5 $\pm$ 4	6 $\pm$ 3	8 $\pm$ 11	10 $\pm$ 17	5 $\pm$ 3
DSM-IV major depressive disorder	11	10	6	0	0	0

*χ^2 = 7.01, d.f. = 2, p = 0.03; **Fisher's exact p = 0.04. Data taken from Robinson *et al.* (2000) reprinted with permission.

These patients were treated with fluoxetine (n = 17), nortriptyline (n = 15), or placebo (n = 16) for 12 weeks and then followed up at 6, 12 and 24 months. Of the 104 total patients enrolled in the study, 23 dropped out before completing the 12-week treatment protocol (13 of 40 fluoxetine, 5 of 31 nortriptyline, and 5 of 33 placebo patients). All patients were followed up between 6 and 9 years following the end of this treatment trial with a mean follow-up duration of survivors of 7.1 $\pm$ 1.2 SD years. During this period, 50 of the 104 patients had died. The background characteristics of the survivors and non-survivors are shown in Table 18.2. At the time of enrollment in the study, there were no significant intergroup differences in race, socio-economic class, education, marital status, personal or family history of psychiatric disorder, severity of impairment, severity of stroke (National Institute of Health (NIH) stroke scale) or time since stroke. The patients who died, however, were significantly older than the survivors (p = 0.0005) (Table 18.2). In addition, there were no significant between group differences in the frequency of arterial hypertension, coronary artery disease, congestive heart failure, atrial fibrillation, chronic pulmonary disease, hypercholesteremia, smoking, obesity, or alcohol use. Patients who died, however, were significantly more likely to have a diagnosis of diabetes mellitus (p = 0.005).

Intention to treat analysis revealed that 42 of 71 patients (59.2%) initially assigned to received antidepressants, were alive at the 9-year follow-up compared with 12 of

Table 18.2. Baseline characteristics of patients who died and patients who survive

Variable	Alive ($n = 54$)	Dead ($n = 50$)
Age (years, mean (SD))*	64.6 (11.2)	72.5 (11.2)
Sex (% male)	63.0	62.0
Race (% white)	91.7	100
SES (% Classes IV and V)	40.0	40.9
Education (years mean (SD))	12.1 (2.4)	12.1 (2.7)
Marital status (% married)	71.1	55.6
Personal history mood disorder (%)	16.4	8.7
Family history mood disorder (%)	19.6	17.4
Functional independence measure (mean (SD))	56.3 (13.1)	53.2 (11.7)
MMSE (mean (SD))	25.9 (4.3)	26.0 (4.0)
NIHSS (mean (SD))	6.2 (4.5)	6.3 (4.4)
Interval from intake to either death or survival (years, mean (SD))	7.1 (1.2)	3.8 (2.1)

* $p < 0.0005$. Data taken from Jorge *et al.* (2003) reprinted with permission.

33 patients (36.4%) who were assigned to receive placebo ($p = 0.03$). Kaplan–Meier survival analysis show that the probability of survival was significantly greater in the patients assigned to the antidepressant group than the placebo group ($p = 0.03$) (Fig. 18.3). An efficacy analysis of the patients who completed the 12-week treatment protocol ($n = 81$) showed that 36 of 53 patients (67.9%) given antidepressants were alive at the 9-year follow-up compared to 10 of 28 patients (35.7%) who received placebo ($p = 0.005$). Twenty-seven of the 53 patients (52%) treated with antidepressants had major or minor depression at baseline compared to 13 of 28 (46.4%) who received placebo ($p = $ NS). Probability of survival was higher in patients who received antidepressants in both the depressed ($p = 0.02$, Kaplan–Meier survival analysis) and the non-depressed group ($p = 0.02$, Kaplan–Meier survival analysis).

A logistic regression model analyzing the association of mortality with variables that were significantly associated with increased mortality rates (i.e., age, stroke type, comorbid diabetes mellitus, relapsing depression, and antidepressant use), found that antidepressant use was an independent predictor of probability of survival ($p = 0.03$) as was diabetes mellitus ($p = 0.02$).

A subanalysis of our data showed that among 58 patients who were followed for 2 years, 36 received antidepressants during the first 12 weeks of the study. Of these 36 patients, 17 continued to receive therapeutic doses of antidepressants for approximately 12 months (mean $= 11.6$ months ± 5.9 SD). At long-term follow-up, 15 of 17 (88.2%) patients who received continuation therapy with antidepressants were

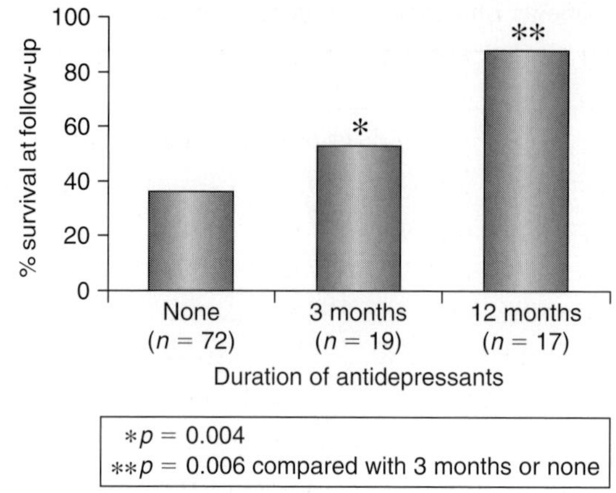

*p = 0.004
**p = 0.006 compared with 3 months or none

Figure 18.4 The percent of patients who survived during 7–9 years of follow-up divided by the duration of time following acute stroke that they received either nortriptyline or fluoxetine antidepressant medication. Among patients with 12 months of treatment, 88.2% (i.e., 15 of 17 patients) survived compared to only 35.7% (10 of 28 patients) who received placebo.

alive compared with 10 of 19 (52.6%) patients who received only 12 weeks of anti-depressant therapy ($p = 0.0006$) (Fig. 18.4). Thus, our preliminary data indicates that the use of antidepressant medication for a minimum of 3 months will significantly increase long-term survival and perhaps extended treatment up to a year or more may promote survival of an even greater degree. This is certainly an area of research which needs to be explored.

The most obvious issue raised by these findings is how antidepressant medication may lead to increased long-term survival. As shown in Chapter 22 (Treatment of poststroke depression) fluoxetine was ineffective in the treatment of poststroke depression but was just as effective as nortriptyline in preventing long-term mortality. This implies that the mechanism of action of the antidepressants in reducing mortality is different than the mechanism of alleviating depression. One possible explanation for how antidepressants might work is the modification of neurotransmission in abnormal feedback loops involving the prefrontal cortex, basal ganglia, and thalamus or in the hypothalamic–pituitary–adrenal axis or noradranergic brain stem nuclei. Abnormalities of these circuits within the brain could lead to medical consequences including hypertension, hyperlipidemia, endothelial injury, and progressive atherosclerosis (Musselman *et al.* 1998). In addition, alterations in autonomic nervous system activity as demonstrated by reduced heart rate variability may be reduced by antidepressant medication (Carney *et al.* 1995). Finally, antidepressant medications might affect serotonin mediated platelet activation or activation of coagulation factors leading to decreased thrombus formation

(Laghrissi-Thode *et al.* 1997). Thus, antidepressants may promote survival through one or several of these pathophysiological mechanisms and this is a topic clearly requiring future research.

In summary, there are at least three publications which have found that depressive disorder including subsyndromal forms of depression are associated with increased mortality as soon as 1 year following stroke and lasting for at least 7 years. Although there are a few studies which have not found, increased mortality in 12–36-month follow-up. I am unaware of any long-term follow-up studies which have failed to show an increased mortality rate associated with poststroke depression. Given this risk associated with depressive disorder, our recent follow-up study examining the results of 3 months of double-blind placebo controlled treatment with fluoxetine or nortriptyline found that active treatment increased survival by approximately 50% at 7–9 years following stroke. These provocative, yet intriguing, findings suggest that antidepressants may represent one of the major advances in the treatment of post-stroke patients. Our data would suggest that all patients who have suffered an acute stroke (both depressed and non-depressed patients) may improve their long-term survival by taking antidepressants medications for 3–12 months or longer.

REFERENCES

Astrom, M., Adolfsson, R., and Asplund, K. Major depression in stroke patients: a 3-year longitudinal study. *Stroke* (1993) 24:976–982.

Avery, D., and Winokur, G. Mortality in depressed patients treated with electroconvulsive therapy and antidepressants. *Arch Gen Psychiatr* (1976) 33:1029–1037.

Burvill, P. W., Johnson, G. A., Jamrozik, K. D., *et al.* Prevalence of depression after stroke: the Perth Community Stroke Study. *Br J Psychiatr* (1995) 166:320–327.

Carney, R. M., Rich, M., TeVelde, A., *et al.* The relationship between heart rate, heart rate variability and depression in patients with coronary artery disease. *J Psychosom Res* (1988) 32:159–164.

Carney, R. M., Saunders, R. D., Freedland, K. E., *et al.* Association of depression with reduced heart rate variability in coronary artery disease. *Am J Cardiol* (1995) 76(8):562–564.

Case, R. B., Moss, A. J., and Case, N. Living alone after myocardial infarction: impact on prognosis. *J Am Med Assoc* (1992) 267:515–519.

Ensinck, K. T. J. L., Schuurman, A. G., van den Akker, M., *et al.* Is there an increased risk of dying after depression? *Am J Epidemiol* (2002) 156(11):1043–1048.

Dalack, G. W., and Roose, S. P. Perspectives on the relationship between cardiovascular disease and affective disorder. *J Clin Psychiatr* (1990) 51(Suppl):4–9.

Glassman, A. H., O'Connor, C. M., Califf, R. M., *et al.* Sertraline treatment of major depression in patients with acute MI or unstable angina. *J Am Med Assoc* (2002) 288(6):701–709.

Gump, B. B., Mastthews, K. A., Eberly, L. E., *et al.* Depressive symptoms and mortality in men. Results from the multiple risk factor intervention trial. *Stroke* (2005) 36:98–102.

House, A., Knapp, P., Bamford, J., *et al.* Mortality at 12 and 24 months after stroke may be associated with depressive symptoms at 1 month. *Stroke* (2001) 32(3):696–701.

Jorge, R. E., Robinson, R. G., Arndt, S., *et al.* Mortality and post-stroke depression: a placebo controlled trial of antidepressants. *Am J Psychiatr* (2003) 160:1823–1829.

Kusumi, I., Koyama, T., and Yamashita, I. Serotonin-stimulated Ca^{2+} response is increased in the blood platelets of depressed patients. *Biol Psychiatr* (1991) 30:310–312.

Laghrissi-Thode, F., Wagner, W. R., Pollock, B. G., *et al.* Elevated platelet factor 4 and beta-thromboglobulin plasma levels in depressed patients with ischemic heart disease. *Biol Psychiatr* (1997) 42(4):290–295.

Lesperance, F., and Frasure-Smith, N. Depression in patients with cardiac disease: a practical review (comment). *J Psychosom Res* (2000) 48(4–5):379–391.

Lesperance, F., Frasure-Smith, N., and Talajic, M. Major depression before and after myocardial infarction: its nature and consequences. *Psychosom Med* (1996) 58(2):99–110.

Maltzberg, B. Mortality among patients with involutional melancholia. *Am J Psychiatr* (1937) 93:1231–1238.

Morris, P. L. P., Robinson, R. G., Andrezejewski, P., *et al.* Association of depression with 10-year post-stroke mortality. *Am J Psychiatr* (1993a) 150:124–129.

Morris, P. L. P., Robinson, R. G., and Samuels, J. Depression, introversion and mortality following stroke. *Aust N Z J Psychiatr* (1993b) 27:443–449.

Murphy, J. M. The epidemiologic face of late-life depression (comment). *J Geriatr Psychiatr* (1989) 22:67–75.

Musselman, D. L., Evans, D. L., and Nemeroff, C. B. The relationship of depression to cardiovascular disease: epidemiology, biology, and treatment. *Arch Gen Psychiatr* (1998) 55(7):580–592.

Pohjasvaara, T., Vataja, R., Leppavuori, A., *et al.* Cognitive functions and depression as predictors of poor outcome 15 months after stroke. *Cerebrovasc Dis* (2002) 14(3–4):228–233.

Robinson, R. G., Schultz, S. K., Castillo, C., *et al.* Nortriptyline versus fluoxetine in the treatment of depression and in short term recovery after stroke: a placebo controlled, double-blind study. *Am J Psychiatr* (2000) 157:351–359.

Tokgozoglu, S. L., Batur, M. K., Topcuoglu, M. A., *et al.* Effects of stroke localization on cardiac autonomic balance and sudden death. *Stroke* (1999) 30(7):1307–1311.

Unutzer, J., Patrick, D. L., Marmon, T., *et al.* Depressive symptoms and mortality in a prospective study of 2558 older adults. *Am J Geriatr Psychiatr* (2002) 10(5):521–530.

Williams, R. B., Barefoot, J. C., and Califf, R. M. Prognostic importance of social and economic resources among medically treated patients with angiographically documented coronary artery disease. *J Am Med Assoc* (1992) 267:520–524.

Williams, L. S., Ghose, S. S., and Swindle, R. W. Depression and other mental health diagnose increase mortality risk after ischemic stroke. *Am J Psychiatry* (2004) 161(6):1090–1095.

19

Suicidal thoughts and plans

Background

Suicide constitutes one of the major public health problems in the USA. Physical illness has been demonstrated to be a significant risk factor for both suicidal ideation and suicide attempts. Mackenzie and Popkin (1987) reported that suicide risk is greater among patients with physical illnesses than among the general population. DeVivo *et al.* (1993) found that 6.3% of all deaths among patients with spinal cord injury (SCI) were caused by suicide and that persons with SCI were 4.9 times more likely to commit suicide than the general population.

Among patients with stroke, suicidal thoughts are relatively frequent but reports of completed suicides are relatively rare. Garden *et al.* (1990) reported on two patients who developed mood disturbance in the acute poststroke period and eventually committed suicide. Although neither patient openly expressed suicidal thoughts to staff or family members, risk factors such as depression, insomnia, and cognitive impairment, may have contributed to these suicides.

Suicidal thoughts after acute stroke

Our first investigation of patients with suicidal thoughts evaluated 301 patients with acute stroke in whom we had systematically asked them about the existence of suicidal thoughts or plans (Kishi *et al.* 1996a). Using the present state examination (PSE), a total of 20 patients (6.6%) reported that they had deliberately considered suicide and that these death wishes were not simply passive death wishes or fleeting thoughts (Fig. 19.1). Background comparisons of the 20 patients who had suicidal intentions and the 281 patients without suicidal intentions are shown in Table 19.1. The suicidal patients were significantly younger than non-suicidal patients ($p = 0.03$). In addition, the patients with suicidal thoughts had a greater frequency of alcohol abuse than non-suicidal patients ($p = 0.03$). The suicidal patients also had a

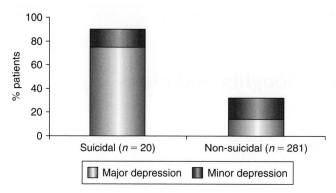

Figure 19.1 The frequency of depression among 301 patients with acute stroke. Note that suicidal patients have a significantly higher prevalence of major depression but not minor depression compared with non-suicidal patients.

Table 19.1. Background characteristics of patients with and without suicidal intentions

Variables	Suicidal group (n = 20) (%)	Non-suicidal group (n = 281) (%)
Age, median years (Q3 − Q1)	50.0 (35.0)*	61.0 (17.0)
Education, median years (Q3 − Q1)	11.5 (4.5)	9.0 (5.8)
Race (n white)	8 (42.1)	92 (33.1)
Married	6 (33.3)	113 (46.3)
Gender (n male)	9 (45.0)	161 (57.3)
Right handedness	15 (88.2)	242 (88.6)
Socioeconomic status, Hollingshead		
Class I–III	3 (16.7)	64 (26.1)
Class IV	8 (44.4)	75 (30.6)
Class V	7 (38.9)	106 (43.3)
Family history of psychiatric disorder	3 (16.7)	24 (8.8)
Personal history		
Psychiatric disorder (excluding alcohol abuse)	4 (21.1)	27 (9.9)
Alcohol abuse	5 (27.8)*	29 (11.2)
Previous cerebrovascular accident	7 (43.8)	34 (17.7)

From Kishi *et al.* (1996a), reprinted with permission.
*$p < 0.05$.
The percentage is based on the n value divided by the total number for whom data are available. Frequently data could not be obtained for all patients.

significantly higher frequency of previous history of stroke than non-suicidal patients (p = 0.01).

On neurological examination, there was no difference in the frequency of motor impairment (67% versus 69%) in the suicidal versus non-suicidal groups. There

Table 19.2. Background characteristics of suicidal and non-suicidal patients with major depression

Variables	Major depression	
	Suicidal ($n = 15$) (%)	Non-suicidal ($n = 42$) (%)
Age, mean years (Q3 − Q1)	58.0 (35.8)	57.0 (25.0)
Education, mean years (Q3 − Q1)	10.0 (6.8)	9.0 (5.0)
Race (n white)	6 (42.9)	19 (45.2)
Married (n male)	6 (42.9)	14 (36.8)
Gender (n male)	7 (46.7)	18 (42.9)
Right handedness	12 (92.3)	36 (87.8)
Socioeconomic status, Hollingshead		
Class IV	6 (42.8)	15 (37.5)
Class V	5 (35.7)	14 (35.0)
Family history of psychiatric disorder	3 (21.4)	6 (14.6)
Prior psychiatric disorder (excluding alcohol abuse)	3 (21.4)	6 (14.3)
Alcohol abuse	4 (28.6)	11 (26.2)
Previous CVA (n positive)	5 (41.7)	5 (17.2)

CVA: cerebrovascular accident.

From Kishi (1996a), reprinted with permission.

The percentage is based on the n value, divided by the total number for whom data are available. Frequently data could not be obtained for all patients.

were also no significant differences in visual field deficits, aphasia, cranial nerve signs, but there was a trend for the suicidal group to have higher frequency of sensory deficit (50%) than the non-suicidal group (27%) ($p = 0.08$).

The patients with suicidal intention had significantly higher scores on the Hamilton depression scale and greater impairments in cognitive function ($p = 0.01$) and social functioning ($p = 0.02$) than the non-suicidal patients. There were no significant differences between groups in terms of the severity of their impairment in activities of daily living.

Among the patients with suicidal intentions, 15 (75%) had major depressive disorder and three (15%) had minor depression (Fig. 19.1). There were only two patients who were non-depressed. The rate of major depression in the non-suicidal patients was 15% and the rate of minor depression was 18%. The two non-depressed suicidal patients were both young females (ages 21 and 25 years from lower socioeconomic classes, one of whom had a past history of stroke).

In an effort to distinguish which clinical factors may have produced the highest risk of suicide, we compared the 15 suicidal patients with major depression with 42 non-suicidal patients with major depression (Table 19.2) (Kishi et al. 1996a). There were no differences in background characteristics, suggesting that younger age, prior stroke, and alcohol abuse were associated with the existence of major depression and not specifically with suicidal thoughts. The suicidal group, however, had a greater frequency of sensory deficit than the depressed non-suicidal patients (55.6% suicidal versus 17.5% non-suicidal) ($p = 0.03$). There were no significant differences between groups in terms of cognitive impairment, activities of daily living, or social functioning, suggesting that these impairment variables associated with suicidal intentions were correlates of major depression and not specifically of suicidal thoughts.

We then compared the two groups based on specific symptoms of depression to see if particular depressive symptoms were associated with suicidal plans (Kishi et al. 1996a). Logistic regression analysis showed no association of any vegetative symptoms with suicidal plans (i.e., autonomic anxiety, anxious foreboding, diurnal variation, weight loss, initial insomnia, loss of energy, loss of libido, terminal insomnia). There was, however, an association of psychological symptoms of depression with suicidal plans ($p = 0.003$). Patients with suicidal intentions had a significantly greater frequency of brooding and social withdrawal compared with the non-suicidal patients. There were no differences in other psychological depressive symptoms (i.e., worrying, loss of interest, hopelessness, self-depreciation, lack of self-confidence, simple or guilty ideas of reference, pathological guilt or irritability).

These data clearly support the conclusion that patients who have major depression following stroke, as with all major depression patients, should be evaluated for suicidal risk. Those who are socially withdrawn and brooding as well as younger, alcoholic, most cognitively and socially impaired, and with prior strokes may be the most at risk. Our study of patients with physical illnesses as well as those carried out by other investigators of patients with physical illnesses (Brown et al. 1986; Liebenluft and Goldberg 1988) suggest that "rational" thoughts of suicide are uncommon in physically ill patients but occur rather in the context of clinically significant depressive disorders. The finding that alcohol abuse is associated with suicidal thoughts has been reported by a number of investigators (Robins et al. 1959; Adams and Overholser 1992).

We have recently compared patients with suicidal intentions following acute stoke with patients having acute traumatic brain injury (TBI) ($n = 65$), myocardial infarction (MI) ($n = 70$), or SCI ($n = 60$) (Kishi et al. 2001a) (Fig. 19.2). A total of 33 patients, among the total group of 496 patients, had suicidal plans and three patients, one with mild MI, one with SCI, and one with stroke, had attempted suicide. Of the 105 patients with major depression, 24.8% had suicidal intentions. This is comparable to the frequency of suicidal plans reported by Asnis et al. (1993) who found that 36% of 178 outpatients with functional major depression had suicidal intentions. There was no difference in the frequency of suicidal thoughts among the four diagnostic groups (MI: 7.1%; SCI: 13.3%; TBI: 4.4%; stroke: 6.6%). There

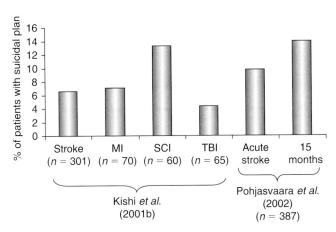

Figure 19.2 The frequency of suicidal thoughts and plans among patients with stroke, MI, SCI, or brain trauma. The frequency of suicidal thoughts was similar across all physical disorders. The strongest association was with major depression.

were no statistically significant differences between patients who were suicidal and those who were not suicidal in terms of gender, race, education, or family psychiatric history. Suicidal patients, however, were significantly younger, had a lower frequency of being married and a greater frequency of personal psychiatric history or substance abuse history compared with the non-suicidal group. Multivariate analysis of demographic characteristics demonstrated that being unmarried was the only demographic characteristic independently associated with suicidal ideas.

Multivariate analysis of neuropsychiatric examination findings demonstrated that the existence of a depressive disorder was the only significant risk factor for suicidal thoughts. Examination of specific vegetative and psychological symptoms of depression among suicidal and non-suicidal patients using logistic regression demonstrated that social withdrawal ($p = 0.01$) and ideas of reference ($p = 0.016$) were independent factors associated with presence of suicidal plan. Hopelessness was found to have a trend association with suicidal plans among patients with major depression ($p = 0.052$).

Among the 33 suicidal patients at the initial in-hospital evaluation, 22 (9 stroke, 2 TBI, 3 MI, and 8 SCI) had at least one follow-up evaluation over the 2 years following onset of illness (Kishi et al. 2001b). Among the 16 patients in this group who were depressed (i.e., 73% of suicidal group), the depression had improved at follow-up in 11 and they were no longer suicidal. The patients whose depressive disorder did not improve continued to have suicidal ideation and the mean duration of suicidal thoughts was 8.7 ± 2.1 SD months.

Table19.3. Background characteristics of patients with acute onset and delayed onset suicidal thoughts following stroke

Variables	Acute-onset suicidal (n = 20) (%)	Delayed-onset suicidal (n = 16) (%)	Non-suicidal (n = 117) (%)	p-value
Age, median years (Q3 − Q1)	50.0 (35.0)	57.5 (23.0)	61.0 (17.0)	<0.10
Education, median years (Q3 − Q1)	11.5 (4.5)	11.0 (5.8)	8.0 (6.0)	<0.12
Race (n white)	8 (42.1)	8 (50.0)	35 (30.2)	NS
Married (n)	6 (33.3)	7 (46.7)	54 (48.2)	NS
Gender (n male)	9 (45.0)	7 (43.8)	70 (59.8)	NS
Right handedness (n)	15 (88.2)	14 (87.5)	102 (89.5)	NS
Socioeconomic status, Hollingshead				
Class IV	8 (44.4)	5 (31.3)	31 (27.7)	
Class V	7 (38.9)	6 (37.5)	55 (49.1)	
Family history of psychiatric disorder (%)	3 (16.7)	2 (12.5)	7 (6.1)	<0.15
Prior psychiatric disorder (excluding alcohol abuse)	4 (21.1)	4 (25.0)	12 (10.5)	<0.14
Alcohol abuse	5 (27.8)	0 (0.0)	11 (9.4)	<0.03
Previous CVA	7 (43.8)	6 (37.5)	15 (12.9)	<0.01

CVA: cerebrovascular accident.
From Kishi et al. (1996b), reprinted with permission.
The percentage is based on the n value divided by the total number for whom data are available. Frequently data could not be obtained for all patients. Q3 − Q1 indicates the third quartile value minus the first quartile value using non-parametric rank order.

We have also examined suicidal intentions among patients who were not suicidal in the acute period following stroke (Kishi et al. 1996b). Follow-up evaluations were obtained from 142 patients seen one or more times during the first 2 years following stroke (Table 19.3). Of the patients who did not have a suicidal plan at the initial evaluation, 16 (11.3%) had developed a suicidal plan at either 3-, 6-, 12-, or 24-month follow-up. There were seven patients found to have suicide plans for the first time at 6 months poststroke, three patients at 12 months, and six patients at 24 months follow-up. Of these 16 patients with delayed-onset suicide plans, two patients attempted suicide during the follow-up period. There was a trend for acute suicidal patients (n = 20) to be younger than non-suicidal patients (n = 117) or delayed-onset suicidal patients (n = 16) but this did not reach statistical difference. Delayed-onset suicide was not associated with prior alcohol abuse but was associated with previous history of stroke compared to non-suicidal patients (p = 0.002).

Using Diagnostic and Statistical Manual, 4th ed. (DSM-IV) diagnostic criteria for major or minor depression, 10 patients (62.5%) with delayed-onset suicide plans had major depression at the time they were suicidal. Two patients (12.5%) had minor depression and four patients (25%) were non-depressed. However, three of the four patients who were non-depressed at the time when suicide plans were elicited had a mood disorder either before or after the onset of the suicide plans (two patients met the criteria before developing suicide plans and one after). Thus, these cases may have represented residual or initial symptoms of depression in patients who did not reach the threshold for diagnosis.

When the lesion location was compared between acute- and delayed-onset suicidal patients, the acute-onset patients had significantly more anterior lesions than the delayed-onset group ($p = 0.04$). The caudal border of the lesion was 54% of the anterior–posterior (A–P) distance in acute-onset patients, while it was 81% of the A–P distance in delayed-onset suicidal patients and 60% in non-suicidal patients. This finding may reflect the association between more anterior lesions and acute-onset major depression as well as major depression with suicidal plans.

There was no significant difference in the frequency of suicidal plans during the acute compared to the chronic poststroke period. Furthermore, there was no significant difference in the frequency of major or minor depression between the acute- versus delayed-onset suicidal patients. A logistic regression found that impaired social functioning at the initial in-hospital evaluation was strongly associated with the development of delayed-onset suicidal thoughts (Kishi *et al.* 2001b).

Pohjasvaara *et al.* (2002) have also examined suicidal thoughts in patients with stroke. This study examined 287 patients in Finland aged 55–85 years who were examined at 3 and 15 months after ischemic stroke. Suicide plans were present in 28 patients (9.8%) at 3 months and in 40 patients (14.0%) at 15 months poststroke. At both the 3-month evaluation and the 15-month evaluation, patients with suicidal thoughts were more depressed as measured by the Beck depression inventory compared with the non-suicidal patients. In addition, suicidal patients compared with non-suicidal stroke patients more often had a history of stroke prior to the index stroke (35% versus 18%, $p = 0.015$), right-sided stroke (60% versus 41.9%, $p = 0.03$), were more disabled as measured by the Rankin scale (Rankin score 4.2 versus 1.9, $p = 0.003$) and were more likely to be dependent in living (45% versus 27%, $p = 0.02$). Logistic regression, however, found that the only independent correlate of suicidal ideas at 15 months following stroke was a history of prior stroke (odds ratio: 2.4; 95% confidence interval (CI): 1.1–4.97).

Numerous studies have demonstrated that reduced serotonergic function is associated with suicidal behavior (Asberg *et al.* 1976; Mann 1987; Roy *et al.* 1989). In addition, early morning awakening associated with acute-onset suicidal plans has been related to decreased serotonergic activity (Gaillard 1985; Leysen and Shotle 1992). These data suggest that decreased serotonergic function may play a role at least in the suicidal thoughts of patients with stroke. We have previously demonstrated (see Chapter 22 on the mechanism of depression) that more anterior lesions are associated with more severe depressive symptoms and that the magnitude of depletion of serotonergic 5-hydroxytryptophan, (5-HT$_2$) receptors in the left parietal cortex was correlated with the severity of poststroke depression (Mayberg *et al.* 1988). Our finding that greater in hospital impairment in social functioning was associated with delayed-onset suicidal thoughts suggests that the mechanisms of suicidal plans may be related more to biological mechanisms in the early period following stroke and to psychological or social causes in the chronic period following stroke.

In summary, although completed suicide remains relatively rare following stroke, approximately 10% of patients who have suffered a stroke will develop suicidal thoughts and intentions. The strongest association with suicidal thoughts is the existence of major depression. Suicidal thoughts in the vast majority of patients go away when the patient is no longer depressed. The environmental and personal factors which seem to play an important role in the development of suicidal plans include social isolation, younger age, prior alcohol abuse history, cognitive and social impairment, and prior strokes. Psychological symptoms of despair, brooding, and hopelessness are also associated with increased risk of suicide. Early identification of these risk factors and intervention including improved social support and treatment of depression, seem to be the most important factors in preventing these potential suicides. Future research should examine the mechanisms of this behavior as well as the benefits of prevention of depression.

REFERENCES

Adams, D. M., and Overholser, J. C. Suicidal behavior and history of substance abuse. *Am J Drug Alcohol Abuse* (1992) 18:343–354.

Asberg, M., Traskman, L., and Thoren, P. 5-HIAA in the cerebrospinal fluid: a biochemical suicide predictor? *Arch Gen Psychiatr* (1976) 38:1193–1197.

Asnis, G. M., Friedman, T. A., Sanderson, W. C., *et al.* Suicidal behaviors in adult psychiatric outpatients. I: description and prevalence. *Am J Psychiatr* (1993) 150:108–112.

Brown, J. H., Henteleff, P., Barakat, S., *et al.* Is it normal for terminally ill patients to desire death. *Am J Psychiatr* (1986) 143:208–211.

DeVivo, M. J., Black, K. J., and Stover, S. L. Causes of death during the first 12 years after spinal cord injury. *Arch Phys Med Rehabil* (1993) 74(3):248–254.

Gaillard, J. M. Neurochemical regulation of the states of alertness. *Ann Clin Res* (1985) 17:175–184.

Garden, F. H., Garrison, S. J., and Jain, A. Assessing suicide risk in stroke patients: review of two cases. *Arch Phys Med Rehabil* (1990) 71(12):1003–1005.

Kishi, Y., Kosier, J. T., and Robinson, R. G. Suicidal plans in patients with acute stroke. *J Nerv Ment Dis* (1996a) 184(5):274–280.

Kishi, Y., Robinson, R. G., and Kosier, J. T. Suicidal plans in patients with stroke: comparison between acute-onset and delayed-onset suicidal plans. *Int Psychogeriatr* (1996b) 8(4):623–634.

Kishi, Y., Robinson, R. G., and Kosier, J. T. Suicidal ideation among patients during the rehabilitation period after life-threatening physical illness. *J Nerv Ment Dis* (2001a) 189:623–628.

Kishi, Y., Robinson, R. G., and Kosier, J. T. Suicidal ideation among patients with acute life-threatening physical illness: patients with stroke, traumatic brain injury, myocardial infarction, and spinal cord injury. *Psychosomatics* (2001b) 42(5):382–390.

Leysen, J. E., and Shotle, A. Role and localization of serotonin $5HT_2$ receptors. *Prog Histochem Cytochem* (1992) 26:241–249.

Liebenluft, E., and Goldberg, R. L. The suicidal, terminally ill patient with depression. *Psychosomatics* (1988) 29:379–386.

Mackenzie, T. B., and Popkin, M. K. Suicide in the medical patient. *Int J Psychiatr Med* (1987) 17:3–22.

Mann, J. J. Psychological predictions of suicide. *J Clin Psychiatr* (1987) 48(Suppl):39–43.

Mayberg, H. S., Robinson, R. G., Wong, D. F., *et al*. PET imaging of cortical S_2-serotonin receptors after stroke: lateralized changes and relationship to depression. *Am J Psychiatr* (1988) 145:937–943.

Pohjasvaara, T., Vataja, R., Leppavuori, A., *et al*. Cognitive functions and depression as predictors of poor outcome 15 months after stroke. *Cerebrovasc Dis* (2002) 14(3–4):228–233.

Robins, E., Murphy, G. E., Wilkinson, R. H., *et al*. Some clinical considerations in the prevention of suicide based on a study of 134 successful suicides. *Am J Pub Health* (1959) 49:888–899.

Roy, A., DeJong, J., and Linnoila, M. CSF monoamine metabolites and suicidal behavior in depressed patients. *Arch Gen Psychiatr* (1989) 46:609–612.

20

Biological markers

In spite of brief periods of enthusiasm about the potential diagnostic utility or etiological insights to be gained from neuroendocrine tests associated with depression, there has been an overall lack of success of neuroendocrine testing in primary depression. Similarly, among patients with poststroke depression, neuroendocrine tests have not been successful in establishing either an alternative method of diagnosing poststroke depression or illuminating neuroendocrine abnormalities which may contribute to the mechanism of poststroke depression.

Since the early 1960s, it has been known that patients with depression secrete an excess amount of cortisol (Gibbons and McHugh 1962; Sachar *et al.* 1973). The dexamethasone suppression test (DST) has been used extensively to study states of hypercortisolism (Carroll *et al.* 1981). Patients given 1 mg of dexamethasone orally will suppress serum cortisol secretion over the following 24 h. In a significant number of patients with primary major depression, especially the melancholic form of depression, there is a failure to suppress serum cortisol following dexamethasone administration. This lack of suppression is referred to as a positive DST response. Sensitivity of a positive DST in identifying patients with melancholic depression is determined by dividing the number of DST-positive depressed patients as a percentage of the total number of depressed patients. Among patients without brain injury (i.e., primary depression) the sensitivity of the DST has been no greater than 60–70%. The specificity of the DST, however, is determined by the percentage of DST negative non-depressed patients as a percentage of the total number of non-depressed patients. First reports of the specificity of the DST in primary melancholic depression was greater than 95% (Carroll *et al.* 1981). Subsequent studies, however, found the specificity of the DST in a variety of depressive disorders to be well below 95% which would preclude the use of this test as a diagnostic probe to identify depression in difficult diagnostic cases.

The first use of the DST in patients with poststroke depression was reported by Finkelstein *et al.* (1982). This study examined 25 randomly selected stroke patients and 13 non-stroke control patients hospitalized at a rehabilitation center. Of the

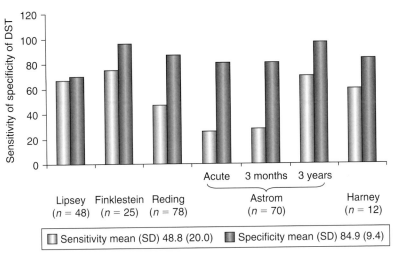

Figure 20.1 The sensitivity and specificity of the DST for major depression in patients with stroke across five separate studies. Across all studies, the mean sensitivity (i.e., the number of depressed, DST-positive patients divided by the total number of depressed patients) was 54% while the mean specificity (i.e., the number of non-depressed, DST-negative patients divided by the total number of non-depressed patients) was 84%. This lack of higher specificity may be explained by lesion volume or poststroke impairment. It prevents the test, however, from being used as a diagnostic test for poststroke major depression.

patients with moderate to severe depressed mood, 75% (9 of 12) failed to suppress serum cortisol levels following dexamethasone suppression compared to 8% (1 of 13) of the control patients ($p < 0.01$). Thus, this study not only found about the expected rate of sensitivity (i.e., 75%) but also a high level of specificity (i.e., 20 of 21 or 96%) (Fig. 20.1).

We also conducted one of the early studies of the DST in poststroke depression (Lipsey *et al.* 1985). The study included 65 patients, not included in any of our acute stroke studies, who were consecutive admissions to a rehabilitation hospital following an acute stroke. The background characteristics of the patients included in the study, grouped according to whether they had a suppressed serum cortisol level following dexamethasone administration (negative DST) or not (positive DST), are shown in Table 20.1. Of the 65 study patients, 10 were removed from the data analysis because of possible drug related false-positive or false-negative DSTs and an additional seven patients were removed since their stroke had occurred more than 1 year prior to evaluation. Of the remaining 48 patients, positive DSTs were significantly associated with presence of major depression. Among 15 patients with major depression, 10 (67%) had positive DSTs compared to only (30%) of the 33 patients without major depression. Thus, we found a 67% sensitivity and a 70% specificity for the DST in identifying major poststroke depression (Fig. 20.1).

Table 20.1. Background characteristics of patients given the DST

Characteristic	Patient group*	
	Positive DST ($n = 29$)	Negative DST ($n = 36$)
Age (years)	64 ± 11	63 ± 9
White (%)	52	58
Male (%)	72	55
Social class[†]		
I–III (%)	21	42
IV–V (%)	79	58
Married (%)	55	50
History of treated psychiatric disorder		
Family (%)	0	14
Personal (%)	7	11
Alcohol abuse		
Recent (%)	17	17
Past (%)	17	14
Time since stroke (mean days $\pm$ SD)	134 ± 319	178 ± 245

* None of the intergroup differences was significant.
[†] Hollingshead.

We also examined the DST response based on lesion location. Among 12 patients with left anterior hemisphere injury, there was no significant increase in the frequency of positive DSTs compared to 36 patients without left anterior hemisphere injury. Similarly, there was no significant difference in the frequency of right or left hemisphere lesions between the positive and negative DST groups. Patients with positive DSTs, however, had larger lesion volumes than patients with negative DSTs ($p = 0.02$). Total lesion volumes were also significantly correlated with 4.00 p.m. serum cortisol levels ($r = 0.48, p < 0.01$). This correlation held even when patients with major depression were excluded from the analysis ($r = 0.42, p < 0.05$), which suggests that non-suppression of cortisol is related to larger lesion volume, independent of depression. Based on this study, we concluded that positive DSTs were not useful diagnostically but were related to both the existence of major depression and the extent of brain injury.

The DST has also been investigated by Bauer *et al.* (1983), Reding *et al.* (1985), Olsson *et al.* (1989), Malec *et al.* (1990), Dam *et al.* (1991), Grober *et al.* (1991), and Astrom *et al.* (1993) (Table 20.2). Reding studied 78 patients in a rehabilitation hospital who were an average of 7 weeks poststroke. Positive DSTs were found in 49% of all patients. There was 87% specificity and a 47% sensitivity of the 8.00 a.m.

Table 20.2. Dexamethasone test results in poststroke depression

Investigator	N	Time since stroke	Depression n (%)	Cortisol sampling	A/A+C sensitivity	D/D+B specificity	A/A+B positive PV	D/C+D negative PV
Finkelstein (1982)	25	37 d mean	12 (48%)	1600; 2300	75	96	90	80
Bauer (1983)	20		3 (15%)		0	83		
Lipsey (1985)	48	160 d mean	15 (31%)	1600; 2300	67	70	50	82
Reding (1985)	61	49 d mean	38 (62%)	800; 1600	63	75	83	56
Malec (1990)	20	8–30 d	6 (30%)	1700; 2300	100	14	33	100
Dam (1991)	76	35 d median	25 (33%)	800; 1600	8	96	50	68
Grober (1991)	29	106 d mean	20 (69%)	1600	15	67	50	26
Astrom (1993)	66	7 d maximum	19 (29%)	700; 1600	26	81	36	73
Harney (1993)	12	21 d maximum	4 (33%)	800; 1600	75	71	60	83
Pooled mean	327		N = 142		42	78	50	69

cortisol determination for the diagnosis of major depression. The test–retest reliability was 84% at 2 weeks. The DST, however, did not predict improvement in the
activities of daily living score at discharge or the duration of rehabilitation therapy
needed. A positive DST was not related to age, gender, or time since stroke. This
study also found that larger, more extensive strokes were associated with an
increased frequency of positive DST independent of depression.

Olsson *et al.* (1989) reported on the DST and its use in evaluating a cohort of
62 patients with acute stroke compared to 25 elderly patients with other acute
medical disorders. During the acute stroke period, postdexamethasone serum cortisol values at 7.00 a.m. were correlated with right-sided lesions ($r = -0.34$), disorientation ($r = 0.29$), and proximity of the lesion to the frontal pole ($r = -0.42$).
Cortisol values, however, did not correlate with the existence of major depression
(Olsson *et al.* 1989).

Astrom *et al.* (1993) reported on a cohort of 70 acute stroke patients who were
followed up at 3 months ($n = 63$) and 3 years ($n = 43$) poststroke. Over the 3 years,
there was an interesting pattern of increasing specificity and sensitivity for the DST.
During the acute phase, the sensitivity of the DST for major depression was only
26% and the specificity was 81% (Fig. 20.1). Cortisol levels following dexamethasone
administration were significantly correlated with disorientation ($r = 0.27$, $p = 0.03$)
and impairment in activities of daily living ($r = 0.35$, $p = 0.003$) but not major
depression. At 3 months follow-up, the sensitivity of the DST for major depression
was 28% and the specificity was 81%. Serum cortisol levels after the DST, however,
were not significantly correlated with either major depression or impairment in daily
activities. At 3 years, the DST sensitivity was 70% and the specificity was 97%.
Cortisol levels following DST administration were significantly correlated with
major depression ($r = 0.57$, $p < 0.001$) but not impairment in activities of daily
living or disorientation.

Another interesting finding from the Astrom study was that non-suppression of
cortisol levels (positive DST) at 3 months was a statistically significant predictor of
major depression at 3 years with an odds ratio of 14 ($p = 0.02$) (Astrom *et al.*
1993). This correlation of DST with outcome at 3 years was maintained even when
age, gender, and impairment in activities of daily living were controlled. Thus,
a positive DST in the early period following stroke may indicate a premorbid or
poststroke pathophysiological vulnerability to depression which plays out by
3 years. It is certainly a finding worthy of further investigation and may be an
indication for long-term antidepressant treatment.

Another study by Harney *et al.* (1993) reported on 12 patients with single lesions
verified by computed tomography (CT) scan given DST at 1 and 3 weeks
poststroke. At 1 week, 9 (75%) of the patients had a positive DST and 6 (50%) continued to have a positive DST at 3 weeks. There was a trend for positive DST to be

associated with Ham-D scores above 10 (three of five DST-positive patients had Ham-D scores >10 while one of six DST-negative had Ham-D scores >10, $p = 0.19$). Larger lesion volume was also associated with a positive DST (post-DST cortisol level at week 1 and week 3 correlated with lesion volume $r = 0.25$ and 0.48 respectively, $p =$ NS). None of the patients had major depression but a positive DST, as in the Astrom study (1993), may predict the late onset of major depression.

Taken together, these studies suggest that major depression following stroke is frequently associated with failure to suppress serum cortisol following dexamethasone administration (i.e., a positive DST). The test may be more useful as time following stroke increases. As specificity in most studies did not exceed 95% and the positive and negative predictive values (PV) were 50% and 69% respectively, the DST does not appear to be a useful instrument for assisting in the diagnosis of depression in the acute stroke patient with aphasia, delirium, or coma. Patients who are unable to communicate verbally are, of course, the patients in which a biological marker such as the DST would be most helpful in establishing a diagnosis of depression. The causes of non-suppression, apart from major depression, appear to be varied, but include lesion characteristics, subclinical depressive symptoms, and impairment characteristics (which may reflect the extent of the lesion).

Several other challenge tests have been assessed in patients with poststroke depression. Barry and Dinan (1990) examined growth hormone (GH) response to desipramine administration. The GH response was measured in 10 patients with poststroke depression, eight age matched poststroke non-depressed patients, and eight healthy controls. Patients scoring greater than 20 on the Center for Epidemiological Studies Depression Scale (CESD) and 17 on the HDS constituted the depressed population. All 10 of the patients with poststroke depression had a blunted GH response to desipramine compared to two of eight of the stroke patients without depression and two of eight control patients ($p < 0.05$). The lack of GH response to desipramine (which increases norepinephrine in the synaptic space) is thought to involve a subsensitive $\alpha2$ adrenergic receptor. The failure to elicit GH following administration of oral desipramine or intravenous clonidine (an $\alpha2$ adrenergic agonist) has been associated with functional depression.

Dam *et al.* (1984) examined 63 stroke patients and 23 control patients using the thyroid releasing hormone (TRH) stimulation test. There was no difference in the thyroid stimulating hormone (TSH) response between stroke patients and control patients as well as no correlation between the frequency of the blunted response to the TRH stimulation and the presence of depression. Similarly, Marchesi *et al.* (1996) examined 13 patients with stroke compared with 10 age and weight matched patients with major depression and 10 age and weight matched controls. Following TRH administration, a blunted TSH response was found in 77% of non-depressed stroke patients, 64% of functionally depressed, and 27% of controls. Thus, blunted

TSH response to TRH was a poor diagnostic marker for depression following stroke and appeared to represent neuroendocrine dysfunction associated with stroke itself rather than depression following stroke.

Ramasubbu *et al.* (1999) examined 12 depressed stroke patients (five major, seven minor depression) eight non-depressed stroke patients who were 18–22 months poststroke and 12 healthy controls. They were given 30 mg of d-fenfluramine or placebo and monitored over a 4 h period. Fenfluramine is a serotonin agonist drug which leads to the release of prolactin (PRL). Although peak PRL responses in depressed stroke patients were significantly greater than in non-depressed patients ($p = 0.005$), when differences in the hemisphere of stroke injury were controlled, differences in PRL response to fenfluramine were not significant between depressed and non-depressed patients.

Morris *et al.* (2003) also gave 30 mg of d-fenfluramine to 9 major and 14 minor depressed patients, and 38 non-depressed patients who were 4–8 weeks following a first ever stroke. PRL secretion over the 6 h following fenfluramine was significantly blunted (i.e., reduced) in patients with major depression compared with minor depression or non-depressed. This finding indicates a diminished serotonergic neurotransmitter response in patients with poststroke major depression. Thus, the d-fenfluramine test may be useful in identifying major depression from non-depressed patients with stroke.

The final laboratory test involved the use of the neurobiochemical markers of brain damage, neuron specific enolase (NSE), and protein S-100B (Wunderlich *et al.* 1999). Protein S-100B is part of a family of calcium binding proteins found in astrocytes and Schwann cells and NSE is found in the cytoplasm of neurons and neuroendocrine cells. Although the authors did not examine the 58 stroke patients for depression, high levels of both NSE and S-100B were associated with larger lesion volumes and greater severity of neurological impairment. In addition, S-100B tended to increase with increasing neuropsychological impairment. Further research will be needed to determine whether these biochemical markers may be correlated with severity of depression.

In summary, the use of biological markers to examine neuroendocrine abnormalities in poststroke depression or to identify the existence of depression in patients who cannot respond to verbal interviews remains in the developmental stage. The use of DST has produced some intriguing results. Most studies have found an association between failure to suppress serum cortisol following dexamethasone administration and the existence of major depressive disorder at some time following a stroke. The sensitivity and specificity with the DST appear to vary over time and positive DSTs have been related to large lesion volumes and severity of impairment independent of depression. The DST, therefore, at the present time, does not appear to be useful in the diagnosis of poststroke depression. Although the TRH test and blunted TSH response as well as the d-fenfluramine test and elevated PRL release did not appear to be useful diagnostically, the lack of GH response to administration of desipramine and blunted PRL release following d-fenfluramine remain potential markers for the identification of poststroke depression. Ultimately, neuroendocrine tests may provide new methods for diagnosing poststroke depression in patients with severe comprehensive aphasia as well as shedding light on the pathophysiological mechanisms of poststroke depression.

REFERENCES

Astrom, M., Olsson, T., and Asplund, K. Different linkage of depression to hypercortisolism early versus late after stroke: a 3-year longitudinal study. *Stroke* (1993) 24:52–57.

Barry, S., and Dinan, T. G. Alpha-2 adrenergic receptor function in post-stroke depression. *Psychol Med* (1990) 10:305–309.

Bauer, M., Gans, J. S., Harley, J. P., *et al.* Dexamethasone suppression test and depression in a rehabilitation setting. *Arch Phys Med Rehabil* (1983) 64(9):421–422.

Carroll, B. J., Feinberg, M., Greden, J. F., *et al.* A specific laboratory test for the diagnosis of melancholia: standardization, validation, and clinical utility. *Arch Gen Psychiatr* (1981) 38:15–22.

Dam, H., Mellerup, E. T., and Rafaelsen, O. J. Diurnal variation of total plasma tryptophan in depressive patients. *Acta Psychiatr Scand* (1984) 69(3):190–196.

Dam, H., Pedersen, H. E., Damkjaer, M., *et al.* Dexamethasone suppression test in depressive stroke patients. *Acta Neurol Scand* (1991) 84(1):14–17.

Finklestein, S., Benowitz, L. I., Baldessarini, R. J., *et al.* Mood, vegetative disturbance, and dexamethasone suppression test after stroke. *Ann Neurol* (1982) 12:463–468.

Gibbons, J. L., and McHugh, P. R. Plasma cortisol in depressive illness. *J Psychiatr Res* (1962) 1:162.

Grober, S., Gordon, W., Silwinski, M., *et al.* Utility of the dexamethasone suppression test in the diagnosis of post-stroke depression. *Arch Phys Med Rehabil* (1991) 72:1076–1079.

Harney, J. H., Fulton, C., Ross, E. D., *et al.* Dexamethasone suppression test and onset of post-stroke depression in patients with ischemic infarction. *J Clin Psychiatr* (1993) 54:343–348.

Lipsey, J. R., Robinson, R. G., Pearlson, G. D., *et al.* Dexamethasone suppression test and mood following stroke. *Am J Psychiatr* (1985) 142:318–323.

Malec, J. F., Richardson, J. W., Sinaki, M., *et al.* Types of affective response to stroke. *Arch Phys Med Rehabil* (1990) 71(5):279–284.

Marchesi, C., Silvestrini, C., Ponari, O., *et al.* Unreliability of TRH test but not dexamethasone suppression test as a marker of depression in chronic vasculopathic patients. *Biol Psychiatr* (1996) 40(7):637–641.

Morris, P., Hopwood, M., Maguire, K., *et al.* Blunted prolactin response to D-fenfluramine in post-stroke major depression. *J Affect Disord* (2003) 76(1–3):273–278.

Olsson, T., Vitanen, M., Hagg, E., *et al.* Hormones in "young" and "old" elderly: pituitary-thyroid and pituitary-adrenal axis. *Gereontology* (1989) 35:144–152.

Ramasubbu, R., Flint, A., Brown, G., *et al.* A neuroendocrine study of serotonin function in depressed stroke patients compared to non depressed stroke patients and healthy controls. *J Affect Disord* (1999) 52(1–3):121–133.

Reding, M., Orto, L., Willensky, P., *et al.* The dexamethasone suppression test: an indicator of depression in stroke but not a predictor of rehabilitation outcome. *Arch Neurol* (1985) 42:209–212.

Sachar, E. J., Hellman, L., and Raffwarg, H. P. Disrupted 24 hour patterns of cortisol secretion in psychotic depression. *Arch Gen Psychaitr* (1973) 28:19–24.

Wunderlich, M. T., Ebert, A. D., Kratz, T., *et al.* Early neurobehavioral outcome after stroke is related to release of neurobiochemical markers of brain damage. *Stroke* (1999) 30(6):1190–1195.

21

Mechanisms of poststroke depression

In considering the mechanisms of poststroke depression, it should be kept in mind that important clinical findings such as cognitive impairment is associated with major, but not minor depression, following the left, but not right, hemisphere stroke (Chapter 14) need to be integrated or explained by the proposed mechanisms of depression. Additional clinical findings include depression is significantly associated with left frontal and left basal ganglia lesions but not comparable lesions of the right hemisphere during the acute period following stroke (Chapter 10). Furthermore, major depression is associated with proximity of the lesion to the frontal pole while minor depression is associated with posterior lesions of the left hemisphere during the acute poststroke period (Chapter 10). Delayed-onset depression is more strongly associated with social impairment than acute onset depression (Chapter 9). Thus, it seems likely that there are multiple kinds of depression following stroke and that major depression, minor depression, acute onset, delayed onset, left hemisphere lesion induced, and right hemisphere lesion induced depressions may have different mechanisms.

The major debate in the literature, however, is whether poststroke depression results from psychological response to impairment/loss or whether it results from neurophysiological response to brain injury. McHugh and Slavney (1998) have described this as a debate about whether the disease perspective or the life story perspective provides greater insight into the cause of poststroke depression. The disease perspective is based on the assumption that a particular clinical syndrome results from a specific abnormality of brain function while the life story perspective assumes that the clinical syndrome arises from a combination of previous life experiences, intentions of the self and a current stressful circumstance (McHugh and Slavney 1998). Thus, Gainotti et al. (1999) argued that since patients with poststroke depression have a lower frequency of diurnal mood variation, anhedonia and thoughts of suicide than patients with primary (i.e., no known brain lesion) depression that "psychological rather than neurological factors mostly account for this important consequence (i.e., major depression) of strokes". On the other hand, we have argued that poststroke depression, in some cases, fits a disease perspective better than a life story perspective.

Ross *et al.* in 1975 demonstrated that injury to axonal projections of biogenic-amine-containing neurons led to a shut down of neurotransmitter production. We therefore hypothesized that lesions of the left dorsolateral frontal cortex or left basal ganglia may interrupt the biogenic-amine-containing axons as they course through the basal ganglia and cortex (Ross *et al.* 1975; Robinson *et al.* 1984). Injury to these ascending axonal projections may lead to subsequent decrease in the production of norepinephrine (NE) and/or 5-hydroxytryptophan (5-HT) in favor of producing protein for neuronal recovery (e.g., regeneration and sprouting).

The anatomy of the biogenic amine pathways could also potentially explain why there is, during the first 6 months following stroke, a significant correlation between anterior–posterior lesion location and severity of depression (see Chapter 10 on Relationship to lesion location). Many of the neuronal cell bodies containing either NE or 5-HT are located in the locus coeruleus or raphe, respectively. The efferent NE or 5-HT containing axons ascend through the median forebrain bundle, pass through the ventral portion of the basal ganglia, enter the frontal cortex and arc posteriorly over the corpus callosum in the deep layers of cortex. These cortical axonal projections run anteriorly to posteriorly and send branches from deep to superficial layers of cortex (Morrison *et al.* 1979). Thus, lesions of the dorsolateral frontal cortex or basal ganglia could interrupt these biogenic-amine-containing axons in a more downstream position than lesions which involve the parietal or occipital cortex and lead to a decrease in the overall production of NE or 5-HT in uninjured areas of the brain. This may alter the function of strategic limbic structures in frontal and temporal cortex ultimately leading to clinical symptoms of depression.

Data obtained from several of our clinical studies have been consistent with this hypothesis. In one study, we examined a consecutive series of 20 patients admitted to the hospital with an acute stroke who underwent a lumbar puncture (Bryer *et al.* 1992). Samples were obtained after 12 h of overnight fast and bed rest (activity and diet can both affect the concentrations of cerebrospinal fluid (CSF) biogenic amine concentrations). Patients were also examined within 5 days following stroke and CSF specimens were taken from the same lumbar space and from the same aliquot (i.e., 3 ml CSF was taken after the first 20 ml had been removed). Control patients ($n = 7$) were hospitalized at the same time, four with multiple sclerosis and three with seizure disorder. Although depressed and non-depressed stroke patients did not differ significantly in their background characteristics, and none of the patients was taking antidepressant medications, depressed patients ($n = 4$, three major depression, one minor) had significantly lower concentrations of CSF 5-hydroxyindole acetic acid (5-HIAA, the metabolite of serotonin) compared with non-depressed stroke patients ($F = 7.4$, $p = 0.014$) and control patients ($p = 0.03$) (Fig. 21.1). There was also a

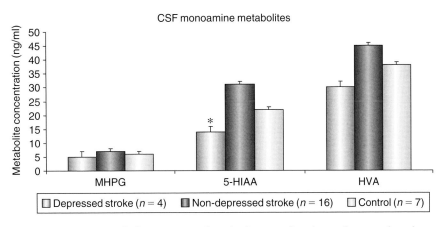

Figure 21.1   Mean ± SEM CSF metabolite concentrations in depressed and non-depressed stroke patients and control subjects. MHPG: 3-methoxy-4-hydroxyphenylglycol. *Depressed patients had significantly lower CSF concentrations of 5-HIAA than non-depressed stroke patients or control patients (reprinted from Bryer *et al.* 1992, with permission).

trend for depressed patients to have lower CSF levels of homovanillic acid (HVA) (the metabolite of dopamine) ($p = 0.06$) compared with non-depressed stroke patients. This finding of significantly lower 5-HIAA in depressed compared with non-depressed patients was maintained even when patients were matched for age, gender, and hemispheric site of the lesion. In addition, there was a trend for lower concentrations of 5-HIAA to be found in patients with lesions closer to the frontal pole ($r = 0.75, p < 0.1$). Thus, data from spinal fluid analysis in patients with acute stroke suggested that abnormalities in the production or metabolism of serotonin may play a role in the etiology of poststroke major depression.

Animal experiments have also supported a possible biochemical basis for the clinical finding that proximity of the lesion to the frontal pole is significantly correlated with severity of depression. Rats were given lesions using a suction probe at one of several positions along the anterior–posterior axis of the lateral cortex (Pearlson *et al.* 1984). Lesions which were more anterior produced a greater amount of spontaneous hyperactivity and depletion of NE than identical lesions which were more posterior (Fig. 21.2). This correlation between proximity of the lesion to the frontal pole and degree of hyperactivity or depletion of NE (i.e., $r = 0.97, p < 0.01$) occurred with lesions of the right hemisphere but not the left hemisphere. Similarly, partial destruction of the nucleus accumbens by electrolytic lesions led to spontaneous hyperactivity following right hemisphere but not left hemisphere lesions (Fig 21.3) (Kubos *et al.* 1987).

Whether spontaneous hyperactivity in the rat has the same underlying pathophysiological mechanism as poststroke mood disorders is uncertain but there are

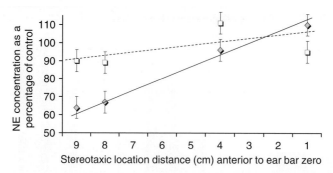

Figure 21.2   The relationship between NE concentration in frontal cortex plus locus coeruleus as a percent of normal control concentration and anterior–posterior location of right hemisphere (closed *diamonds*) or left hemisphere (open *squares*) lesion location. Higher number on the stereotaxic location indicate more anterior lesions. For the two most anterior lesion locations, right-sided frontal cortical lesions produced significantly greater depletion of NE than left lesions and there was a graded effect with anterior producing greater depletion than posterior lesions (reprinted from Pearlson and Robinson 1984, with permission).

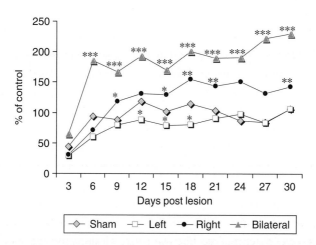

Figure 21.3   Spontaneous activity in daily running wheels expressed as a percentage of preoperative baseline over 30 days following right, left, or bilateral electrolytic lesions of the nucleus accumbens (NA). Right hemisphere NA lesions produced significantly greater activity than identical left hemisphere lesions. Bilateral lesions showed an interaction effect. Asterisks indicate the level of significance compared to control values for that postoperative day, $*p < 0.05$, $**p < 0.01$, $***p < 0.001$ (modified from Kubos *et al.* 1987, with permission from Elsevier).

some interesting parallels. For example, left frontal and basal ganglia lesions are associated with depression in humans while right frontal lesions are significantly associated with the indifference response or sometimes mania (see Chapter 25) (Robinson *et al.* 1984; Starkstein *et al.* 1989). The indifference response is

Table 21.1. Demographic characteristics of patients with left hemisphere or right hemisphere stroke

Characteristics	Left hemisphere stroke ($n = 8$)	Right hemisphere stroke ($n = 9$)
Gender		
Male	7	4
Female	1	5
Race		
Black	1	4
Caucasian	7	5
Marital status		
Married	5	5
Single/widowed	2	1
Divorced/separated	1	3
Hollingshead (class IV or V)	5	9
Other medical illnesses (hypertension, diabetes, or heart disease)	4	7
Prior psychiatric illness	1	0
Smoking history (one pack or more/day)	4	6
Alcohol abuse	0	1
Medications		
Antihypertensives	5	4
Anticonvulsants	0	2
Minor tranquilizers	3	2
Lithium	1	0

characterized by undue cheerfulness, lack of concern, and elevated mood. If the indifference response or mania may be the result of disinhibition which may be manifested as spontaneous hyperactivity in the rat, this could provide an animal model of poststroke mood disorders based on similarities in lesion location.

In another clinical study implicating serotonin in poststroke depression, we examined postsynaptic serotonergic receptors in patients with stroke using positron emission tomography (PET) (Mayberg *et al.* 1988). Patients with right hemisphere stroke ($n = 9$) were compared to patients with left hemisphere stroke ($n = 8$) and age-comparable normal controls ($n = 17$). The background characteristics of the patients based on lesion hemisphere are shown in Table 21.1. There were no statistically significant differences in background characteristics, previous medical history, use of medications at the time of the PET scan study, or neurological findings. Similarly, there were no statistically significant differences in the volume of the lesion, the anterior or posterior borders of the lesion, frequency of subcortical involvement or frontal cortical involvement. Clinical evaluations and PET scans were done 18 ± 14 (SD) months poststroke for left hemisphere lesion patients and 15 ± 9 months poststroke for right hemisphere lesion patients ($p =$ NS). There were no significant intergroup differences in activities of daily living scores or degree of cognitive impairment.

Patients were administered [3-N–^{11}C]methylspiperone (NMSP) intravenously over 10–20 s. It has been demonstrated in other studies that NMSP binding in human cerebral cortex is predominantly serotonin S_2 receptors (or 5-HT$_2$ receptors) (Lyon *et al.* 1986). Although 5-HT$_2$-receptor binding was significantly decreased in several brain regions that included the stroke site (e.g., for right hemisphere strokes, the number of radioactive counts in the area of cortex which included the stroke lesion compared to uninjured cortex was 0.67 ± 0.32 and for left hemisphere strokes it was 0.76 ± 0.13, indicating significantly less binding in the injured compared with uninjured cortex). In *uninjured* areas of temporal and parietal cortex, however, right hemisphere stroke led to increased 5-HT$_2$-receptor binding in the ipsilateral compared with the symmetrical area of cortex (Fig. 21.4). Left hemisphere strokes, however, did not produce an increase in binding ratio (i.e., ipsilateral radioactive counts divided by radioactive counts in symmetrical contralateral area) compared to controls or patients with left hemisphere stroke. Using either non-parametric

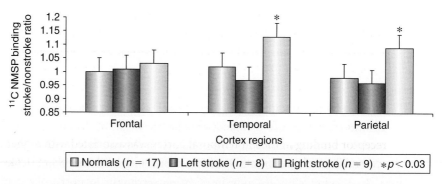

Figure 21.4 PET measurements of NMSP binding to cortical S_2 serotonin receptors in non-injured areas of frontal, temporal and parietal cortex following first ever right or left stroke. Binding was measured by comparing radioactive counts in the region of interest to non-specific binding in the cerebellum and then comparing the stroke hemisphere to an identical area of the opposite hemisphere. Although left hemisphere stroke ($n = 8$) produced slightly decreased binding in temporal and parietal cortex, there was a significant *increase* in S_2 receptors in temporal and parietal cortex following right hemisphere lesions ($n = 9$). The control subjects ($n = 17$) were age and sex distribution comparable normals (data from Mayberg *et al.* 1988).

or parametric statistics, NMSP activity (i.e., ratio of ipsilateral to contralateral radioactivity counts) was significantly higher in the temporal cortex ($p = 0.029$) and parietal cortex ($p = 0.018$) among patients with right hemisphere stroke compared to patients with left hemisphere stroke or normal controls. There were no significant differences, however, in the number of 5-HT$_2$ receptors in the frontal cortex among patients with right or left hemisphere stroke and normal controls.

As an increase in 5-HT$_2$ binding ratio could result from either increased binding in the injured hemisphere or a decreased binding in the uninjured hemisphere, we compared uninjured (normal) cortex with binding in the cerebellum (there are no known 5-HT$_2$ receptors in cerebellum so this represents nonspecific binding). Patients with left hemisphere stroke had cortical to cerebellar binding ratios in the right (i.e., contralateral uninjured) frontal, temporal, and parietal cortices which were not significantly different to binding ratios in the contralateral hemisphere among patients with right hemisphere stroke. This finding indicates that the higher degree of 5-HT$_2$-receptor binding in patients with right hemisphere stroke compared with left hemisphere stroke is due to greater binding in the right (i.e., ipsilateral cortex) rather than less binding in the left (i.e., contralateral cortex). The amount of cortical serotonergic binding, both ipsilateral and contralateral to the stroke, however, was lower in patients with ischemic brain lesions compared to normal controls. This generalized decrease in 5-HT$_2$ receptors in patients with stroke was probably due to generalized cerebrovascular disease which decreased the overall number of serotonin receptors throughout the brain.

Among patients with left hemisphere strokes, the ipsilateral to contralateral NMSP binding ratio (i.e., 5-HT$_2$ binding) in the left temporal cortex was highly correlated (using either Spearman's correlations or Pearson's correlations) with the Zung depression score (Fig. 21.5). Furthermore, correlations between left temporal cortical binding and Hamilton depression score or present state examination (PSE) total score were also significant or nearly significant (Hamilton: $r = 0.62$, $p < 0.1$; PSE: $r = 0.76$, $p < 0.05$). This finding showed that a lower level of 5-HT$_2$-receptor binding in the left temporal cortex was associated with higher depression scores. This only held, however, for patients with left hemisphere stroke (i.e., there were no significant correlations between depression scores and 5-HT$_2$-receptor binding in frontal, temporal, or parietal cortex following right hemisphere stroke or frontal or parietal cortex following left hemisphere stroke).

In summary, this study demonstrated that, at approximately 16 months after injury, right hemisphere lesions were associated with an increase in serotonin 5-HT$_2$-receptor binding in uninjured areas of temporal and parietal cortex while left hemisphere strokes were not. Furthermore, among patients with left hemisphere stroke, a decreased quantity of 5-HT$_2$ receptors in the left temporal cortex was found to be associated with an increased severity of depressive symptoms.

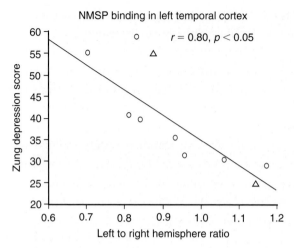

Figure 21.5 Relationship between Zung depression score PET measures of NMSP binding to S$_2$ serotonin receptors in the temporal cortex following a left hemisphere stroke (n = 8) (open circles). The binding is expressed on the horizontal axis as a ratio of binding in the left temporal cortex to binding in an identical region of the right temporal cortex. Lower numbers indicate less S$_2$ serotonin receptor binding. Lower S$_2$ receptors were associated with higher depression scores. The triangles indicate receptor changes in one patient who had spontaneous remission of a major depression. As the depression score fell from 55 to 25, the amount of serotonin S$_2$ receptor binding increased from 0.86 to 1.15. This patient with a small left basal ganglia infarct demonstrated that S$_2$ receptor binding may be a state marker for poststroke depression (data from Mayberg *et al.* 1988).

We have also examined some of the anatomical structures which play an important role in poststroke depression using measures of metabolic activity derived from [^{18}F] fluorodeoxyglucose (FDG) PET imaging (Mayberg 1993). For many years it has been known that lesions in one area of the brain are capable of producing dysfunction in remote areas, a phenomenon referred to as diaschisis (Baron 1989). A group of six patients with single lesions of the basal ganglia restricted to the head of the caudate with or without extension into the anterior limb of the internal capsule were studied using FDG PET imaging. When the three patients with depression were compared to three patients with comparable lesions of the caudate nucleus but without mood disorder, bilateral hypometabolism in orbitofrontal cortex, anterior temporal cortex, and cingulate cortex was seen in patients with depression but not in the controls (Fig 21.6). The controls only showed decreased metabolic activity in the frontal cortex, presumably as a result of interruption of the frontal to caudate neuronal projections with decreased activity of the frontal neurons. The most pronounced changes, however, occurred in the temporal lobes of depressed patients. Patients with depression had marked bilateral decreases in the metabolic rate of

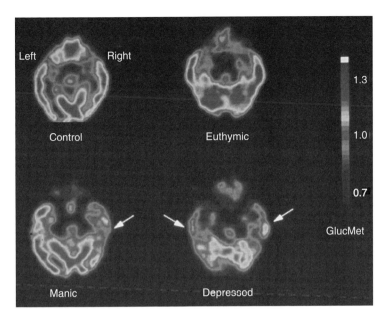

Figure 21.6   FDG PET scans in patients with single caudate lesions and varying mood states. Scans at
the level of the temporal lobe are shown in four subjects. Patients with euthymia have
normal and symmetric temporal lobe metabolism; in contrast, patients with mania show
unilateral (right-sided) temporal hypometabolism and patients with depression show
bilateral temporal hypometabolism. GlucMet: glucose metabolism.

the inferior temporal lobe and also cingulate cortex hypometabolism. In contrast,
patients with euthymia had normal temporal and cingulate metabolism. Thus,
although depressed and non-depressed patients had frontal cortex hypometabolism, the depressed patients had additional areas of decreased activity in temporal and cingulate cortices.

Before discussing the implications of these findings to suggest an anatomical
substrate for poststroke depression, it is worthwhile to examine the literature on
depression in the elderly (without overt stroke lesions) for findings which may illu-
minate the mechanisms of depression in patients with stroke. Since 1990 (Coffey
et al. 1993), it has been reported that deep white matter hyperintensities (DWMH)
and periventricular hyperintensities (PVH), as identified on magnetic resonance
imaging (MRI) scan, have been associated with late, compared with early, onset of
major depression (Hickie *et al.* 1995). Krishnan *et al.* (1997) compared 32 elderly
patients with major depressive disorder and encephalomalasia with 57 patients
with major depressive disorder without encephalomalasia. After controlling for
age, the group characterized by hyperintensities on MRI had later age at onset of
depression and tended to have lower frequency of positive family history of mood
disorder. Greenwald *et al.* (1998) demonstrated an association between major

depression in the elderly and left frontal deep white matter ($p < 0.005$) and left putamenal ($p < 0.04$) hyperintensities. A recent MRI study of 88 elderly depressed patients and 47 age and gender matched non-depressed controls revealed, using statistical parametric mapping, two major regions of increased lesion density in depressed patients. One in the medial–orbital–prefrontal white matter and one in a region of the left internal capsule (MacFall et al. 2001).

Thomas et al. (2002) conducted the first study which examined the neuropathology of the white matter hyperintensities among patients with a history of major depressive disorder. MRI scans of three brain regions were done in 20 elderly patients with a history of major depression and 20 matched controls. Neuropathological examination found that all of the DWMH in the depressed sample were ischemic compared to the controls where less than a third of the DWMH were ischemic ($p < 0.001$). The non-ischemic DWMH were primarily small lesions (less than 3 mm) while larger lesions reflected ischemic damage in both groups. Furthermore, ischemic lesions in the depressed patients were more likely to be in the dorsal–lateral–prefrontal cortex compared with the controls.

Using PET brain imaging in non-elderly patients, Drevets et al. (1998) have found reduced regional cerebral blood flow and regional cerebral metabolic rate for glucose in the subgenual area of prefrontal cortex in patients with unipolar or bipolar depression. Subsequent neuropathological investigations found a pronounced loss of gray matter in this region in both unipolar and bipolar mood disorder. Using xenon ^{133}XE inhalation in 20 elderly outpatients with major depressive disorder who had a minimum of 14 days off all psychotropic medications and 20 age, sex, and blood pressure matched normal controls. Nobler et al. (2000) found decreased cerebral blood flow in prefrontal, superior temporal and anterior parietal regions in the depressed groups. Subsequent study using PET found a mismatch between cerebral blood flow and cerebral metabolic rate for glucose with greater deficits relative to controls in cerebral blood flow suggesting that depression in the elderly is more closely related to changes in vascular supply than to changes in neuronal activity (Sackeim et al. 1993).

Based on these studies of primary and poststroke depression, we have proposed the following hypothesis about the anatomical basis of some poststroke depressions (i.e., acute onset depression following left frontal or basal ganglia lesions). The left prefrontal cortex appears to play a central role in the etiology of these depressions (Fig. 21.7). Although it must be acknowledged that observed abnormalities in left prefrontal cortical brain function may be the distant effect of another more central abnormality, such as interruption of the biogenic amines projecting to the frontal lobe, or by genetic abnormalities, the convergence of data provides a strong argument that this region plays a central role in the etiology of depression. The temporal polar cortex is connected with the anterior orbitofrontal

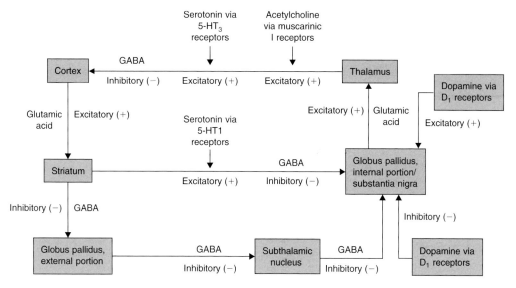

Figure 21.7 Circuit diagram showing the pathways which may mediate the mechanism of poststroke depression. These circuits could explain why both cortical and striatal lesions can lead to depression. GABA: gamma aminobutyric acid.

cortex through the uncinate fasciculus which maintains inhibitory input to the amygdala (Crosby *et al.* 1962). The frontal and prefrontal cortices also have efferent connections with the anterior cingulate cortex and caudate nucleus, as well as with the orbitofrontal cortex (Alexander *et al.* 1986). The dorsal lateral cortex, the lateral orbital frontal cortex and cingulate all project to the basal ganglia, as does the amygdala. These subcortical basal ganglia projections then project to the internal or external globus pallidus and then to the subthalamic nucleus or the dorsal medial nucleus of the thalamus. The dorsal medial nucleus in turn projects back to the prefrontal and orbitofrontal cortex (Fig. 21.7). These neuronal circuits appear to mediate cognitive (i.e., executive functions), inhibitory, motivation, and mood symptoms. If frontal abnormalities as well as dysfunction of another brain region such as the temporal pole, amygdala, basal ganglia, or thalamus are needed to produce depression, the cyclical nature of most depressions could be explained by distant episodic effects of a lesion in one area and chronic (i.e., direct brain lesion) effects in another area.

Recently, an alternative hypothesis for the etiology of poststroke depression has been proposed. This hypothesis is based on the release of proinflammatory cytokines due to ischemic neuronal damage was proposed by Spalletta *et al.* (in preparation). This hypothesis was based on the findings that Thomas *et al.* (2000) assayed intercellular adhesion molecule-1 (ICAN-1) in the dorsal–lateral–prefrontal cortex and occipital cortex in 20 deceased individuals over age 60 with a history of major depressive disorder and 20 comparison subjects. Expression of ICAN-1 was significantly greater in the dorsal lateral prefrontal cortex gray and white matter of the depressed group with no difference in the occipital cortex compared with controls. Subsequently, it was hypothesized that cytokines may suppress serotonin by activating the enzyme indoleamine-2,3-dioxygenase (IDO) that catabolizes tryptophan. Thus, IDO activation would prevent tryptophan from being converted to serotonin, leading to decreased levels of serotonin (Capuron and Dantzer 2003). Furthermore, cerebral ischemia has been shown to lead to increases in the proinflammatory cytokine interleukin-1β (IL-1β) (Tarkowski *et al.* 1995). Thus stroke may lead to increased production of cytokines such as ICAN-1 or IL-1β which then leads to decreases in the production of biogenic amines and subsequently to clinical symptoms of depressive disorder.

Finally, we have recently investigated another alternative hypothesis for the etiology of poststroke depression involving the ability of patients with stroke lesions of the basal ganglia to experience positive and negative emotion (Paradiso *et al.* 2002). Ten patients with focal right basal ganglia lesions were compared with eight patients with focal left basal ganglia lesions and 27 age-comparable controls with no brain lesions. The patients with right basal ganglia lesions had a significant decrease in their reported feelings of sadness or fear following the presentation of standardized photographs showing sad or fearful faces or scenes compared to patients with left basal ganglia lesions or controls. Patients having right lesions who were approximately 8 months following stroke also had a decreased perception of positive emotion compared with patients having left lesions or controls. These findings suggested that the inability to perceive positive or negative emotion could lead to the indifference reaction (associated with decreased perception of negative stimuli) or depression (associated with decreased perception of positive stimuli) in patients with stroke. This impaired mediation of emotion hypothesis implicates the same anatomical structures as the PET and MRI lesion findings but suggests that the impaired processes may not specifically involve the biogenic amines but rather the perception or interpretation of emotional feelings.

Other hypotheses may also be proposed but the preponderance of evidence both from poststroke depression studies as well as depression in the elderly have consistently implicated a similar set of neural structures as outlined in Fig. 21.7.

In summary, although the etiology of poststroke depression, like all depressive disorders, is not known, our findings that metabolites of serotonin are decreased in the spinal fluid of depressed stroke patients and that serotonin receptors are decreased in the left temporal cortex of depressed stroke patients, suggests an important role of serotonin depletion in the cause of poststroke major depression. We have hypothesized that the cortical-thalamic circuits described by Alexander *et al.* (1990) are disrupted by direct ischemic injury or altered serotonergic modulation to produce the symptoms of poststroke depression. Recent work has also suggested some modifications to this hypothesis. For example, ischemic brain injury could lead to increased production of proinflammatory cytokines which in turn activate or inhibit enzymes leading to decreased production of brain serotonin. Furthermore, the disruption of certain frontal-thalamic circuits could be manifested by decreased perception of emotional stimuli. This phenomenon could be mediated by serotonergic dysfunction. The inability to experience happy (i.e., positive) emotional feelings could lead to depression. This is an area desperately needing further research.

REFERENCES

Alexander, G. E., Crutcher, M. D., and DeLong, M. R. Basal ganglia-thalamocortical circuits: parallel substrates for motor, oculomotor, "prefrontal" and "limbic" functions. *Prog Brain Res* (1990) 85:119–146.

Alexander, G. E., DeLong, M. R., and Strick, P. L. Parallel organization of functionally segregated circuits linking basal ganglia and cortex. *Annu Rev Neurosci* (1986) 9:357–381.

Baron, J. C. Depression of energy metabolism in distant brain structures: studies with positron emission tomography in stroke patients. *Semin Neurol* (1989) 9:281–285.

Bryer, J.B., Starkstein, S.E., Votypka, V., *et al.* Reduction of CSF monoamine metabolites in poststroke depression. *J Neuropsychiatr Clin Neurosci* (1992) 4:440–442.

Capuron, L., and Dantzer, R. Cytokines and depression: the need for a new paradigm. *Brain Behav Immun* (2003) 17(Suppl 1):S119–S124.

Coffey, C. E., Wilkinson, W. E., Weiner, R. D., *et al.* Quantitative cerebral anatomy in depression. A controlled magnetic resonance imaging study. *Arch Gen Psychiatr* (1993) 50(1):7–16.

Crosby, E., Humphrey, T., and Laner, E. *Correlative Anatomy of the Nervous System.* MacMillan, New York, 1962.

Drevets, W. C., Ongur, D., and Price, J. L. Reduced glucose metabolism in the subgenual prefrontal cortex in unipolar depression. *Mol Psychiatr* (1998) 3(3):190–191.

Gainotti, G., Azzoni, A., and Marra, C. Frequency, phenomenology and anatomical–clinical correlates of major post-stroke depression. *Br J Psychiatr* (1999) 175:163–167.

Greenwald, B. S., Kramer-Ginsberg, E., Krishnan, R. R., *et al.* Neuroanatomic localization of magnetic resonance imaging signal hyperintensities in geriatric depression. *Stroke* (1998) 29:613–617.

Hickie, I., Scott, E., Mitchell, P., *et al.* Subcortical hyperintensities on magnetic resonance imaging: clinical correlates and prognostic significance in patients with severe depression. *Biol Psychiatr* (1995) 37:151–160.

Krishnan, K. R. R., Hays, J. C., and Blazer, D. G. MRI-defined vascular depression. *Am J Psychiatr* (1997) 154:497–501.

Kubos, K. L., Moran, T. H., and Robinson, R. G. Differential and asymmetrical behavioral effects of electrolytic or 6-hydroxydopamine lesions in the nucleus accumbens. *Brain Res* (1987) 401:147–151.

Lyketsos, C.G., Treisman, G.J., Lipsey, J.R., et al. Does stroke cause depression? *J Neuropsychiatr Clin Neurosci* (1998) 10: 103–107.

Lyon, R. A., Titeler, M., and Frost, J. J. H-3-N-methylspiperone labels D2-dopamine receptors in basal ganglia and S2 serotonin receptors in cerebral cortex. *J Neurosci* (1986) 6:2941–2949.

MacFall, J. R., Payne, M. E., Provenzale, J. E., et al. Medial orbital frontal lesions in late onset depression. *Biol Psychiatr* (2001) 49:803–806.

Mayberg, H. S. Neuroimaging studies of depression in neurologic disease. In S. E. Starkstein and R. G. Robinson, eds., *Depression in Neurologic Disease*. Johns Hopkins Press, Baltimore, 1993.

Mayberg, H. S., Robinson, R. G., Wong, D. F., et al. PET imaging of cortical S_2-serotonin receptors after stroke: lateralized changes and relationship to depression. *Am J Psychiatr* (1988) 145:937–943.

McHugh, P. R., and Slavney, P. R. *Perspectives of Psychiatry*. Johns Hopkins University Press, Baltimore, London, 1998.

Morrison, J. H., Molliver, M. E., and Grzanna, R. Noradrenergic innervation of the cerebral cortex: widespread effects of local cortical lesions. *Science* (1979) 205:313–316.

Nobler, M. S., Roose, S. P., Prohovnik, I., et al. Regional cerebral blood flow in mood disorders, V: Effects of antidepressant medication in late-life depression. *Am J Geriatr Psychiatr* (2000) 8(4):289–296.

Paradiso, S., Hansen, R., and Robinson, R. G. Affective dementia? Age associated reduction of blood flow in limbic areas associated with impaired appraisal of unpleasant stimuli. Presented at *Second International Congress on Vascular Dementia Conference*, Salzburg, Austria, 2002.

Pearlson, G. D., and Robinson, R. G. Suction lesions of the frontal cerebral cortex in the rat induce asymmetrical behavioral and catecholaminergic responses. *Brain Res* (1981) 218:233–242.

Pearlson, G.D., and Robinsn, R.G. Effect of anterior–posterior lesion location on the asymmetrical behavioral and biochemical response to cortical suction ablations in the rat. *Brain Res* (1984) 293: 241–250.

Robinson, R. G., Kubos, K. L., Starr, L. B., et al. Mood disorders in stroke patients: importance of location of lesion. *Brain* (1984) 107:81–93.

Ross, R. A., Joh, T. H., and Reis, D. J. Reversible changes in the accumulation and activity of tyrosine hydroxylase and dopamine B hydroxylase in neurons of the locus coeruleus during the retrograde reaction. *Brain Res* (1975) 92:57–72.

Sackeim, H. A., Prohovnik, I., Moeller, J. R., et al. Regional cerebral blood flow in mood disorders. II. Comparison of major depression and Alzheimer's disease. *J Nucl Med* (1993) 34(7):1090–1101.

Starkstein, S. E., Robinson, R. G., Hoing, M. A., et al. Mood changes after right hemisphere lesion. *Br J Psychiatry* (1989) 155:79–85.

Tarkowski, E., Rosengren, L., Blomstrand, C., et al. Early intrathecal production of interleukin-6 predicts the size of brain lesion in stroke. *Stroke* (1995) 26:1393–1398.

Thomas, A. J., Ferrier, I. N., Kalaria, R. N., et al. Elevation in late-life depression of intercellular adhesion molecule-1 expression in the dorsolateral prefrontal cortex. *Am J Psychiatr* (2000) 157(10):1682–1684.

Thomas, A. J., O'Brien, J. T., Davis, S., et al. Ischemic basis for deep white matter hyperintensities in major depression: a neuropathological study. *Arch Gen Psychiatr* (2002) 59(9):785–792.

22

Treatment of poststroke depression

Background

Although our use of treatment modalities in medicine has been driven by studies demonstrating efficacy of treatment, our choice among competing treatment is often influenced by our conceptualization of the cause of the disorder. Poststroke depression may be viewed from either a social–psychological perspective or a physiological–biological perspective. These two perspectives could lead to different and sometimes mutually exclusive treatment approaches. As evidenced by the number of studies of poststroke depression, both psychological and family interventions have been proposed or utilized, although the great majority of studies have examined pharmacological treatment. Clinicians, however, who view poststroke depression as an understandable consequence of unwanted physical dependency or inadequate social support may have little enthusiasm for pharmacological approaches. It is unlikely, however, that these conceptualizations are mutually exclusive and the most pragmatic approach is probably a combination of both pharmacological treatment and psychological assistance in addressing the patient's response to stroke related impairments.

In spite of increasing empirical support for the importance of pharmacological treatment in poststroke depression, there continue to be reports of patients who have not received adequate treatment or whose depression has not been treated. Patients whose depressions following stroke have not been recognized, in general, have failed to receive an assessment for poststroke depression. The US Department of Health and Human Services Guidelines for Stroke Rehabilitation (Gresham *et al.* 1995), however, documents the need to evaluate poststroke patients for depression. As early as 1982, Feibel and Springer (1982) reported that although 31 of 85 acute stroke patients had moderate to severe depressive symptoms, depression was diagnosed and treated in only three of these cases. These authors referred to this lack of treatment of depression, as one of the great unmet needs of stroke survivors. More recent studies have also documented the continued failure of some treating physicians to recognize and treat poststroke depressive disorders (Schubert *et al.* 1992).

During the past decade there have been a significant number of studies published on the treatment on poststroke depression. This literature has increased to a size that, I believe, makes the treatment of poststroke depression the most extensively researched treatment in psychosomatic medicine. The published studies, organized by design, are shown in Table 22.1.

Pharmacological treatments

In contrast to the sparse literature on psychological intervention, pharmacological treatment has a large empirical database to support its efficacy in poststroke depression. The available data is of sufficient volume to document that the failure to include appropriate pharmacological treatment in the management of poststroke depression if there are no contraindications, withholds an important treatment modality which could improve the patient's psychological, as well as physical, recovery from stroke. The previous findings presented in Chapters 13 and 14 document the importance of pharmacological treatment in the improved recovery of both physical impairment, as measured by activities of daily living (ADL), and cognitive impairment following stroke. In addition, in Chapter 18 we presented data which showed the possible role of pharmacological intervention in decreasing mortality following stroke. These findings together present a strong case for the use of pharmacological treatment in the care of patients with poststroke depression.

Anecdotal reports in the literature since the early 1980s have suggested the efficacy of antidepressant treatment for poststroke depression (Ross and Rush 1981). The first controlled treatment trial was conducted by our group and published in 1984 (Lipsey *et al.* 1984). The study included 39 patients who were in an acute stroke hospital, a rehabilitation hospital or were outpatients who met Diagnostic and Statistical Manual (DSM-III) diagnostic criteria for either major or minor (dysthymic) depressive disorder who were treated with nortriptyline ($n = 17$) or placebo ($n = 22$). The patients were not significantly different in their mean age, racial mix, social class, gender, marital status, or time since stroke. Mean age was 62 ± 9 years in the nortriptyline and 60 ± 12 years in the 20 placebo patients. The mean time since stroke was 261 days $\pm$ 437 SD in the nortriptyline group and 128 ± 190 SD in the placebo group.

The patients received 25 mg of nortriptyline for week 1, 50 mg during weeks 2 and 3, 75 mg during weeks 3 and 4 and 100 mg during weeks 5 and 6. In the nortriptyline group, 100% of the patients had mono or hemiparesis compared to 95% in the placebo group. Similarly, 21% of the nortriptyline and 10% of the placebo group had aphasia. In addition, CT scan analysis demonstrated that there were no significant

Table 22.1. Treatment studies of poststroke depression

Author (year)	n	Medication (n) (maximum dose)	Duration	Evaluation method	Results	Response rate	Completion rate
Double-blind placebo-controlled studies							
Lipsey et al. (1984)	34	Nortriptyline (14) (maximum 100 mg)	6 weeks	Ham-D, ZDS,	Nortriptyline > placebo intention to treat and efficacy	Completers: 100% Nortriptyline 33% Placebo	11 of 14 Nortriptyline 15 of 20 Placebo
Reding et al. (1986)	27	Trazodone (7) (maximum 200 mg) Placebo (9)	32 + 6 days	ZDS	Efficacy: trazodone > placebo on Barthel ADL for patients with abnormal DST	NR	
Andersen (1994b)	66	Citalopram (33) (20 mg, 10 mg > 65 years) Placebo (33)	6 weeks	Ham-D, MES	Intention to treat Citalopram > placebo	Completers: 61% Citalopram 29% Placebo	26 of 33 Citalopram 31 of 33 Placebo
Grade et al. (1998)	21	Methylphenidate 30 mg (maximum 30 mg)	3 weeks	Ham-D	Intention to treat Methylphenidate > placebo	NR	9 of 10 Methylphenidate Placebo 10 of 11 Placebo
Wiart et al. (2000)	31	Fluoxetine (20 mg) Placebo	6 weeks	MADRS	Intention to treat Fluoxetine > placebo	62% Fluoxetine 33% Placebo	14 of 16 Fluoxetine 15 of 15 Placebo
Robinson et al. (2000)	56	Fluoxetine (23) (40 mg) Nortriptyline (16) (100 mg) Placebo (17)	12 weeks	Ham-D	Intention to treat Nortriptyline > both Fluoxetine = placebo	14% Fluoxetine 77% Nortriptyline 31% Placebo	14 of 23 Fluoxetine 13 of 16 Nortriptyline 13 of 17 Placebo
Fruehwald (2003)	54	Fluoxetine (28) (20 mg) Placebo (26)	12 weeks	Beck (BDF) Ham-D	Ham-D > 15 Fluoxetine = placebo Ham-D scores	69% Fluoxetine Ham-D ≤ 13 75% Placebo	26 of 28 Fluoxetine 24 of 26 Placebo

Table 22.1. (*Continued*)

Author (year)	n	Medication (n) (maximum dose)	Duration	Evaluation method	Results	Response rate	Completion rate
Double-blind studies without placebo control							
Miyai et al. (2000)	24	Desipramine (13) (100 mg); Trazodone (6) (100 mg); Fluoxetine (5) (20 mg)	4 weeks	Ham-D	Desipramine = Trazodone = Fluoxetine No placebo comparison	NR	8 of 13 Desipramine; 6 of 6 Trazodone; 4 of 5 Fluoxetine
Lauritzen et al. (1994)	20	Imipramine (mean 75 mg) + Mianserin (mean 25 mg); Desipramine (mean 66 mg) + Mianserin (mean 27 mg)	6 weeks	Ham-D, MES	Intention to treat Imipramine + Mianserin > Desipramine + Mianserin on MES not Ham-D	Ham-D no difference MES 81% Imipramine + mianserin; 13% Desipramine + Mianserin	8 of 10 Imipramine + Mianserin; 5 of 10 Desipramine + Mianserin
Open label/Retrospective							
Gonzalez-Torrecillas (1995)	37	*Open label* Fluoxetine (26) (20 mg); Nortriptyline (11) (75+ mg); Untreated (11)	4 weeks	Ham-D, MADRS, BDI	Efficacy analysis Fluoxetine = Nortriptyline = Nortriptyline > no treatment	NR	25 of 26 Fluoxetine; 10 of 11 Nortriptyline; 10 of 11 Uuntreated
Lazarus et al. (1992)	58	*Retrospective* Methylphenidate (28) (26 mg); Nortriptyline (30) (58 mg)	5 days; 4 weeks	Clinical evaluation	Methylphenidate = Nortriptyline in response rate	Remission 53% Methylphenidate; 43% Nortriptyline	NA

Study	N	Design/Treatment (dose)	Duration	Measure	Results		
Balunov (1990)	90	*Open label* Amitriptyline (30) (75 mg) Seduxene (30) (1.5 mg) Untreated (30)	4 weeks	Ham-D	Amitriptyline > Seduxene = nc treatment	Response 100% Amitriptyline NSR NR no treatment	NR
Shima (1997)	20	*Open label* Not specified e.g., Imipramine Amoxapine	4 weeks	Clinical evaluation	10 of 10 < age 65 significantly or moderately improved 3 of 10 > 65 improved	NR	100%
Stamenkovic et al. (1996)	10	*Open label* Fluoxetine (10) (20 mg)	8 weeks	Ham-D, BDI	Mean Ham-D 32.4–11.4 Mean BDI 46.6–11.2	NR	50%
Finklestine et al. (1987)	60	*Retrospective* cyclic drugs (42) No treatment (18)	6 weeks	Clinical	40% of treated patients improved versus 17% of untreated	NR	NA
Lazarus (1992)	10	*Open label* Methylphenidate (10) (17 mg mean)	3 weeks	Ham-D	4 of 10 had >50% reduction of Ham-D	40%	100%
Masand et al. (1991)	17	*Retrospective* Methylphenidate (6) (9.2 mean) Dextroam (11) (8.4 mean)	3 days	CGI	2 of 6 Methylphenidate 6 of 11 Dextroamphetamine improved moderately	NR	NA
Dam (1996)	52	*Open label* Fluoxetine (16) (20 mg) Maprotiline (17) (150 mg) Placebo (17)	3 months	Ham-D	No group difference in final Ham-D Maprotiline and Fluoxetine significantly decreased initial to final	NR	16 of 18 Fluoxetine (89%) 14 of 17 Maprotiline (82%) 16 of 17 placebo (94%)

Table 22.1. (*Continued*)

Author (year)	n	Medication (n) (maximum dose)	Duration	Evaluation method	Results	Response rate	Completion rate
Paolucci (2001)	136	*Open label* Fluoxetine (120) (20 mg) Paroxetine (16)	NR	Ham-D	Significantly decreased Ham-D for both Fluoxetine and Paroxetine	80.6% Response to overall no group difference	116 of 120 Fluoxetine 15 of 16 Paroxetine
Spalletta et al. (2002)	48	*Open label* Fluoxetine (24) (20–40 mg) Sertraline (21) (50–100 mg)	8 weeks	Ham-D	Right stroke Ham-D improved more than left	88% right stroke 40% left stroke responded	45 of 48 no description of drug received
Martensson et al. (1997)	8	*Open label* Buspirone (8) (30–60 mg)	8 weeks	MADRS CGI	Significantly decreased over 8 weeks in MADRS	75%	100%
Johnson et al. (1992)	10	*Retrospective* Methylphenidate (10 mg)	5 days–1 month	Clinical assessment	7 of 10 patients improved	NR	100%
Kimura et al. (2002)	12	*Open label* Milnacipram (30–75 mg bid)	6 weeks	Ham-D	7 of 10 with Ham-D < 7	70% remission	83%
Zifko et al. (2002)	267	*Open label* Sertraline (267) (50 mg)	12 weeks	WHO-Well being CGI	CGI 88% improved with significance WHO-WI score	NR	97%
Murray (1986)	14	*Retrospective* ECT (14) (non-dominant unilateral)	3–18 days	Clinical	12 of 14 improved	NR	NR

Study	N	Treatment	Dose/sessions	Measures	Outcome		
Currier (1992)	20	*Retrospective* ECT (20) (19 non-dominant unilateral)	5–20 Rx	Clinical	19 of 20 marked or moderate improvement, 7 of 19 relapsed	NR	100%
Stamenkovic (1996)	10	Fluoxetine (20 mg) Paroxetine (16) (20 mg)	8 weeks	Ham-D, BDI, CGI	Fluoxetine produced significantly decreased in MD, BDI, CGI	NR	5
Hougaku et al. (1994)	20	*Open label* Lisuride maleate (0.075 mg)	12 weeks	SRQ-D, Ham-D	47% marked or moderate improvement, 88% more than mild improvement	NR	17 of 20 completed
Psychological treatment							
Lincoln (1997)	19	Open CBT (19)	10 sessions: 3 months (mean 8 sessions)	Beck Depression Hospital Anxiety and Depression	8 patients improved BDI score, 11 no improvement	NR	16 of 19 (84%)
Lincoln (2003)	123	Open CBT (39) Attention: Placebo (43) No treatment (41)	10 sessions: 3 months 10 sessions: 3 months No contact	Beck Depression, Wakefield depression	60 patients with depression Dx, no group difference at 3 or 6 months	NR	NR
Transcranial magnetic stimulation							
Jorge (2003)	20	*Double-blind* Active rTMS (10) Sham rTMS (10)	3 weeks 10 Rx 3 weeks 10 Rx	Ham-D	Active group significantly greater reduction in Ham-D than sham	30% active 0%	100% both groups 100% both groups

CGI: clinical global impression; Dx: diagnostic; NSR: National schedule of rates; Rx: treatment; SRQ-D: self-rating questionnaire for depression; WI: Wakefield Depression Inventory; ZDS: zung depression scale; not reported.

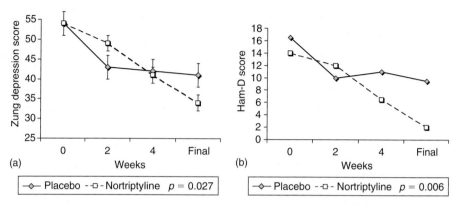

Figure 22.1   Hamilton (a) and Zung (b) depression scores over 6 weeks of double-blind treatment with nortriptyline (dose 20–100 mg/day) (n = 11) or placebo (n = 15). Although placebo-treated patients showed some improvement, the nortriptyline-treated patients had significantly lower Ham-D scores at 4 weeks, and significantly lower Hamilton and Zung depression scores at 6 weeks compared with the placebo group [modified from Lipsey *et al.* (1984), reprinted with permission].

differences between the active and placebo groups in their frequency of right or left hemisphere lesions, lesion volume or in mean distance of lesion from the frontal pole. Placebo and active treatment groups were also not significantly different in their ADL scores (i.e. Johns Hopkins functioning inventory (JHFI) scores were 11.5 ± 4.5 for the nortriptyline groups versus 9.1 ± 5.9 for the placebo group). Patients, however, differed in their cognitive impairment with the nortriptyline group being more impaired than the placebo group (mini-mental state examination (MMSE) scores nortriptyline 20.4 ± 6.2, placebo 24.4 ± 4.7, $p = 0.04$). Of the 17 nortriptyline patients, 11 were completers while 15 of the 22 placebo patients completed the study. Intention-to-treat analysis of Hamilton depression (Ham-D) scores versus time with last observation carried forward found a significant time-by-treatment interaction. The nortriptyline group showing significantly greater improvement than the placebo group (Fig. 22.1, $p = 0.026$). Similarly efficacy analysis demonstrated that among the 26 patients who completed the entire study the nortriptyline group improved in Ham-D scores more than the placebo group ($p = 0.006$).

Treatment response was determined by having a >50% reduction in Ham-D score while remission rate was determined by having a final Ham-D score below 8. Intention-to-treat analysis showed that 14 of 17 (82%) nortriptyline patients were both responders and remitters compared to 8 of 22 (36%) placebo patients who were both responders and remitters ($p = 0.002$). Efficacy analysis showed a 100% response and remission rate among active treatment patients and a 40% response and remission rate among the placebo patients ($p = 0.0002$).

Serum nortriptyline levels at week 2 following 1 week of 50 mg of nortriptyline were 63 ± 44 ng/ml SD and at week 4, after 1 week of 75 mg, the mean serum concentration mean was 74 ± 38 ng/ml and at week 6, after 2 weeks of 100 mg, mean serum level was 116 ± 40 ng/ml SD. Mean nortriptyline levels between weeks 4 and 6 were significantly different. Repeated measures analysis of variance (ANOVA) failed to show any significant difference between active and placebo groups in terms of improvement of cognitive function (i.e. MMSE) or ADL (i.e., JHFI score) over the 6 week treatment period.

The second double-blind treatment trial for poststroke depression was conducted by Reding *et al.* in 1986. In this study 27 patients approximately 6 weeks poststroke who were participants in a stroke rehabilitation program were randomly assigned to treatment with either trazodone hydrochloride or placebo (Reding *et al.* 1986). Major findings from the study were that patients who scored higher than 50% on the Zung scale (% score was based on the number of items answered) ($n = 9$) or who had a clinical diagnosis of depression ($n = 8$) tended, although not statistically significant, to have a greater improvement in their Barthel ADL score when treated with trazodone compared to placebo. When only patients with abnormal dexamethasone suppression tests (DST) were considered, the seven patients who were treated with trazodone had a significantly greater improvement in Barthel ADL scores than the nine patients treated with placebo. There was no report of the improvement in Zung depression scores in the trazodone-treated patients compared with the placebo patients as the only outcome measure in this study was the Barthel ADL score.

The first study utilizing the new selective serotonin reuptake inhibitor (SSRI) drugs and using double-blind methodology for the treatment of poststroke depression was reported by Andersen *et al.* (1994a). There were 33 patients treated with 20 mg HS of citalopram, or 10 mg HS in patients over 65, and 33 patients given placebo. Entrance criteria for the study included a Ham-D score of 13 or greater. If the patient did not respond to treatment by 3 weeks, the dose was doubled and outcome was measured after 6 weeks. The mean time since stroke was 10 ± 10 SD weeks for citalopram and 13 ± 11 SD weeks for placebo patients. There were six dropouts within 3 weeks from the citalopram group (one died of an aortic aneurysm, one suffered a new stroke, one developed a rash, one violated the protocol, one complained of dizziness and one complained of headache), and one dropout from the placebo group (dizziness). There were two late dropouts; one was from the citalopram group (uneasiness) and one from the placebo group (died of cardiac failure). Results of both the intention-to-treat and the efficacy analysis (early dropouts excluded) demonstrated that there was a significantly greater reduction in Ham-D scores in the citalopram compared with the placebo-treated group at both 3 and 6 weeks. This was also true when the Melancholia Scale (MES)

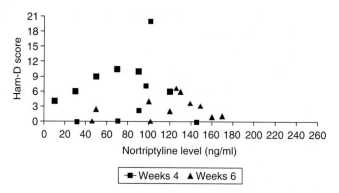

Figure 22.2 Ham-D scores in individual patients related to their serum level of nortriptyline. After 4 weeks of treatment (75 mg oral dose for 1 week), serum levels were lower and depression scores higher than after 6 weeks (100 mg dose for 2 weeks). Whether higher serum levels or the additional 2 weeks of treatment were the most important element in lowering the Hamilton scores cannot be determined from these data [modified from Robinson and Forrester (1987), reprinted with permission].

was used to measure depression severity ($p = 0.005$) (Fig. 22.2). Response to treatment was indicated by 50% reduction in the Hamilton score. Of 27 patients who received citalopram and completed the study, 16 responded, compared with 9 of 32 placebo patients ($p < 0.05$). Time-since-stroke analysis revealed that response to treatment was better in patients who were 7 or more weeks poststroke than those who were less than 7 weeks poststroke. Side effects associated with the SSRI medication during the first week were nausea, vomiting, and fatigue.

Treatment trials utilizing other SSRI medications includes our study which compared fluoxetine, nortriptyline and placebo as shown on Table 22.1. There were 23 patients who received fluoxetine, 16 nortriptyline and 17 placebo using a double-blind methodology (Robinson et al. 2000). The patients were admitted to the study if they had a diagnosis of major or minor depression based on the present state examination (PSE) and DSM-IV diagnostic criteria. There were nine withdrawals in the depressed fluoxetine group, six dropped out within the first 3 weeks, two between weeks 4 and 6 and one between weeks 7 and 9. Three complained of gastrointestinal symptoms and 6 simply refused treatment with no reason given. Of the depressed nortriptyline patients, one dropped out during the first 3 weeks, one during weeks 7–9 and one between weeks 10 and 12. Two had medical deterioration and one refused treatment without giving explanation. In the placebo group, four patients dropped out during the first 3 weeks. One patient died due to pulmonary embolism, one deteriorated medically and two refused treatment without explanation. Using an intention-to-treat analysis, repeated measures ANOVA comparing Ham-D scores for all patient groups demonstrated a significant time-by-treatment

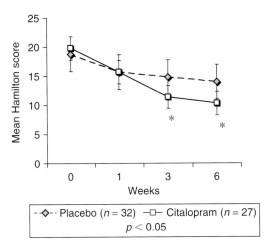

Figure 22.3 Efficacy analysis of Ham-D scores over 6 weeks of double-blind treatment with citalopram (dose 10 or 20 mg). Patients treated with the SSRI, citalopram ($n = 27$) had significantly lower Hamilton scores at 4 and 6 weeks of treatment compared with placebo-treated patients ($n = 32$) (data extracted from Andersen *et al.* 1994a).

interaction ($p = 0.004$). *Post hoc* analysis of group depression scores indicated no intergroup difference at the initial evaluation between the nortriptyline and fluoxetine groups, although the placebo group had a significantly lower mean score than the nortriptyline group ($p < 0.05$). At 12 weeks the nortriptyline group had significantly lower mean Ham-D score than the fluoxetine group or the placebo group ($p < 0.05$), Fig. 22.3. A non-parametric analysis of direction of change in Ham-D scores (i.e., trajectories) also revealed a significant difference between groups, indicating that the nortriptyline group had more consistent improvement in Ham-D score than the fluoxetine or placebo group. Analysis of time-by-treatment interaction covarying for baseline scores also revealed a significant time-by-treatment interaction ($p = 0.01$). There were no differences between the fluoxetine and placebo groups. The response and remission rates were 10 of 16 (63% response) and 8 of 16 (50% remission) for the nortriptyline group, 2 of 23 (9% response) and 0 of 23 (0% remission) for the fluoxetine group and 4 of 17 (24% response) and 1 of 17 (6% remission) for the placebo group.

Efficacy analysis utilizing only study completers showed the same effect and a response rate which was 10 of 13 (77% for nortriptyline) 2 of 14 (14% for fluoxetine) and 4 of 13 (31% for placebo). Analysis of potentially confounding variables in this study also failed to change the treatment results. Five of the nortriptyline patients, three of the fluoxetine patients and one placebo patient had been treated in an identical protocol in Argentina. Reanalysis of results removing these patients, however, and utilizing only patients examined in Iowa revealed the same results.

Similarly, an analysis of patients treated with fluoxetine for the first 6 weeks when a maximum dose of 20 mg was administered revealed a significantly greater improvement in the nortriptyline compared with the fluoxetine and placebo-treated groups at 6 weeks of treatment ($p = 0.04$). We also examined the results when the increased number of male patients in the fluoxetine group was controlled. Again, both intention-to-treat and efficacy analysis demonstrated a time-by-treatment interaction with nortriptyline-treated patients having significantly lower Ham-D scores.

The results of treatment on ADL and cognitive function showed no significant treatment effects. These findings have been discussed in Chapter 13 on the effect of depression on ADL, Chapter 14 on the effect of and depression on cognitive impairment.

Since fluoxetine was not found to be superior to placebo in this treatment study, this raises the issue of whether other studies would find similar results. The data are mixed. As indicated in Table 22.1, there were two other double-blind treatment trials with placebo controls which evaluated the efficacy of fluoxetine. The study by Wiart *et al.* (2000) included 31 patients, 16 administered fluoxetine and 15 placebo. The patients were selected from those who had been hospitalized following acute stroke in a neuro-rehabilitation center. All patients were less than 3 months post-stroke and all patients had major depression based on a clinical examination and the International Classification of Diseases (ICD-10) diagnostic criteria and a Montgomery Asberg depression rating scale (MADRS) score greater than 19. Two patients in the fluoxetine group dropped out, one for elevated alanine amino transferase (ALT) levels and the other for non-compliance. There were no dropouts from the placebo group. The fluoxetine-treated patients demonstrated significantly greater mean change (baseline to endpoint) in MADRS scores than did the placebo-treated patient. A response indicated by greater than 50% drop in MADRS scores indicated the fluoxetine-treated group had a 62% response rate versus 33% in the placebo group ($p = 0.1$). This study did not report an intention-to-treat analysis nor did they demonstrate a significant repeated measures ANOVA showing a significant time-by-treatment interaction.

The second study to examine fluoxetine in a double blind 12-week study using placebo control was reported by Fruehwald *et al.* (2003). In this study, there were 28 patients treated with fluoxetine (2 dropped out) and 26 patients treated with placebo (2 dropped out). Patients were included if their Ham-D score was greater than 15 and there was no significant impairment in verbal communication. Patients were less than 2 weeks poststroke with a mean time since stroke of 11.0 ± 3.9 days, and 11.1 ± 3.5 days in the fluoxetine and placebo groups, respectively. One patient receiving fluoxetine died a few days before the end of the study and one had a pulmonary embolism; one patient receiving placebo dropped out because of an intra dermatological disease, one was removed because she developed suicidal ideation.

The patients given active fluoxetine decreased their Ham-D scores from 32.8 ± 12.7 to 9.5 ± 7.9 while the placebo patients decreased from 30.3 ± 15.0 to 11.2 ± 12.4. There were no significant intergroup differences in the change of Ham-D scores or Beck depression scores over the 3 months of double-blind treatment. The response rate in the active treated patients was 18 of 26 (69%) and in the placebo-treated patients was 18 of 24 (75%). This study did include an 18-month open label follow-up in which 22 patients received fluoxetine and 18 received placebo. At the end of the 18-month follow-up, the Ham-D score in the fluoxetine-treated group was 10.8 ± 1.6; significantly lower than the placebo-treated patients whose mean Ham-D score was 22.2 ± 15.0. The 18-month response rate was 18 of 22 (81%) in the fluoxetine-treated group and 5 of 18 (28%) in the placebo group. Thus, at long-term open label follow-up there appeared to be a treatment response to fluoxetine greater than placebo. When the placebo patients relapsed and whether there was any mid-point deterioration in the patients on fluoxetine is not clear.

Based on the available data from double-blind placebo-controlled trials, two of three studies failed to show a significant treatment effect of fluoxetine. The reason why fluoxetine was not effective in treating poststroke depression in these studies is unclear. In our study, we believe that the doses above 20 mg of fluoxetine may have led to gastrointestinal side effects. For example, we examined weight change in patients receiving fluoxetine. Ten of 12 fluoxetine patients lost 10 lbs or more (mean 15.1 ± 8.1 SD lbs or 8% of initial body weight) while only 2 of 13 nortriptyline patients and one of 11 placebo-treated patients lost 10 lbs or more ($p = 0.0004$). Fluoxetine, thus, induced significant weight loss in the majority of these elderly patients. There was, however, no significant correlation between the amount of weight loss and change in Ham-D scores. Similarly, there was an increase in the pulse rate of the patients treated with nortriptyline from 78 bpm to 87 bpm while the fluoxetine and placebo-treated groups showed no significant change (e.g. fluoxetine 72 bpm prior to treatment and 73 bpm following 12 weeks of treatment).

There have been a total of 27 studies including double-blind treatment trials as well as open label and retrospective studies of poststroke depression. Although the majority of these studies examined standard antidepressant medications, there are several studies which have reported clinical improvement associated with stimulant medications such as methylphenidate. Although there is only one double-blind treatment trial, there are a total of 4 studies which have evaluated the use of stimulant medications. The double-blind trial was conducted by Grade *et al.* (1998). This study included 10 patients given methylphenidate and 11 given placebo. Patients were entered in the study if they agreed to participate. There was no requirement that the patient have a depression diagnosis by diagnostic criteria or a particular score on the Ham-D scale. Although the mean dose was 22.2 ± 1.9 SEM, patients were given a maximum dose of 30 mg of methylphenidate. In the methylphenidate group, only five patients completed the 3-week trial. Of the five patients who discontinued before 3 weeks, four had completed 1 or 2 weeks and reportedly had already achieved significant improvement of their depression and rehabilitation scores. Only one patient withdrew because of abdominal pain related to peptic ulcer disease. In the placebo group, 8 of 11 patients completed 3 weeks. Of the two patients who dropped out at 2 weeks, there was reported improvement in depression and rehabilitation scores and one patient dropped out due to worsening depression. Analysis of covariance revealed that patients receiving methylphenidate treatment scored lower on the Ham-D and the Zung depression scale at the end of treatment compared with the placebo group. The Ham-D scores went from 20.0 ± 20.9 SEM to 6.7 ± 1.5 SEM in the methylphenidate-treated group. There was no report of response rate and no indication of how many patients met diagnostic criteria for major or minor depression.

This study, although the first to use double-blind controls in the assessment of stimulants, did not fulfill the requirements for an assessment of the utility of methylphenidate for the treatment of poststroke depression. Thus, although the psychostimulants may provide a rapid response of depression to treatment, their short-term and long-term efficacy and safety as well as utility in a clearly diagnosed population of poststroke depression has yet to be demonstrated and further treatment trials evaluating the effectiveness of stimulant medication are needed.

The efficacy of psychotherapy has been examined in a number of non-controlled trials but two reports by Lincoln *et al.* (1997) and Lincoln and Flannaghan (2003) have evaluated, in controlled trials, the utility of cognitive behavioral psychotherapy. The most recent study involved 123 patients of whom 39 received 10 sessions of cognitive behavioral therapy (CBT) over 3 months. The second group of 43 patients received an individual meeting with the investigators, (attention placebo group) the third group of 41 patients received no contact. The patients recruited for this study responded to a letter sent to them while they were living at home 1 month after an acute stroke. Patients were entered if their Beck Depression Inventory (BDI) was greater than 10 or the Wakefield Depression Inventory was greater than 18. Of the 123 patients involved in the study, 60 patients had a diagnosis of depressive disorder. During the course of treatment there were five patients who dropped out of the CBT group (three refused treatment and one patient died). Two dropped from the attention placebo group (one refused treatment and one patient died) and five patients dropped out (of the no intervention group two refused and three died). After 3 months of treatment, the BDI went from 17 to 12 in the CBT group, from 15 to 13 in the attention placebo group and from 18 to 14.5 in the no intervention group (p = NS). The authors concluded that CBT in the treatment of depression following stroke was ineffective. Thus, although one might expect that psychological treatment would be effective in the treatment of patients with poststroke depression, the available evidence thus far suggests that CBT does not appear to be effective in this condition.

Electroconvulsive treatment

Electroconvulsive therapy (ECT) has also been reported to be effective in some cases of poststroke depression. The first study to report a beneficial effect of ECT was Murray *et al.* (1986) who conducted a retrospective study of 14 cases of poststroke depression (nine developed depression within 1 year of stroke and five developed depression after 1 year) treated with ECT. All of the patients who developed depression after 1 year and seven of the nine who developed depression before 1 year were significantly improved. The number of treatments ranged from 3 to 18 with an average of 7.7. None of the patients had an exacerbation of their neurological symptoms or a recurrence of stroke.

A second retrospective study of 20 patients with unipolar major depression (n = 14) or major depression with psychosis (n = 6) found that 19 (95%) showed a marked or moderate improvement with ECT (Currier *et al.* 1992). The mean number of treatments was 10 and 19 patients had non-dominant unilateral ECT. There were five patients with significant complications including hypertension (one patient), delirium requiring neuroleptics (two patients), pulmonary edema (one patient), and arrhythmia (one patient). Thus ECT is not contraindicated in patients with poststroke depression and appears to produce a good response in the majority of patients. Controlled trials of treatment efficacy for ECT in poststroke depression are clearly needed.

Transcranial magnetic stimulation therapy

We have recently completed a small study of rapid transcranial magnetic stimulation (rTMS) in the treatment of poststroke depression. This study included 10 patients given rTMS and 10 given sham rTMS using double-blind methodology (Jorge *et al.* 2004) (Table 22.1). There were no significant intergroup differences in either their background characteristics or risk factors for depressive disorder. Patients were entered in the study only if they had failed treatment on at least one occasion. In fact, the active treatment patients had failed a mean of 3.8 ± 1.4 SD prior treatment trials with adequate doses of antidepressant medications while the sham-treated group had failed a mean of 3.8 ± 1.1 SD prior treatments. The initial

Ham-D scores were 20.1 ± 6.7 in the active treated group and 20.8 + 6.0 in the sham-treated group. Eighty percent of the active treated patients (8 of 10) had major depressive disorder as did 90% of the sham-treated group. The remaining three patients met DSM-IV criteria for minor depression.

Transcranial magnetic stimulation (rTMS) was administered at 10 Hz, 110% of motor threshold, 20 trains of 5 s duration for 10 sessions over the left prefrontal cortex. The center of the stimulation coil was held at the midpoint of the middle frontal gyrus in the left hemisphere using markings on a skull cap and based on structural Magnetic Resonance Imagings (MRIs) and distance measurements.

The Ham-D scores between baseline and final assessment at week 3 (1 week after discontinuation of the rTMS) showed a mean reduction of 7.3 points (38%) in the active treated group and 2.7 points (13%) in the sham-treated group (Fig. 22.4). Analysis of covariance demonstrated a significantly greater reduction in Ham-D scores in the active than the sham-treated group. This was also confirmed using non-parametric statistical analysis. Of the 10 patients who received active rTMS, three responded to treatment (i.e., greater than 50% reduction in Ham-D score) and one patient remitted (i.e., final Ham-D score 7 or less). None of the patients who received sham stimulation met criteria for either response or remission.

In addition to the response to treatment, we found a significant positive correlation between the decrease in Ham-D scores and both left frontal gray matter and

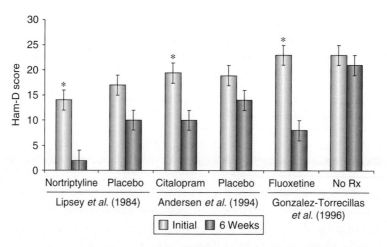

Figure 22.4 Comparison of treatment outcome findings in three studies, all of 6 weeks duration, that utilized Ham-D scores as an outcome measure. The Lipsey *et al.* (1984) and Andersen *et al.* (1994a) studies were double-blind controlled. Gonzalez-Torrecillas *et al.* 1995 did not report standard deviations of mean scores but ANOVA demonstrated significantly greater improvement at 6 weeks in the fluoxetine-treated group compared to those who received no treatment. Rx: treatment, *$p < 0.05$.

left frontal white matter volumes (Spearman's rho = 0.51, $p < 0.03$ and 0.52, $p < 0.03$, respectively). The greater the left prefrontal brain volume, the greater the reduction in Ham-D scores with rTMS treatment. We did not find a significant correlation between the change in Ham-D score and age, total cerebral volume, total left frontal lobe volume, or the distance from the middle frontal gyrus to the stimulating coil (Spearman's rho = -0.25, $p < 0.30$). Although there were no significant adverse events. Six patients developed transient headaches that were relieved with acetaminophen and five patients complained of local discomfort. There were no significant differences in the frequency of these adverse events between the active and sham-treated group, however.

This is the first study to demonstrate the potential utility of rTMS for the treatment of poststroke depression. Although the response and remission rates were only modest, this was probably related to the refractory nature of the depressive disorders that we were treating. In addition, it is possible that some of our patients would have shown further reduction in depressive symptoms if we had given them more than 10 sessions of rTMS. Although the response rates to ECT appear to be greater than 60%, the use of rTMS has the advantage of not producing memory disturbance and other complications of seizures and general anesthesia.

SUMMARY

All of the 27 treatment studies published to date have reported some benefit of either pharmacological treatment, ECT treatment, or rTMS treatment for poststroke depression. The only treatment modality which has not, thus far, demonstrated a significant efficacy is psychotherapy treatment. A comparison of the double-blind treatment trials which utilized the Ham-D as an outcome variable is shown in Fig. 22.4. In each study, there were side effects which occurred in the medication-treated group. It is unclear, however, whether the side effects were related to the underlying illness in combination with medication. Among the 7 double-blind treatment trials there was a 19% dropout rate among the actively treated patients compared to 11% among the placebo-treated patients ($p = 0.0826$). Thus, the use of antidepressant medications in this population must be done with care and with an effort to minimize any possible adverse consequences. Patients with cardiac conduction abnormalities, narrow angle glaucoma, or significant urinary retention should not be treated with nortriptyline. On the other hand, the benefits of antidepressant medication have been demonstrated in both double-blind as well as open label and retrospective studies. There can be little doubt that poststroke depression in most cases can be effectively treated and should be rigorously treated because of its utility in alleviating depressive symptoms. In addition, Chapter 13 on ADL and Chapter 14 on cognitive impairment have demonstrated the utility of antidepressant treatment on physical recovery and intellectual recovery. In addition, Chapter 19 on mortality and its treatment provides another strong argument for the great benefit to risk ratio associated with the use of antidepressants even in an elderly stroke population. Further studies are needed to determine which are the most effective, as well as the safest, treatments for depressive disorder following stroke and to determine their effect on recovery and survival. At the present time, patients without a strong contraindication to antidepressant medication who develop a depression should clearly be started on antidepressant treatment. Even among patients with contraindications to antidepressants, a decision about the benefit risk ratio of antidepressant therapy should be undertaken with their primary care physician.

REFERENCES

Andersen, G., Vestergaard, K., and Lauritzen, L. Effective treatment of poststroke depression with the selective serotonin reuptake inhibitor citalopram. *Stroke* (1994a) 25:1099–1104.

Andersen, G., Vestergaard, K., Riis, J. O., *et al.* Incidence of post-stroke depression during the first year in a large unselected stroke population determined using a valid standardized rating scale. *Acta Psychiatr Scand* (1994b) 90:190–195.

Balunov, O. A., Sadov O. G., and Alemasova, A. Y. Therapy of depression in post-stroke patients. *Alaska Med* (1990) 32:20–29.

Currier, M. B., Murray, G. B., and Welch, C. C. Electroconvulsive therapy for post-stroke depressed geriatric patients. *J Neuropsychiatr Clin Neurosci* (1992) 4:140–144.

Dam, M., Tonin, P., De Boni, A., *et al.* Effects of fluoxetine and maprotiline on functional recovery in poststroke hemiplegic patients undergoing rehabilitation therapy. (comment). *Stroke* (1996) 27(7):1211–1214.

Feibel, J. H., and Springer, C. J. Depression and failure to resume social activities after stroke. *Arch Phys Med Rehabil* (1982) 63:276–278.

Finklestine, S. P., Weintraub, R. J., Karmouz, N., *et al.* Antidepressant drug treatment for post-stroke depression: retrospective study. *Arch Phys Med Rehabil* (1987) 68:772–776.

Fruehwald, S., Gatterbauer, E., Rehak, P., *et al.* Early fluoxetine treatment of post-stroke depression – a three-month double-blind placebo-controlled study with an open-label long-term follow up. *J Neurol* (2003) 250(3):347–351.

Gonzalez-Torrecillas, J. L., Mendlewicz, J., and Lobo, A. Effects of early treatment of poststroke depression on neuropsychological rehabilitation. *Int Psychogeriatr* (1995) 7(4):547–560.

Grade, C., Redford, B., Chrostowski, J., *et al.* Methylphenidate in early poststroke recovery: a double-blind, placebo-controlled study. *Arch Phys Med Rehabil* (1998) 79(9):1047–1050.

Gresham, G., Duncan, P., Stason, W., *et al. Post-Stroke Rehabilitation.* Vol. 16. Department of Health and Human Services, Rockville MD, 1995.

Hougaku, H., Matsumoto, M., Hata, R., *et al.* Therapeutic effect of lisuride maleate on post-stroke depression. *Nippon Ronen Igakkai Zasshi* (1994) 31(1):52–59.

Johnson, M. L., Roberts, M. D., Ross, A. R., *et al*. Methylphenidate in stroke patients with depression. *Am J Phys Med Rehabil* (1992) 71:239–241.

Jorge, R. E., Robinson, R. G., Arndt, S., *et al*. Mortality and post-stroke depression: A placebo controlled trial of antidepressants. *Am J Psychiatr* (2003) 160:1823–1829.

Jorge, R. E., Robinson, R. G., Tateno, A., *et al*. Repetitive transcranial magnetic stimulation as treatment of poststroke depression: A preliminary study. *Biol Psychiatr* (2004) 55(4): 398–405.

Kimura, M., Kanetani, K., Imai, R., *et al*. Therapeutic effects of milnacipran, a serotonin and noradrenaline reuptake inhibitor, on post-stroke depression. *Int Clin Psychopharmacol* (2002) 17(3):121–125.

Lauritzen, L., Bendsen, B. B., Vilmar, T., *et al*. Post-stroke depression: combined treatment with imipramine or desipramine and mianserin: a controlled clinical study. *Psychopharmacology* (1994) 114:119–122.

Lazarus, L. W., Winemiller, D. R., Lingam, V. R., *et al*. Efficacy and side effects of methylphenidate for post-stroke depression. *J Clin Psychiatr* (1992) 53:447–449.

Lincoln, N. B., and Flannaghan, T. Cognitive behavioral psychotherapy for depression following stroke: a randomized controlled trial. *Stroke* (2003) 34(1):111–115.

Lincoln, N. B., Flannaghan, T., Sutcliffe, L., *et al*. Evaluation of cognitive behavioural treatment for depression after stroke: a pilot study. *Clin Rehabil* (1997) 11(2):114–122.

Lipsey, J. R., Robinson, R. G., Pearlson, G. D., *et al*. Nortriptyline treatment of post-stroke depression: a double-blind study. *Lancet* (1984) i(8372):297–300.

Martensson, B., Murray, V., von Arbin, M., *et al*. Alternative treatment for poststroke depression. *Am J Psychiatr* (1997) 154(4):583–584.

Masand, P., Murray, G. B., and Pickett, P. Psychostimulants in post-stroke depression. *J Neuropsychiatr Clin Neurosci* (1991) 3:23–27.

Miyai, I., Suzuki, T., Kang, J., *et al*. Improved functional outcome in patients with hemorrhagic stroke in putamen and thalamus compared with those with stroke restricted to the putamen or thalamus. *Stroke* (2000) 31(6):1365–1369.

Murray, G. B., Shea, V., and Conn, D. K. Electroconvulsive therapy for poststroke depression. *J Clin Psychiatr* (1986) 47(5):258–260.

Paolucci, S., Antonucci, G., Grasso, M. G., *et al*. Post-stroke depression, antidepressant treatment and rehabilitation results. A case-control study. *Cerebrovasc Dis* (2001) 12(3):264–271.

Rampello, L., Alvano, A., Chiechio, S., *et al*. An evaluation of efficacy and safety of reboxetine in elderly patients affected by "retarded" post-stroke depression. A random, placebo-controlled study. *Arch Gerontol Geriatr* (2005) 40(3):275–285.

Reding, M. J., Orto, L. A., Winter, S. W., *et al*. Antidepressant therapy after stroke: a double-blind trial. *Arch Neurol* (1986) 43:763–765.

Robinson, R. G., and Forrester, A. W. Neuropsychiatric aspects of cerebrovascular disease. In R. E. Hales and S. C. Yudofsky, eds., *Textbook of Neuropsychiatry*. American Psychiatric Press, Inc, Washington, DC, 1987.

Robinson, R. G., Schultz, S. K., Castillo, C., *et al*. Nortriptyline versus fluoxetine in the treatment of depression and in short term recovery after stroke: a placebo controlled, double-blind study. *Am J Psychiatr* (2000) 157:351–359.

Ross, E. D., and Rush, A. J. Diagnosis and neuroanatomical correlates of depression brain damaged patients. *Arch Gen Psychiatr* (1981) 38:1344–1354.

Schubert, D. S. P., Taylor, C., Lee, S., *et al.* Detection of depression in the stroke patient. *Psychosomatics* (1992) 33:1–5.

Shima, S. The efficacy of antidepressants in post-stroke depression. *Keio J Med* (1997) 46(1):25–26.

Spalletta, G., Guida, G., De Angelis, D., *et al.* Predictors of cognitive level and depression severity are different in patients with left and right hemispheric stroke within the first year of illness. *J Neurol* (2002) 249(11):1541–1551.

Stamenkovic, M., Schindler, S., and Kasper, S. Poststroke depression and fluoxetine. *Am J Psychiatr* (1996) 153:446–447.

Wiart, L., Petit, H., Joseph, P. A., *et al.* Fluoxetine in early poststroke depression: a double-blind placebo-controlled study. *Stroke* (2000) 31:1829–1832.

Zifko, U. A., Rupp, M., and Schwarz, S. Sertraline in the treatment of post-stroke depression – results of an open multicenter study. *Wien Med Wochenschr* (2002) 152(13–14):343–348.

23

Prevention of poststroke depression

Within the past few years, several studies have been published examining the question of whether depression following stroke can be effectively prevented. Given the data that was presented in Chapters 13 on depression and physical impairment, Chapter 14 on depression and cognitive impairment and Chapter 19 on depression and mortality, the obvious conclusion is that methods need to be developed to prevent poststroke depression.

The first study which attempted to prevent poststroke depression was published by Palomaki *et al.* (1999). This study involved a placebo-controlled trial of mianserin in 100 patients under age 71 admitted to hospital for an acute ischemic stroke. Patients were included if their stroke had occurred <30 days prior to admission and if there was no evidence of other diseases which would confound the assessment. Patients were randomized to mianserin and placebo and stratified according to hemisphere of infarction or brain stem infarction and presence or absence of severe aphasia. The initial dose of mianserin was 10 mg at bedtime and the dosage was increased as tolerated over 10 days to a maintenance level of 60 mg per day. Treatment was continued for 12 months and then gradually withdrawn over 4 weeks.

The mean interval from stroke to beginning of the study was 14.3 days. Ten patients on placebo and 9 on mianserin discontinued the treatment study prematurely. The 10 patients on placebo stopped due to lack of efficacy (3 patients), lack of compliance (3 patients), side effects (3 patients) and death (1 patient). Nine patients on mianserin discontinued the treatment prematurely due to lack of efficacy (one patient), lack of compliance (one patient), side effects (six patients) and death (one patient). At the time of enrollment in the study, three patients receiving mianserin and two patients receiving placebo had a major depressive disorder. During the course of the treatment study, there were no significant differences between the treatment groups in the frequency of major depression. At 2 months, two patients receiving mianserin and five on placebo had major depression, at 6 months, four patients on mianserin and three on placebo had major depression and, at 12 months, five mianserin and five placebo patients had major depression. In addition, there was no significant difference between groups in the number of patients with dysthymia which was found in 4.5% of the mianserin treated and 6.5% of the placebo treated patients during the 18 months.

Using the clinical global impression assessment (CGIA), 21% of patients had some degree of depression at the initial evaluation. The prevalence of patients with at least mild depression according to the CGIA, increased from a total of 11% at the 12-month follow-up to a total of 32% (29 of 91) at 18 months. There were no significant differences between groups in the Hamilton depression (Ham-D) scale or the Beck depression inventory at the 12-month follow-up.

In addition to not finding any difference between the mianserin and placebo treated patients in depression scores at any of the follow-up intervals, there were no differences in severity of impairment as measured by the Rankin scale or the Barthel index of activities of daily living. Similarly, the mean duration of hospital stay was not significantly different (18.3 days for placebo 24.6 days for mianserin).

The second study examining the prevention of poststroke depression was done by our group (Narushima *et al.* 2002). Patients who were not depressed following acute stroke were assigned to nortriptyline ($n = 15$), fluoxetine ($n = 17$), or placebo ($n = 16$) treatment as part of the study described in Chapter 23 on treatment. This study included both depressed and non-depressed patients who were analyzed separately. Patients were admitted to the non-depressed protocol if they did not have a diagnostic and statistical manual (DSM-IV) diagnosis of either major or minor depression based on the semistructured present state examination (PSE). In addition, all patients in the non-depressed group had Ham-D scores <10. Patients were treated for 3 months and then followed for an additional 21 months after discontinuation of the study medication.

The background characteristics of the patients are shown in Table 23.1. There were no significant differences among the three groups in age, education, time since stroke, marital or socioeconomic status and personal or family psychiatric history. There were, however, fewer female patients in the fluoxetine group (i.e., 2 of 17 patients on fluoxetine compared to 8 of 15 on nortriptyline and 4 of 16 on placebo, $p = 0.04$). There were six patients on fluoxetine who withdrew from the study; four dropped out during the 3-month treatment period, one reported gastrointestinal symptoms, two deteriorated medically and one refused treatment. Three patients died during the 21-month follow-up and one patient dropped out. In the nortriptyline group, two patients dropped out during the treatment period, one refused treatment, and one reported sedative effects. After treatment, five patients dropped out; four refused participation and one reported side effects. One placebo patient dropped out during the treatment period due to a rash. One patient died between months 6 and 9. There were no significant differences among the three treatment groups in the rate of discontinuation.

Table 23.1. Background characteristics of patients (intention-to-treat analysis)

	Depressed			Non-depressed		
	Fluox	Nortrip	Placebo	Fluox	Nortrip	Placebo
n	23	16	17	17	15	16
Age (year $\pm$ SD)	65 $\pm$ 14	64 $\pm$ 10	73 $\pm$ 8	66 $\pm$ 13	65 $\pm$ 13	67 $\pm$ 9
Sex (% F)	26*	69	47	12**	53	25
Race (% Caucasian)	83	69	94	94	87	87
Education (year $\pm$ SD)	12 $\pm$ 3	12 $\pm$ 3	11 $\pm$ 3	13 $\pm$ 3	13 $\pm$ 2	11 $\pm$ 4
Married (%)	74	75	59	76	67	63
Hollingshead (%)						
I–III	70	60	65	47	73	69
IV–V	30	40	35	53	27	31
Prior psychiatric history (%)	9	12	18	12	6	0
Family psychiatric history (%)	13	31	12	18	13	6
Since stroke (week $\pm$ SD)	16 $\pm$ 35	5 $\pm$ 4	6 $\pm$ 3	8 $\pm$ 11	10 $\pm$ 17	5 $\pm$ 3
DSM-IV major depression	11	10	6	0	0	0

*$\chi^2 = 7.01$, d.f. $= 2, p = 0.03$; **Fisher's exact $p = 0.04$.

During the 12-week treatment period, minor depression developed in five (33%) of the placebo patients, while minor depression developed in three (20%) of the fluoxetine treated, and one (7.7%) of the nortriptyline treated patients. Using intention-to-treat analysis, there were no significant differences in the incidences of depression during the treatment period, however, two of the three depressed fluoxetine patients dropped out during the treatment study. Thus, using an efficacy analysis, the rate of depression was significantly higher in the placebo group (5 of 15) compared with the combined active treatment groups (2 of 26; $p = 0.036$).

Using an intention-to-treat analysis, there was no significant between group differences in mean scores on the 17-item Ham-D scale during the first 3 months of treatment. Based on efficacy analysis, however, there was a significant time-by-treatment interaction between the active and the placebo treated patients ($p = 0.026$). This analysis found that the active treatment group (nortriptyline plus fluoxetine) had a significantly greater decline in Ham-D scores compared with patients receiving placebo.

During the follow-up period from 3 to 24 months, the active treated patients had a significantly greater frequency of depression than the placebo patients ($p = 0.047$) indicating that depression was more likely to develop in actively treated patients compared with placebo treated patients 6 months after the treatment was discontinued

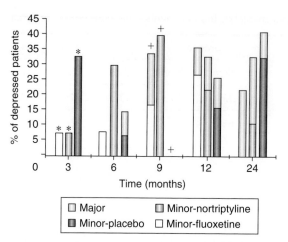

Figure 23.1 Diagnostic outcomes of poststroke patients entered in the follow-up study comparing fluoxetine (*n* = 17), nortriptyline (*n* = 15), and placebo (*n* = 16). Note that after treatment for the first 3 months, nortriptyline and fluoxetine reduced the incidence of poststroke minor depression. By 9 months (i.e., 6 months after stopping antidepressants), the patients given antidepressants had a significantly higher rate of depression than the patients given placebo. *χ^2 = 4.42, d.f. = 1, *p* = 0.036 (active versus placebo treatment); $^+$Fisher's exact test (two-tail), *p* = −0.028 (difference among the three treatment groups); $^+\chi^2$ = 3.95, d.f. = 1, *p* = 0.047 (active versus placebo treatment).

(Fig. 23.1). Using an intention-to-treat analysis, from 3 to 9 months after active treatment had been discontinued, there was a significant time-by-treatment interaction in mean scores on the 17-item Ham-D scale (*p* = 0.038). This finding demonstrated that Ham-D scores among the fluoxetine and nortriptyline treated patients increased at a significantly faster rate than the placebo group (Fig. 23.2). *Post hoc* comparisons demonstrated significant differences between the nortriptyline and placebo groups (*p* = 0.022) as well as the fluoxetine and placebo group (*p* = 0.09) (Fig. 23.2). At 1- and 2-year follow-up, there were no significant differences among the three treatment groups.

This study demonstrated that poststroke depression might be prevented, particularly by administering nortriptyline in non-depressed patients during the first 3 months following stroke. Since the treatment period only extended for 3 months, it was impossible to say if this was truly prevention of depressive disorder and longer term studies need to be conducted. In addition, this study demonstrated that discontinuation of antidepressant treatment in patients who are at risk for developing poststroke depression may, in fact, precipitate depressive disorder. Although it is unclear why patients who were treated with fluoxetine or nortriptyline would develop more depressive symptoms after discontinuation of the medication than

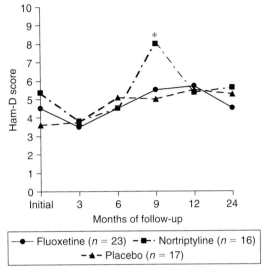

Figure 23.2 Mean Ham-D scores for poststroke patients entered in the follow-up study comparing fluoxetine, nortriptyline, and placebo. After medications had been stopped at 3 months, note the increasing mean depression scores in the nortriptyline treated patients from 3- to 9-month follow-up. There was a significant time-by-treatment interaction between 3 and 9 months for nortriptyline versus placebo treatment ($F = 4.28$, d.f. = 2, 35, $p = 0.022$). By 12-month follow-up there were no inter-group differences suggesting that the increased vulnerability to depressive symptoms lasts about 6 months after discontinuation of antidepressants.
*From 0 to 3 months, there was a significant time by treatment interaction between the active and the placebo treated patients (efficacy analysis: $F = 5.56$, d.f. = 1, 27, $p = 0.026$).
*From 3 to 9 months, a comparison between active and placebo treatment revealed a significant time by treatment interaction (intention-to-treat analysis: $F = 3.45$, d.f. = 2.66, $p = 0.038$; efficacy analysis: $F = 2.60$, d.f. = 4, 52, $p = 0.046$).

patients treated with placebo, it is possible that these represent withdrawal effects from medication. As early as 1959, Andersen and Kristiansen (1959) reported discontinuation symptoms associated with tricyclic antidepressants. Tricyclic withdrawal symptoms including anorexia, nausea, diarrhea, sleep disturbance and movement disturbance (e.g., akathesia). An alternative explanation is that depression may have been aborted because of the treatment and relapse occurred when the protective drugs were discontinued. Whatever the explanation, the important question which arises from this phenomenon of increased depressive diagnosis and symptoms, within 6 months following discontinuation of treatment, is whether this could have been prevented by a longer course of antidepressant medication.

The third prevention study did extend treatment for 12 months. Rasmussen *et al.* (2003) examined the utility of sertraline in preventing depression in 137 patients

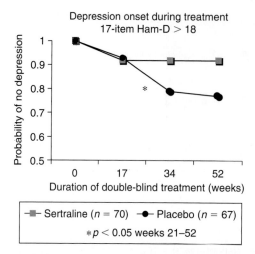

Figure 23.3 Survival curves for patients treated with sertraline or placebo to prevent poststroke depression. Patients given sertraline had a significantly lower frequency of depression than the placebo patients from weeks 21 to 52 (from Rasmussen *et al.* 2003, reprinted with permission).

randomly assigned to 12 months of sertraline ($n = 70$) or placebo ($n = 67$). Patients were enrolled if they were within 4 weeks of having had an acute stroke without comprehension impairment or serious comorbid illness and if their score on the 17-item Ham-D scale was <13. Patients were administered 50 mg of sertraline or matching placebo and were randomly assigned using double-blind methodology. The dose of sertraline was increased flexibly according to clinical need, at any time after 2 weeks, in 50 mg increments up to a maximum dose of 150 mg/day. Of the 70 patients assigned to sertraline, 35 (50%) completed the 12-month study, while 32 (47.8%) of the 67 patients assigned to placebo completed the study. Using Ham-D score of >18 as an indication of clinically significant depression, the frequency of depression at the end of 52 weeks of treatment was 8.2% (95% confidence interval (CI): 2.4–13.9%) in the sertraline treated group and 22.8% (95% CI: 13.7–32.0%) in the placebo group (Fig. 23.3). The 17-item Ham-D scores were significantly lower in the sertraline group than the placebo treated group from 21 to 52 weeks following treatment. A repeated measure analysis of variance (ANOVA) found a significant treatment-by-time interaction between 21 and 52 weeks of therapy using the scores on the geriatric depression scale. An intention-to-treat analysis (last observation carried forward) showed that the percent of patients rated as having a clinical global impression (CGI) severity score ≥ 3 (mild to severe range) was 18% among those given sertraline and 29.8% among those given placebo ($p = 0.012$). The mean sertraline dose was 62.9 mg with 78.6% of the patients (55) treated with 50 mg of sertraline.

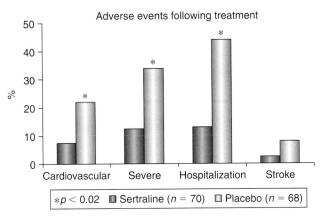

Figure 23.4 The frequency of adverse medical events among patients treated for 1 year following acute stroke with sertraline or placebo. Cardiovascular events and hospitalization were significantly lower in the sertraline treated patients compared with the placebo group (from Rasmussen *et al.* 2003, reprinted with permission).

The frequency of adverse events was significantly influenced by the presence or absence of sertraline (Fig. 23.4). Using an intention-to-treat analysis, there was a significantly higher frequency of adverse cardiovascular events, including severe adverse events and rehospitalization for physical illness in the placebo, compared with the sertraline treated patients. Although this study did not report the death rate among sertraline versus placebo treated patients, it is unlikely that in a period of 1 year significant differences in treatment related death rate would have been discovered. This study is one of the most important studies to be reported in the treatment or prevention of poststroke depression because it is the first study to demonstrate both the ability of antidepressant treatment to prevent poststroke depression and decrease the frequency of comorbid physical illnesses particularly cardiovascular disorders. This finding is similar to that reported in patients with major depression following myocardial infarction in which the use of sertraline significantly reduced the number of adverse physical illnesses following myocardial infarction (Glassman *et al.* 2002).

The most recent prevention study was reported by Niedermaier *et al.* (2004). Patients with ischemic stroke received either mirtazapine (30 mg) ($n = 35$) or no medication ($n = 35$) in an open randomized design. Patients were started 1 day following stroke and re-examined 7, 44, 90, 180, 270 and 360 days later. Of the non-treated group, 144 of 233 completers (42%) developed DSM-IV major depression while only 2 of 31 (6%) completers in the treated group became depressed.

For many years, psychiatrists have been interested in prevention. There are numerous trials in the literature demonstrating the efficacy of antidepressant medication as well as psychological treatment in preventing recurrence of depressive disorder among patients who have had previous episodes of depression (Frank *et al.* 1990). This type of secondary prevention has been highly beneficial to patients with mood disorders. The ability to prevent the first onset of depression, however, has not previously been achieved in psychiatry because a high-risk population of patients could not be identified with sufficient risk to justify the administration of antidepressants in patients who had never experienced depression. Poststroke depression, however, represents a relatively unique population because of the high risk of developing depression within the first several years following stroke. The combined prevalence of major and minor depressive disorder as demonstrated in Chapter 6 is approximately 40% during the acute stroke period. In addition, among patients who have not developed a depression during the acute poststroke period, approximately 40% will develop depression between 3 months and 2 years following stroke (see Chapter 9 on delayed onset depressions). This indicates that over 2 years, there is a high risk for developing depression. Thus, the poststroke population is at sufficiently high risk for developing depression that primary prevention strategies are justified. The four studies presented in this chapter suggest that sertraline, nortriptyline, mirtazapine and perhaps fluoxetine may be effective in preventing the development of depression in patients who would otherwise have developed poststroke depression. This represents the first time, to my knowledge, that primary prevention has been successful in psychiatry. As indicated in Chapters 13 and 14, successful treatment of poststroke depression improves both physical and cognitive recovery from stroke and as shown in Chapter 19, antidepressant treatment may reduce the death rate over 7 years following stroke by as much as 50%.

In summary, four studies have examined prevention of poststroke depression and three of the studies have provided evidence of the utility of preventing this disorder using nortriptyline, sertraline, mirtazapine or fluoxetine. Based on the adverse consequences of developing depression following stroke, these studies support the contention that all patients who have suffered an acute stroke should be placed on antidepressants to prevent the development of depression and enhance physical and cognitive recovery and reduce mortality. Furthermore the available data suggest that sertraline does not lead to adverse side effects or complication but, on the contrary, leads to fewer adverse events compared with the natural course of poststroke events. Thus, the benefit-to-risk ratio appears to be very large. Future studies will need to examine other pharmacological and non-pharmacological interventions to prevent the development of poststroke depression and to determine which treatments are most effective and have the greatest benefit-to-risk ratio. Treatments such as transcranial magnetic stimulation, psychological treatment (e.g., problem solving therapy), and a wide range of selective serotonin reuptake inhibitors or selective norepinephrine and serotonin reuptake inhibitors need to be examined to determine their efficacy in the prevention of poststroke depression. Prevention of poststroke depression may represent one of the major advances in the care of stroke patients.

REFERENCES

Andersen, H., and Kristiansen, E. S. Tofranil treatment of endogenous depressions. *Acta Psychiatr Scand* (1959) 34:387–397.

Frank, E., Kupfer, D. J., Perel, J. M., *et al.* Three-year outcomes for maintenance therapies in recurrent depression. *Arch Gen Psychiatr* (1990) 47(12):1093–1099.

Glassman, A. H., O'Connor, C. M., Califf, R. M., *et al.* Sertraline treatment of major depression in patients with acute MI or unstable angina. *J Am Med Assoc* (2002) 288(6):701–709.

Narushima, K., Kosier, J. T., and Robinson, R. G. Preventing post-stroke depression: a 12 week double-blind randomized treatment trial with 21 month follow-up. *J Nerv Ment Dis* (2002) 190(5):296–303.

Niedermaier, N., Bohrer, E., Schulte, K., *et al.* Prevention and treatment of poststroke depression with mirtazapine in patients with acute stroke. *J Clin Psychiatr* (2004) 65:1619–1623.

Palomaki, H., Kaste, M., Berg, A., *et al.* Prevention of poststroke depression: 1 year randomized placebo controlled double blind trial of mainserin with 6 month followup after therapy. *J Neurol Neurosurg Psychiatr* (1999) 66:490–494.

Rasmussen, A., Lunde, M., Poulsen, D. L., *et al.* A double-blind, placebo-controlled study of sertraline in the prevention of depression in stroke patients. *Psychosomatics* (2003) 44(3):216–221.

Part III

Poststroke mania

24

Prevalence and clinical symptoms

Since the first edition of this text in 1998, the literature on mania following stroke continues to be dominated by anecdotal reports and small series of cases examining risk factors for secondary mania. Secondary mania is generally defined as mania following a precipitating causative event such as head injury, stroke, or drug exposure (Rosenbaum and Barry 1975; Krauthammer and Klerman 1978; Forrest 1982). Cohen and Niska (1980) first reported on lesion location associated with secondary mania and suggested an association with right hemisphere injury. Two cases of poststroke mania were reported by Jampala and Abrams (1983) in which one patient with a left and one with right hemisphere cortical infarction developed mania. Cummings and Mendez (1984) also reported two cases of mania occurring within a few days following right hemispheric thalamic infarctions. Both patients were in their 60s with no previous history of psychiatric disorder and no family history of mood disorder. After a review of the literature, Cummings and Mendez suggested that right hemisphere lesions appear to be frequently associated with the onset of secondary mania. In addition, case reports have suggested that patients with "secondary" mania are older than those with "primary" (i.e., no associated organic precipitant) mania and have a lower frequency of positive family history of psychiatric disorder (Krauthammer and Klerman 1978; Starkstein et al. 1987).

We have conducted a series of studies of patients with secondary mania. The total number of patients that have been identified and examined in our studies is 27. Different groups of these patients were used to examine various aspects of mania. The secondary mania group consisted of patients with brain lesions due to stroke ($n = 17$), traumatic injury ($n = 4$), or brain tumors ($n = 6$). Patients were sometimes selected based on our ability to determine the onset of the brain pathology or to identify a single focal lesion visible on computed tomography (CT) or magnetic resonance (MR) scan.

Due to the relatively rare occurrence of secondary mania, the prevalence of poststroke mania has never been examined. The Oxfordshire Community Stroke Project (House et al. 1991) examined 128 patients, 95 seen for the first time at

1-month poststroke and 33 seen for the first time at 6 months poststroke. None of the patients were diagnosed with manic disorder. Similarly, the Perth Community Stroke Study (PCSS) (Burvill *et al.* 1995) examined 294 patients during the acute poststroke period. None of the patients were diagnosed with mania although the study focused primarily on depressive disorder. In our studies of 379 patients hospitalized following an acute stroke, we have seen only two cases of mania, neither of which, however, developed during the first few days following stroke. One case began at 3-month poststroke and the other at 6 months poststroke as part of our follow-up evaluations. However, in our series of 27 patients with secondary mania, there are several cases of patients who developed mania within a few days following traumatic head injury or stroke. Furthermore, we have examined two separate populations of patients with acute traumatic brain injury (TBI), 6 of 66 patients (9%) in the first study (Jorge *et al.* 1993) and 9 of 96 (10%) in the second study (Jorge *et al.* in preparation) met Diagnostic and Statistical Manual, 4th ed. (DSM) IV diagnostic criteria for mania. None of the patients had post-TBI mania during the initial evaluation, but three developed mania at 3 months, two at 6 months, three at 9 months and one at 1 year. Thus, the prevalence of secondary mania depends on the time following brain injury as well as the etiology of injury. It appears that TBI produces a significantly higher frequency of mania than stroke. This suggests that the nature of the injury or more likely the location of traumatic injury involving anterior orbital–frontal cortex basal temporal lobe are more common after TBI and may explain the higher frequency of mania in this condition.

Epidemiological studies of patients with primary mania (i.e., patients with no known etiological agent) have found the lifetime prevalence of mania to be approximately 1%. The national comorbidity survey (Kessler *et al.* 1994) examined 8098 respondents using the "Composite International Diagnostic Interview" (CIDI). Manic episodes were identified in 1.3% of the respondents during the previous 12 months and 1.6% of respondents during lifetime assessment. Given this 12-month prevalence of approximately 1%, the prevalence in poststroke patients appears to be no higher than in the general population. Although this might suggest that mania is not specifically associated with stroke or with other types of head injury and simply occurs spontaneously in some patients, analysis of the clinical correlates of mania following brain injury suggests that there are specific factors which increase the likelihood of mania developing following brain injury.

Although the prevalence of mania does not appear to be significantly increased among patients with stroke as compared to the general population, one might wonder whether the clinical phenomenology of mania following brain injury is significantly different than that of primary mania. We have combined the clinical data obtained from 25 of our 27 patients with secondary mania and compared the frequency of specific clinical symptoms of mania to the frequencies found in

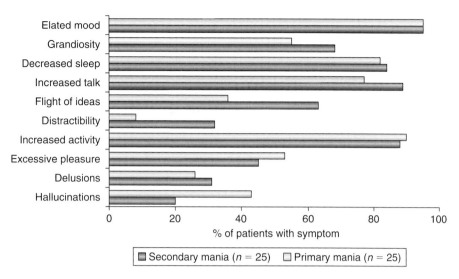

Figure 24.1 The frequency of manic symptoms found in patients with mania following brain injury (secondary) compared to patients with mania not associated with brain injury (primary). There were no significant differences in the frequency of any of the symptoms, which suggests that the clinical presentation of secondary mania is very similar to that of primary mania.

25 patients with primary mania (Fig. 24.1) (Starkstein *et al.* 1987). The age of the patients with primary mania was significantly younger than those with secondary mania (i.e., primary mania 26 ± 12 years (SD) versus secondary mania 52 ± 20 years (SD), $p = 0.001$). There were no differences in the frequency of females (primary mania 52%, secondary mania 36%). We then compared the frequency of each manic symptom between patients with post-brain injury mania and primary mania (Fig. 24.1). There were no significant differences between primary and secondary manias in the frequency of any manic symptom. A case presentation of a patient with poststroke mania will illustrate some of the typical clinical symptoms seen in these patients.

CASE STUDY

The patient was a 79-year-old widowed woman who had worked for many years as a newspaper reporter. She had no previous personal history or family history of psychiatric disorder. In addition, the patient had no significant previous medical history and remarkably, she was not taking any medications.

   The patient had recently retired and was on a vacation trip overseas. After one week abroad, fellow travelers noted a sudden change in her behavior. Following an evening in which she complained of confusion, difficulty in thinking, and memory lapse, she was noted on the next day to become hyperactive and euphoric. She was hypertalkative with increased energy and began writing almost constantly throughout the day. She mailed writings to her family which they found to be disorganized and incoherent. She began to fear that foreign government agents were watching her and trying to prevent her from exposing to the world failures of that government to protect human rights. In spite of these beliefs, she called the local police to protect her while she hurriedly tried to return to the USA. After returning to the USA, she called her relatives from an airport that was not on her itinerary and far out of the way. Her relatives picked her up at the airport, found her to be in a confused and agitated state and admitted her to the hospital. Medical workup test results, including toxicology, chemistry, and blood cell counts, (Venereal Disease Research Laboratories, VDRL), thyroid, B12 measurements, were all normal. A CT scan showed a recent ischemic infarction involving the head of the right caudate nucleus and anterior arm of the internal capsule.

At the time of admission, the patient was elated and hyperactive with flight of ideas, pressured and excessive speech, decreased need for sleep, and increased sexual interest. She continued to be convinced that government spies had been watching her and were trying to prevent her from fulfilling her humanitarian role to expose human rights abuses under that government.

The patient was treated with lithium (300 mg/day) and gradually over several weeks returned to a euthymic state. Six months later, however, the patient discontinued her lithium and within a few weeks had a recurrence of mania. A new CT scan showed only the original right caudate infarct with no new lesions. At the time of the second admission, the patient was grandiose, hypertalkative, had flight of ideas, decreased need for sleep, increased interest in sex and moderately increased activity. She was placed back on lithium and again gradually improved. There were no paranoid delusions at the time of her second admission but she had grandiose beliefs about her imminent fame from a book that she was writing.

In summary, the prevalence of poststroke mania appears to be about 1% and to have the same symptoms as mania without brain injury. Traumatic brain injury produces a significantly higher frequency of mania compared with stroke which is probably due to the prefrontal and anterior temporal lesions produced by TBI.

REFERENCES

Burvill, P. W., Johnson, G. A., Jamrozik, K. D., et al. Prevalence of depression after stroke: the Perth Community Stroke Study. Br J Psychiatr (1995) 166:320–327.

Cohen, M. R., and Niska, R. W. Localized right cerebral hemisphere dysfunction and recurrent mania. *Am J Psychiatr* (1980) 137:847–848.

Cummings, J. L., and Mendez, M. F. Secondary mania with focal cerebrovascular lesions. *Am J Psychiatr* (1984) 141:1084–1087.

Forrest, D. V. Bipolar illness after right hemispherectomy. *Arch Gen Psychiatr* (1982) 39:817–819.

House, A., Dennis, M., Mogridge, L., *et al.* Mood disorders in the year after first stroke. *Br J Psychiatr* (1991) 158:83–92.

Jampala, V. C., and Abrams, R. Mania secondary to left and right hemisphere damage. *Am J Psychiatr* (1983) 140:1197–1199.

Jorge, R. E., Robinson, R. G., Starkstein, S. E., *et al.* Secondary mania following traumatic brain injury. *Am J Psychiatr* (1993) 150:916–921.

Kessler, R. C., McGonagle, K. A., Zaho, S., *et al.* Lifetime and 12-month prevalence of DSM-III-R psychiatric disorders in the United States. *Arch Gen Psychiatr* (1994) 51:8–19.

Krauthammer, C., and Klerman, G. L. Secondary mania: manic symptoms associated with antecedent physical illness or drugs. *Arch Gen Psychiatr* (1978) 35:1333–1339.

Rosenbaum, A. M., and Barry, M. J. Positive therapeutic response to lithium in hypomania secondary to organic brain syndrome. *Am J Psychiatr* (1975) 132:1072–1073.

Starkstein, S. E., Pearlson, G. D., Boston, J., *et al.* Mania after brain injury: a controlled study of causative factors. *Arch Neurol* (1987) 44:1069–1073.

25

Clinical and lesion correlates of poststroke mania

Family history

Clinical correlates of poststroke mania have not been clearly identified because of the small number of cases identified in the literature. There are several factors which have been identified in some cases but not all. We attempted to investigate clinical correlates of poststroke mania by comparing patients with secondary mania to patients with poststroke major depression or no mood disturbance following stroke (Robinson *et al.* 1988). The patients with secondary mania used in this study were the first 17 patients we identified with secondary mania, 9 of whom had mania following stroke. The 31 patients with major depression consisted of a consecutive series of patients with single-acute stroke lesions which preceded the onset of depression and who had no history of premorbid psychiatric disorder or other neurological or medical illness. Similarly, the group with no mood disturbance represented a consecutive series of patients examined following a single-acute stroke lesion with at least 6 months of follow-up and no prior history of neurological or physical illness. These patients had no diagnosis of mania, depression, or anxiety disorder either at the time of the acute stroke or at follow-up. The background characteristics of the three groups of patients are shown in Table 25.1.

There were no significant differences among the three groups in terms of background characteristics except that patients with secondary mania were slightly, but not significantly, younger than those in the other two groups. There was a significantly longer period of follow-up for the patients with no mood disturbance compared to patients with secondary mania or depression.

Although we did not obtain multi-informant family histories, single- or double-informant family histories revealed that four (24%) of the secondary mania patients had a first-degree relative with a definite history of mood disorder (defined as a history of hospitalization or other medical treatment for a depressive or manic disorder). In addition, three (18%) of the secondary mania patients had a first-degree relative with a "possible" history of affective disorder (defined as a history of hospitalization

Table 25.1. Data on patients with mania secondary to brain injury and patients with and without depression after stroke

	Poststroke patients					
	Mania secondary to brain injury ($n = 17$)		Major depression ($n = 31$)		Non-depressed ($n = 28$)	
	n	%	n	%	n	%
Age (mean years ± SD)	53.3 ± 20		59.8 ± 12.5		63.7 ± 9.4	
Female	8	47	14	45	6	21
Black	4	24	15	48	19	68
Education (mean years ± SD)	9.35 ± 3.5		9.2 ± 3.1		8.5 ± 3.3	
Married	8	47	15	48	11	39
Right handed	15	88	27	87	24	86
Possible or definite family history of mood disorder	7*	41	3	10	1	4
Personal history of mood disorder before index episode	7*	41	0	0	0	0
Time since brain injury (mean months ± SD)	5.8 ± 7.2		6.7 ± 8.7		17.8 ± 7.5	

*$p < 0.01$ compared to major depression and non-depressed.

or medical care for an unknown type of psychiatric disorder). Among the major depression patients, only two (6%) had a definite family history and one had a possible family history of mood disorder. Of the non-depressed patients, one had a possible history of mood disorder and none had a definite history (Fig. 25.1). The frequency of a definite or possible family history of mood disorder among patients with secondary mania was significantly greater than patients with major depression or no mood disturbance ($p = 0.002$).

When the patients with secondary mania were limited to those with mania following stroke, there continued to be a significant association of a definite or possible family history of mood disorder and poststroke mania (i.e., 4 of 9 manic patients versus 3 of 31 poststroke major depression patients had a family history of mood disorder) ($p < 0.05$).

In order to validate this finding in a new group of patients, we added an additional 8 patients with secondary mania studied after the original 17. There was only one patient with a positive family history of mood disorder among 6 additional patients with stroke. Using the overall group of 25 manic patients, however, family history of mood disorder continued to be a significantly more frequent finding among patients with secondary mania compared to those with poststroke depression or no mood disorder ($p = 0.05$).

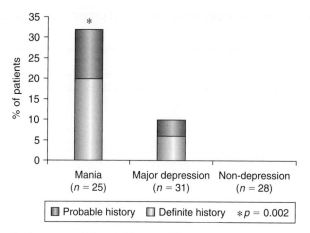

Figure 25.1 The frequency of family history (definite or probable) of mood disorder in the primary relatives of patients with mania following stroke (*n* = 15), tumors (*n* = 6), or trauma (*n* = 4) compared to poststroke major depression or no mood disorder following stroke. Patients with mania were significantly more likely to have a family history of mood disorders than the other two groups.

Vascular disease and age of onset

Another risk factor for late-onset mania was identified by Cassidy and Carroll (2002). The records of 366 bipolar patients were reviewed and divided at age 47 based on the bimodal distribution of age at first psychiatric hospitalization. Using that threshold, 23 (6.3%) were classified as late onset and 343 (93.7%) as early onset. The vascular risk factors included hypertension, hyperlipidemia, and history of smoking, atrial fibrillation, coronary artery disease, and cerebrovascular accident. In order to compare patients who were matched for sex, race, and age within 3 years, there were 18 patients with late-onset mania who could be matched to patients with early-onset mania and five patients with late-onset mania who could not be matched. Of the 18 late-onset patients, 16 had 2 or more vascular risk factors and 8 had 3 or more. This is compared to the 18 matched controls where 11 had 2 or more and only 3 had 3 or more risk factors. The late-onset mania group had significantly more vascular risk factors than the early-onset group (*p* = 0.026).

Fujikawa *et al.* (1995) examined 20 patients who developed bipolar disorder after age 50 (late-onset mania) who were prospectively identified. These patients were compared with 20 age- and sex-matched patients who developed affective disorder before age 50 and 20 patients who developed major depression after age 50. Patients with focal neurological symptoms were excluded as the authors were interested in looking for evidence of silent cerebral infarction on magnetic resonance (MR) scan. The incidence of silent cerebral infarction in patients with late-onset mania was 65% which was significantly higher than patients with early-onset mania ($p < 0.05$). The incidence of mixed type silent cerebral infarction (involving both the cortex and perforating arteries (subcortical regions) was 50% in patients with late-onset mania which was significantly higher than patients with late-onset depression ($p < 0.05$). The authors concluded that as many as half of all cases of late-onset mania may be secondary to cerebral infarction. In addition, the mixed type of silent cerebral infarction involving both cortical and subcortical brain regions was significantly more prevalent in the patients with late-onset mania than in those with late-onset major depression. This may suggest the importance of both cortical and subcortical mechanisms in the etiology of mania or may simply reflect the differences in brain areas which are associated with the onset of mania following injury.

Movement disorder

Berthier *et al.* (1996) examined 9 patients with bipolar affective disorder with cerebrovascular lesions. Of the 9 patients with bipolar disorder, 8 had no family history of bipolar disorder in first-degree relatives. One patient had a father who committed suicide during a stress-induced depression. Two patients had a personal history of depressive disorder prior to the onset of stroke and the mean age at onset of mood disorder was 51.2 ± 9 years. In 8 of the 9 cases, the first affective episode was depressive (89%) while, in the remaining case the onset of the disorder could not be determined. Furthermore, the mean time from the stroke to the onset of mania was 8.6 ± 7 SD months (range 2–24). The mean duration of follow-up was 4.8 ± 7 SD years. In addition, 7 of the 8 patients who had neurological findings had evidence of movement disorder with or without associated motor or sensory deficit. Three patients had hemidystonia, one patient oral-lingual dystonia, one patient hemichorea, two patients had a postural tremor, one patient had bradykinesia, and another patient had unilateral Parkinsonism. The patients often had rapid cycling mood disorder defined as four episodes of mood disorder within 1 year, two of the four patients with bipolar type I and two patients with bipolar type II disorders were rapid cyclers.

Right hemisphere lesion location

The lesion location in the Berthier *et al.* study (1996) was restricted to the right hemisphere in 7 of the 9 cases (78%) while the remaining two patients had bilateral hemispheric damage. Thus, the Berthier study demonstrated that patients may develop bipolar disorder without having a family history of mood disorder. Secondly, there were a significant number of patients who had rapid cycling disorder and movement disorders associated with their stroke. This may suggest the importance of subcortical lesions in rapid cycling mood disorder. The most common site (in 7 of the 9 cases) was the putamen and the periventricular white matter (6 cases). The internal capsule (4 cases) and the caudate nucleus (3 cases) (Berthier *et al.* 1996).

In our previously described study of patients with mania, poststroke depression, and no stroke-related disorder (Robinson *et al.* 1988), patients were also compared for the nature, localization, and volume of brain injury associated with mania or depression. Patients with secondary mania included those with brain tumors ($n = 6$) predominantly frontal meningiomas) or closed head injuries ($n = 2$). There were, however, no statistically significant differences in the volumes of the lesions between the patients with secondary mania, depression, and no mood disturbance. The hemispheric location of lesion was established by means of computed tomographic (CT) or MR scan, or clinical neurological examination. In the secondary mania group, 12 of the 17 patients had a lesion restricted to the right hemisphere while only one patient had a left hemisphere lesion (Fig. 25.2). Of the patients with major depression, 19 of the 31 had lesions involving the left hemisphere, while 9 of the 28 patients in the non-depressed group had lesions localized to the left hemisphere and 10 had lesions localized to the right hemisphere. Mania was significantly more commonly associated with right hemisphere injury and depression was more commonly associated with left hemisphere lesions ($p = 0.0001$). If the analysis only

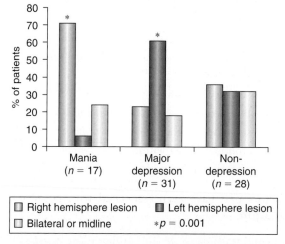

Figure 25.2 Frequency of right or left hemisphere lesion location in patients with mania following stroke ($n = 9$), tumors ($n = 6$), or traumatic brain injury ($n = 2$) compared to patients with acute poststroke major depression or no mood disturbance following stroke. Mania was strongly associated with right hemisphere lesion location while major depression following acute stroke was associated with left hemisphere lesions. The association of diagnosis with lesion location was highly significant ($p = 0.0001$) (data from Robinson *et al.* 1988).

included patients with stroke, this finding still held true (i.e., eight of nine patients with poststroke mania had right hemisphere lesions compared to 7 of 31 depressed patients ($p = 0.01$)).

The strength of this association between mania and right hemisphere lesions also held true when the additional eight patients with secondary mania were added. Of the eight new patients with secondary mania, seven had unilateral involvement of the right hemisphere and one had a bilateral frontal lesion (four had right basotemporal lesions, one had orbitofrontal, and three had basal ganglia lesions). When only patients with poststroke mania were considered, 14 of 15 patients had right hemisphere stroke.

The lesion locations of 13 of our patients with secondary mania and 22 patients with poststroke major depression are shown on schematic templates from CT or MR scans in Fig. 25.3. Patients with secondary mania had cortical lesions predominantly involving the right basotemporal or orbitofrontal cortex. In addition, there were subcortical lesions associated with secondary mania involving the right thalamus or right basal ganglia. These regions are all part of, or are connected to the limbic system.

Patients with poststroke depression, on the other hand, had lesions involving the left basal ganglia, left frontal insular cortex, and left basotemporal cortex (Fig. 25.3). Although some of the lesions associated with depression involved limbic areas, they were more widely distributed than those associated with mania and involved areas only indirectly connected to limbic structures. In addition, although some of the depressed patients had right hemisphere lesions, there was virtually no overlap of the right hemisphere lesions associated with mania and those associated with major depression (Fig. 25.3). In contrast, the poststroke non-depressed patients had lesions scattered equally between the left, right, and brain stem regions (Fig. 25.2).

In summary, both anecdotal and case series of poststroke mania have identified numerous factors associated with this disorder. Probably the most consistent findings were the onset of mania after age 50 and the association with right hemisphere lesions particularly the right basal ganglia and other limbic-related structures. Other factors that have been associated with poststroke mania are family history of mood disorder, risk factors of vascular disease, such as hypercholesterolemia and hypertension, and finally, an association with movement disorders.

Subcortical atrophy

As indicated previously, mania is a relatively rare complication of stroke and it seems likely that factors other than lesion location would play a role in the development of

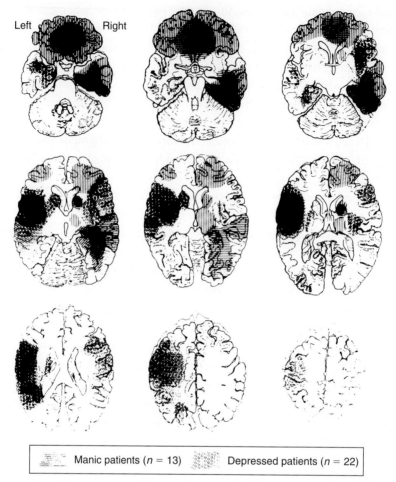

Left   Right

Manic patients ($n = 13$)   Depressed patients ($n = 22$)

Figure 25.3 Areas displaying evidence of injury on CT or MR scan are shown in templates of axial brain slices for both mania and depression. Locations of lesions are indicated by horizontal and vertical lines for manic patients and circles for depressed patients. Mania was associated primarily with orbitofrontal, thalamic, caudate, and basotemporal lesions in the right hemisphere; major depression was associated with left frontal and left caudate lesions. Although right hemisphere lesions are sometimes associated with depression, there was no overlap of the areas of injury in the depressed patients and the manic patient (reprinted from Robinson *et al.* 1988 with permission).

mania. This chapter has identified factors such as family history of mood disorder or movement disorder which may be important secondary factors in the development of mania. In an effort to identify other non-lesion factors in the etiology of post-stroke mania, we conducted a study of secondary mania controlling for lesion location using a two-by-two design (i.e., presence or absence of mania and presence or absence of brain lesion). Patients with secondary mania were compared to patients

Table 25.2. Characteristics of study group

	Secondary mania (n = 11)	Primary mania (n = 25)	Lesion controls (n = 11)	Normal controls (n = 11)
Age, years (mean ± SD)	52 (20)	26 (12[a])	50 (16)	54 (19)
Sex (% female)	37	52	37	33
Handedness (% right)	82	96	100	93
Time since injury (mean months ± SD)[b]	10 (9)		15 (15)	
Time from first affective symptoms to CT scan (mean years ± SD)	0.9 (1.3)	16 (8)		
Family history of mood disorder (% positive)	27	60	9	0

[a]$F = 14.9$; d.f. $= 3.67$; $p < 0.001$.
[b]Months from brain lesion (excluding patients with tumor) or months of follow-up (for lesion controls).

with primary mania and were also compared with lesion-matched patients with no mood disorder (Table 25.2).

The patients with secondary mania were a consecutive series of 11 patients from our first 17 who had CT or MR scans which demonstrated a single-focal lesion that could be dated for onset (i.e., stroke or post-surgical rather than meningioma). The primary mania group consisted of 25 patients who met criteria for bipolar mood disorder for whom a CT scan had been obtained. There was no history of prior brain injury or CT scan evidence of a brain lesion. The lesion control group consisted of 11 patients with brain lesions documented by brain imaging who were matched to the secondary mania patients for age (± 2 years), lesion type (vascular or traumatic), lesion size (small <5% of the brain volume, medium 5–15% of brain volume, or large >15% of the brain volume), and lesion location (both patients had partial or complete involvement of the same brain regions as specified by Levine and Grek 1984). This is the same technique that was used for the investigation of patients with depression as described in Chapter 17 on premorbid risk factors and poststroke depression.

The non-lesion control group consisted of patients who were matched (± 2 years) in age with the secondary mania group who had no previous history of psychiatric disorder, or CT or MR scan evidence of brain injury. There were no significant differences in gender distribution or handedness. The patients with primary mania, however, were significantly younger than those in the other three groups ($p = 0.001$) (Table 25.2). As expected, patients with primary mania had a significantly greater frequency of family history of mood disorder than the patients with secondary mania or the lesion controls ($p = 0.005$).

Among the 25 patients with primary mania, all of them had a prior history of depressive disorder. Among the 11 patients with secondary mania, 6 had a prior history of depressive episodes, defined as depression that led to medical treatment or significantly disrupted daily activities prior to the onset of mania. The depressive episode began after brain injury in five of the patients while one patient had a history of depression prior to the brain lesion.

In addition to the analysis of lesion size and location, a number of structural brain measurements were made on CT scan. The lesion locations for patients with secondary mania and controls were as follows: seven exclusively located in the right hemisphere, two bilateral, and two midline. The causes of injury were as follows: five post-surgical tumors, four strokes, and two trauma. Measurements taken from the CT scans included the following: bifrontal ratio (BFR), distance between the tips of the frontal horns divided by the distance between the inner tables of the skull along the same line; bicaudate ratio (BCR), minimal distance between caudate indentations of the frontal horns divided by the distance between the inner tables of the skull along the same line; lateral ventricular to brain ratio (VBR2), multiple of the minimal coronal distance between the lateral walls of the lateral ventricle at the waist level and the sagittal distance between the extreme anterior–posterior extent of the lateral ventricle divided by the multiple of coronal inner table diameter and midsagittal inner table diameter; third ventricular to brain ratio (VBR3), multiple of the maximal sagittal and coronal diameters of the third ventricle divided by the multiple of the trans-pineal and midsagittal inner table diameters; frontal fissure ratio (FFR), maximal width of the interhemispheric fissure at the frontal level divided by the trans-pineal coronal inner table diameter; sylvian fissure ratio (SFR), the average of the maximum sylvian width divided by the trans-pineal coronal inner table diameter; and the four cortical sulci ratio (4CSR), sum of widths of the four widest sulci divided by the trans-pineal coronal inner table diameter (Gomori *et al.* 1984).

The findings of these measurements are shown in Fig. 25.4 (Starkstein *et al.* 1987). Patients with secondary mania had significantly higher values for BFR and VBR3, and a nearly significant higher value for BCR compared with the other three groups. There were no statistically significant intergroup differences in the remaining CT scan measurements.

Previously in this chapter, I demonstrated that some patients with mania following brain injury had a positive family history of mood disorder. Since this CT scan study found that subcortical atrophy, as indicated by increased BFR and VBR3, was associated with post-injury mania, we examined whether subcortical atrophy and family history of mood disorder occurred in the same patients. We therefore examined CT measurements from patients with and without a family history of mood disorders and the results are shown on Fig. 25.5. Patients without a family history of psychiatric disorder had larger bifrontal and BCR than patients with a

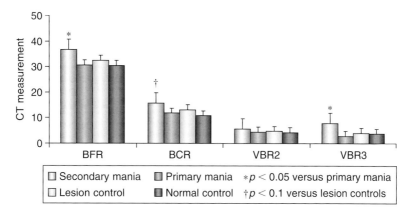

Figure 25.4   Measurements taken from CT scans (mean ± SEM) of patients with mania after brain injury (secondary), of patients with mania without brain injury (primary), of patients matched with secondary manics for age, lesion size, and location and of non-lesion, age-matched (to secondary manics) controls. The BFR and third ventricle to brain size ratio (VBR3) were significantly greater in the secondary mania patients compared to each of the other groups. This suggests that patients who developed mania following brain injury had subcortical atrophy which was probably present before the injury and made them more vulnerable to becoming manic following injury (data taken from Starkstein *et al.* 1987).

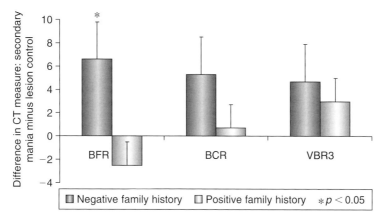

Figure 25.5   CT measurements in patients with secondary mania minus the same CT measurement in their lesion-matched control, comparing patients with and without a family history of psychiatric disorder. A positive number means the secondary mania patient had a larger measurement (more atrophy) than a patient with the same lesion but without mania. Secondary mania patients who did not have a family history showed greater differences from their controls (this was statistically significant for the BFR) for all measures. This suggests that patients who developed mania had a right hemisphere lesion plus either a family history of mood disorder or greater subcortical atrophy compared to patients with the same lesions who did not become manic (data taken from Starkstein *et al.* 1987).

family history of mood disorder. This reached statistical significance for the BFR and suggested that following a lesion of a limbic-connected area of the right hemisphere, patients who develop mania may have either a family history of mood disorder or subcortical atrophy. In other words, our data suggests a "2 hit" hypothesis for the rare occurrence of poststroke mania. A premorbid genetic vulnerability or a premorbid brain atrophy, followed by an injury to limbic connected region of the right hemisphere.

Perhaps the most relevant question in relation to this finding is "What is the cause of the subcortical atrophy found in a significant number of patients with secondary mania?" Although the answer to this question can only be based on speculation, this is a finding that has been reported in studies of a number of psychiatric disorders, including primary mood disorders (Nasrallah *et al.* 1982), schizophrenia (Swayze *et al.* 1992), anorexia (Herzog and Copeland 1985), and others (Jacoby and Levy 1980). The increased BFR and VBR3 ratios in the secondary mania group indicate significant frontal, subcortical, and diencephalic brain atrophy that cannot be explained on the basis of either the focal lesion or the patient's age since the age-matched lesion control patients were not significantly different than the age-comparable non-lesion controls. In addition, all but one of the CT scans were done soon after the focal brain lesion or in the case of patients with brain tumors after their first neurological symptoms began. Thus, it is likely that the subcortical atrophy predated the focal lesion. Although the cause of the subcortical atrophy in any of the conditions in which it has been identified has not been determined, factors such as perinatal anoxia, exposure to toxins in the environment or other environmental factors have been implicated (Nasrallah *et al.* 1982). A study of monozygotic twins who were discordant for schizophrenia found that the affected twin had enlarged ventricles (Berman *et al.* 1992), which suggests that environmental factors may play an important role in the development of subcortical atrophy.

Since genetic vulnerability was one of the significant associations with poststroke mania, it might be argued that these patients had bipolar mood disorder and the brain lesion before the mania was simply a coincidence. The finding that argues most strongly against this hypothesis, however, is the highly significant association between secondary mania and a right hemisphere lesion. If patients were destined to develop mania based on genetic vulnerability one would not expect an association with a particular lesion location.

Another possible explanation for these findings might be that increased VBR are associated with depression rather than mania. The findings that argue against this interpretation are that only six of the 11 patients with mania had prior depressive episodes and CT scan measurements were not significantly different between those patients with and without prior depression (see Chapter 27 on bipolar disorder following stroke). Furthermore, based on the comparison with lesion controls as well as patients with primary mania, the increased VBR cannot be explained by any of the following variables: duration of mood disorder, the existence of a right hemisphere lesion, or the length of follow-up since brain lesion (i.e., the lesion control patients were followed up for a greater period of time after their injury compared to the secondary mania patients).

These findings, as well as our previous findings of major depression associated with left basal ganglia lesions and enlarged VBR (see Chapters 10 and 17), suggest that an important contribution can be made by subcortical mechanisms in the pathogenesis of mood disorders following stroke. Finally, our finding that subcortical atrophy probably predated the mood disorder suggests that a mild degree of subcortical atrophy may play an important "permissive" role in mediating poststroke mood disorders, albeit a strategic lesion is also necessary to initiate that particular clinical syndrome.

REFERENCES

Berman, K. F., Torrey, E. F., Daniel, D. G., *et al.* Regional cerebral blood flow in monozygotic twins discordant and concordant for schizophrenia. *Arch Gen Psychiatr* (1992) 49:927–934.

Berthier, M. L., Kulisevsky, J., Gironell, A., *et al.* Poststroke bipolar affective disorder: clinical subtypes, concurrent movement disorders, and anatomical correlates. *J Neuropsychiatr Clin Neurosci* (1996) 8(2):160–167.

Cassidy, F., and Carroll, B. J. Vascular risk factors in late onset mania. *Psychol Med* (2002) 32(2):359–362.

Fujikawa, T., Yamawaki, S., and Touhouda, Y. Silent cerebral infarctions in patients with late-onset mania. *Stroke* (1995) 26(6):946–949.

Gomori, J. M., Steiner, I., Melamed, E., *et al.* The assessment of changes in brain volume using combined linear measures: a CT scan study. *Neuroradiology* (1984) 26:21–24.

Herzog, D. B., and Copeland, P. M. Eating disorders. *New Engl J Med* (1985) 313(5):295–303.

Jacoby, R. J., and Levy, R. Computed tomography in the elderly. 2. Senile dementia: diagnosis and functional impairment. *Br J Psychiatr* (1980) 136:256–269.

Levine, D. N., and Grek, A. The anatomic basis of delusions after right cerebral infarction. *Neurology* (1984) 34:577–582.

Nasrallah, H. A., Whitters, M., and Jacoby, C. G. Cerebral ventricular enlargement in bipolar affective disorder. *J Affect Disord* (1982) 4:15–19.

Robinson, R. G., Boston, J. D., Starkstein, S. E., *et al.* Comparison of mania with depression following brain injury: causal factors. *Am J Psychiatr* (1988) 145:172–178.

Starkstein, S. E., Pearlson, G. D., Boston, J., *et al.* Mania after brain injury: a controlled study of causative factors. *Arch Neurol* (1987) 44:1069–1073.

Swayze, V., Andreasen, N. C., Randall, J., *et al.* Subcortical and temporal structures in affective disorder and schizophrenia: a magnetic resonance imaging study. *Biol Psychiatr* (1992) 31:221–240.

26

Bipolar disorder following stroke

As indicated in the previous chapter, a significant number of patients with secondary mania were also found to have episodes of depression. In contrast, however, other patients with secondary mania did not have episodes of depression within the period of study or prior to the stroke. We examined patients with bipolar disorder and compared them to patients with secondary mania but no evidence of depressive episodes (Starkstein *et al.* 1991).

The most obvious concern in patients with mania but without episodes of depression is whether sufficient follow-up had been obtained to identify the existence of a bipolar disorder. The diagnostic categories of Diagnostic and Statistical Manual of Mental Disorder (DSM-IV) (see Chapter 5) do not include unipolar mania and once a patient has had an episode of mania they are presumed to have a bipolar disorder. Although one cannot be sure that a patient with a single or recurrent episodes of mania will not have depression (similarly one cannot be sure that patients with unipolar depression will not have an episode of mania in the future), all of the patients included in the bipolar disorder associated with brain injury had depression *prior* to the onset of mania. Patients with mania had variable amounts of follow-up but none of them had depression prior to onset of mania or at any time following the episode of mania.

We included in this study all of the 25 patients from our secondary mania studies who had a demonstrable lesion on computed tomographic (CT) scan with focal neuropathology. There were a total of 19 patients with lesions that could be localized on CT scan. Of these patients, seven had at least one episode of depression prior to the onset of mania while 12 patients had no history of depression either prior to or following the identified episode of mania.

The background characteristics of bipolar and mania-only patients are shown in Table 26.1. There were no significant differences in age or in personal or family history of mood disorders. Among the bipolar patients, one had a family history of bipolar disorder and one had a family history of alcoholism. Among the 12 mania-only patients, three had a family history of mood disorder ($p = $ NS).

Table 26.1. Demographic data

	Bipolar	Mania only
Number of patients	7	12
Age (mean years) (SD)	61.2 (15.9)	50.1 (16.9)
Sex (% females)	43	33
Handedness (% right-handed)	86	83
Education (mean years) (SD)	8.7 (2.2)	11.4 (3.6)
Family history of psychiatric disorder (% positive)	29	25
Personal history of psychiatric disorder (% positive)	0	0

From Starkstein *et al.* (1991) reprinted with permission.

Among the patients with bipolar disorder, six of seven (85%) developed depression within the 1st week following brain lesion. Only one patient was given antidepressant medication. The onset of mania occurred within the 1st month following brain injury in three patients while the other three patients developed mania within the first 6 months (in one patient, the time from brain injury to onset of mania could not be determined). Patients with mania only developed manic symptoms within the 1st week following brain lesion in 5 of 12 cases (40%), while 3 of 12 patients (25%) developed mania between 18 months, and 4 years following brain injury. In the remaining four patients, the time of the mania was documented but the age of the brain lesion was uncertain. Thus, there was some variability in the time from brain injury to the onset of mania. About half of the cases occurred within the first month following brain injury. The onset of mania in bipolar disorder patients appeared to be somewhat closer to the time of injury (i.e., within the first 6 months) compared to the mania-only patients (i.e., from several days to 4 years after the injury).

Neurological findings were not significantly different in the bipolar and mania-only patients; motor deficits were found in 71% of the bipolar patients and 42% of the mania-only patients; visual field deficits were present in 29% and 50% respectively; sensory deficits were present in 14% and 17% respectively.

There were no significant differences in the frequency of symptoms of mania between the bipolar and mania-only patients. Grandiose delusions were found in 71% of the bipolar patients and 83% of the mania-only patients; hyperactivity was found in 86% and 83% respectively; pressure of speech in 86% and 92% respectively; irritability in 14% and 50% respectively; overspending in 57% and 50% respectively. Patients with bipolar disorder, however, had significantly greater impairment of cognitive function than the mania-only patients (25.2 ± 4.7 SD versus 28.6 ± 1.8 SD, $p < 0.05$). The reason for the greater degree of cognitive impairment in the bipolar group is unclear.

The lesions for the bipolar and mania-only patients are shown in Fig. 26.1. Of the seven bipolar patients, six had lesions restricted to the right hemisphere which involved the head of the caudate in two patients, the thalamus in three patients, and ischemic infarction of several cortical and subcortical regions (head of the caudate, dorsolateral frontal cortex), and basotemporal cortex in one patient.

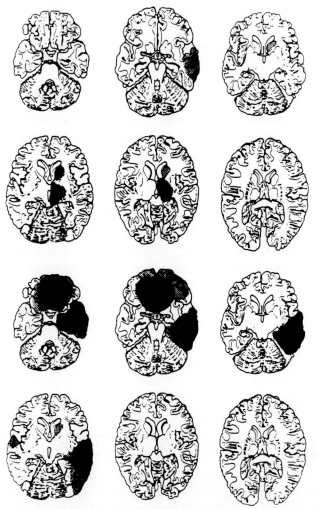

Figure 26.1 Upper panel—bipolar group: schematic templates of CT scan slices showing the largest cross-sectional area of lesion for manic-depressive patients. Lesions mainly involved the right head of the caudate and right thalamus. Lower panel—mania-only group: schematic templates of CT scan slices showing the largest cross-sectional area of lesion for mania-only patients. Lesions mainly involved the orbitofrontal cortex and the right basotemporal cortex. Reprinted from Starkstein *et al.* (1991), with permission.

Stroke lesions occurred in five of these six patients while one had a bleed secondary to trauma. The remaining patient developed bipolar disorder following removal of a pituitary adenoma.

Among the mania-only patients, 8 of 12 had lesions restricted to the right hemisphere (Fig. 26.1). Three patients with mania only had stroke lesions involving the basal temporal cortex, amygdala, and hippocampus including the head of the caudate (one case), and the occipitotemporal cortex (one case). Two patients had gliomas involving the inferior temporal lobe (one case), or the temporal and parietal lobes (one case). Three patients had orbitofrontal meningiomas. Two patients had closed head injury involving orbitofrontal cortex, one patient had an arteriovenous malformation in the inferior temporal lobe, and one patient had a post-traumatic hematoma in the inferior temporal lobe.

The frequency of cortical versus subcortical lesions are shown in Fig. 26.2. Patients with bipolar disorder had a significantly higher frequency of subcortical lesions compared to patients with mania only who had a higher frequency of cortical lesions.

In addition, patients with mania only had significantly larger lesions than the bipolar patients (12.6 ± 9.5 SD % for those with mania only versus 2.8 ± 4.2 SD % for the bipolar group $p < 0.05$, where the lesion volume is calculated as the percent of the largest cross-sectional area of the lesion divided by the area of the whole brain at the level of the body of the lateral ventricle). This finding probably reflects the fact that bipolar disorders were found to be associated with subcortical lesions, which are usually smaller than cortical lesions, and cortical lesions are associated with mania only. No significant differences were observed in the distance of anterior or posterior lesion borders from the frontal pole.

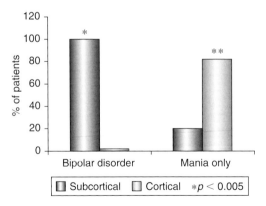

Figure 26.2 The frequency of subcortical and cortical lesions in patients with bipolar disorder or mania-only following brain lesions. Bipolar disorder was strongly associated with lesions of the basal ganglia or thalamus in the right hemisphere while mania-only was associated with right cortical lesions. Data from Starkstein *et al.* (1991).

The course of the unipolar and bipolar disorders, including the length of follow-up in each case is shown in Fig. 28.1. Although most episodes of mania appeared to respond to treatment with lithium, some episodes were non-responsive and were treated with carbamazepine or neuroleptic medication. This issue will be discussed in Chapter 28. These longitudinal courses of mood disorder demonstrate, however, that both bipolar disorder and mania alone can be characterized by recurrent episodes of mood disorder. These episodes may be variable in duration and present with either manic or hypomanic symptoms. There have been no systematic studies of poststroke mania that have examined the duration of the disorder or frequency of relapse but anecdotal cases of this type have demonstrated that both poststroke mania and depression may recur and preventive treatment is an important goal of poststroke mood disorder research (see Chapter 23).

The finding of greater cognitive impairment in bipolar compared with mania only-patients was surprising given the association of bipolar disorder with subcortical lesion location and the smaller lesion volumes compared with those of mania-only patients. As discussed in Chapter 14 on "Relationship of depression to cognitive impairment", poststroke major depression has been found to be associated with greater cognitive impairment. Thus, the presence of a previous episode of depression may have led to more severe cognitive impairments in the bipolar group. Alternatively, the fact that lesions were predominantly of the right hemisphere and the mini-mental state examination is a language based examination could have led to a greater degree of language impairment associated with right subcortical as compared with right cortical structures. Caudate and thalamic lesions have been reported to produce intellectual and language deficits (Graff-Radford *et al.* 1984). Whatever the explanation, this phenomenon is worthy of further investigation.

The major question raised by this study is why some patients developed mania only (unipolar mania) while others developed bipolar disorder. Shukla *et al.* (1987) reported a similar frequency of depression (30%) in their series of patients with mania after closed head injury. The finding of significantly different frequencies of cortical versus subcortical lesion location in the bipolar versus mania-only groups suggests that mania may be associated with orbitofrontal and basotemporal mechanisms which lead to limbic dysfunction in the right hemisphere. Subcortical lesions, on the other hand, may have produced hypometabolic effects in both ipsilateral and contralateral brain regions (i.e., crossed and uncrossed hemisphere diaschises) (Takano *et al.* 1985; Pozzili *et al.* 1987). If depression was mediated through left ventral lateral limbic dysfunction, right subcortical lesions may have induced these changes in the left hemisphere with mania developing only when this left hemisphere effect ceases and right hemisphere limbic dysfunction emerges.

Although the mechanisms of bipolar versus unipolar mood disorder following brain injury will need further investigation, the fact that unipolar and bipolar mood disorders following brain injury can be distinguished based in part on lesion location suggests that there may be different etiologies for unipolar versus bipolar mania and that the course and treatment of these disorders may be unique.

In summary, our study of secondary unipolar disorder showed that 37% of patients with mania following brain injury had a prior episode of depression and, therefore, a bipolar course. Bipolar disorder was found to be associated with subcortical lesions while mania only was associated with cortical lesions (mainly involving the right orbitofrontal and right inferior temporal cortices) and significantly larger lesion volumes. Although the bipolar and mania-only groups showed similar deficits in neurological examination, bipolar patients had significantly lower mini-mental state examination scores.

REFERENCES

Graff-Radford, N. R., Eslinger, P. J., and Damasio, A. R. Nonhemorrhagic infarction of the thalamus: behavioral, anatomic, and physiologic correlates. *Neurology* (1984) 34:14–23.

Pozzili, C., Passafiume, D., Bastianello, S., *et al*. Remote effects of caudate hemorrhage: a clinical and functional study. *Cortex* (1987) 23:341–349.

Shukla, S., Cook, B. L., Mukherjee, S., *et al*. Mania following head trauma. *Am J Psychiatr* (1987) 144:93–96.

Starkstein, S. E., Fedoroff, J. P., Berthier, M. D., *et al*. Manic depressive and pure manic states after brain lesions. *Biol Psychiatr* (1991) 29:149–158.

Takano, T., Kimura., K., Nakamura, M., *et al*. Effect of small hemispheric infarction on the ipsilateral cortical blood flow in man. *Stroke* (1985) 16:64–69.

27

Mechanism of mania following stroke

Injury to the inferior temporal cortex, orbital frontal cortex, caudate, and thalamus have all been demonstrated to lead to the development of mania in vulnerable patients. These constitute the major elements of the lateral orbital frontal circuit as described by Alexander *et al.* (1990) and the association of mania with injury to these structures suggests that these right hemisphere regions may play an important role in the mediation of mania following stroke.

One of the main factors, however, which must be taken into account in understanding the mechanism of poststroke mania is the lateralized effect of lesions. Hemispheric specialization and, therefore, the association with unilateral hemispheric lesions in secondary mania, appears to be even stronger than the lateralized effect in acute poststroke depression. Although the number of secondary mania cases is significantly less than the number of secondary depression cases, 21 out of 27 (78%) secondary mania cases that we have seen have had exclusively right hemisphere involvement compared to about 56% of patients with major depression who had exclusively left hemisphere lesions (see Chapter 10: "Relationship of depression to lesion location"). Five manic patients had midline or bilateral hemisphere involvement and only one patient had a localized left hemisphere lesion. These findings suggest that there is a strong association between mania and right hemisphere injury, one that is stronger than the association between major depression and acute left hemisphere lesions.

The second previously described finding from the studies of secondary mania is intrahemispheric lesion location. Lesions in all of the secondary mania cases involved either the basal portion of the frontal lobes, basal and medial portions of the temporal lobes, or the subcortical basal ganglia or thalamic nuclei. These structures are part of the ventral lateral limbic circuit described in Chapter 21 "Mechanism of poststroke depression." Output from the orbitofrontal cortex projects to the caudate nucleus and to basotemporal cortex (Fig. 27.1). The caudate nucleus has multisynaptic projections to the putamen, globus pallidus, and dorsomedial thalamic nucleus. The dorsal medial thalamic nuclei project back to the prefrontal cortex

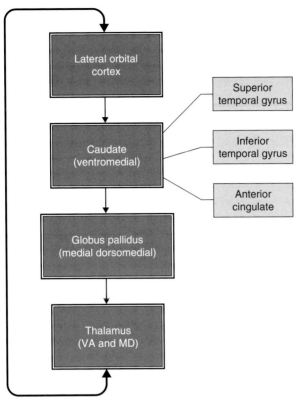

Figure 27.1   Cortical-basal ganglia-thalamic loop described by Alexander *et al.* (1986). Note that decreased input from the inferior temporal gyrus due to lesion or decreased metabolic activity could alter function within the entire circuit.

and orbitofrontal cortex. The basotemporal cortex projects to the amygdala, basal ganglia, and dorsomedial thalamus (Nauta 1971).

In addition to the orbitofrontal projections to the basotemporal cortex and caudate nucleus, the orbitofrontal cortex also projects to a subcortical limbic region known as the septo-hypothalo-mesencephalic continuum (Nauta 1971). This septo-hypothalamic region connects to the pituitary and visceral motor system. Thus, by way of multiple efferent projections, the orbitofrontal cortex may affect not only the emotion circuitry of the limbic system but it may also modulate vegetative symptoms and body rhythms through the hypothalamic and pituitary adrenal axis.

Previous investigators have suggested that the frontal lobe may play a central role in the mediation of emotion. Welt (1888) suggested that injuries to the medial orbital surface of the frontal lobes might cause a change in character expressed by restlessness, euphoria, over talkativeness, and lowered ethical and moral standards. Jastrowitz (1888) described several patients with frontal lobe tumors, some of whom showed euphoric mood with pressured speech and a tendency to pun and use obscene language. He used the term "moria" to describe these symptoms. Oppenheim (1890) noted similar symptoms in patients with frontal brain lesions and referred to them as "witzelsucht." Kleist (1931) hypothesized that the orbitofrontal cortex was the center of emotional life while the frontal convexity was associated with psychomotor and intellectual activity. Apathy and lack of motor activity was associated with lesions of the frontal convexity while orbitofrontal lesions were associated with euphoria and lack of social inhibitions. Poetzl (1924 as cited in Rylander in 1939) reported on one patient with a lesion of the frontal convexity who had an akinetic syndrome and on another patient with an orbitofrontal lesion who had symptoms of euphoria and disinhibition. Rylander (1939) described personality changes in 32 patients following frontal lobe surgery. Euphoria developed in 20 patients (18 of whom had orbitofrontal surgically removal), 17 developed hyperactivity, and 10 developed hypersexuality. Finally, Blumer and Benson (1975) described two syndromes associated with frontal lobe damage consistent with Kleist's proposal. One syndrome, termed "pseudodepressive," was characterized by slowness, indifference, and apathy associated with lesions of the prefrontal convexity. The other syndrome, called "pseudopsychopathic," was characterized by grandiose thoughts, hyperactivity, and disinhibition and was associated with orbitofrontal lesions. Thus, there is a long history of clinical observation indicating that changes in mood, psychomotor activity, and social behavior are disrupted by lesions of the frontal lobe. It is certainly possible (if not likely) that many of these cases represented secondary mania.

In addition to this assessment of lesion location and hypothesized neural circuitry, we have undertaken an assessment of metabolic activity in different brain regions in three individual patients with mania following subcortical lesions (Starkstein *et al.* 1990). Patients were given [^{18}F]fluorodeoxyglucose (FDG) and regional brain metabolic activity was measured using positron emission tomography (PET). One patient had a small hemorrhagic lesion in the white matter under the right frontal lobe at the tip of the horn of the lateral ventricle. The second patient had an ischemic infarction involving the anterior limb of the right internal capsule and the inferior portion of the head of the caudate. The third patient had an ischemic infarction involving the right head of the caudate extending into the anterior limb of the internal capsule. All patients were manic at the time of the PET scan and had mania rating scale scores (Bech *et al.* 1986) of 15 points, 21 points, and 33 points respectively (higher scores indicate greater severity of mania). Patients one and three were taking lithium but no other medications at the time of the scan while patient two was taking no medication.

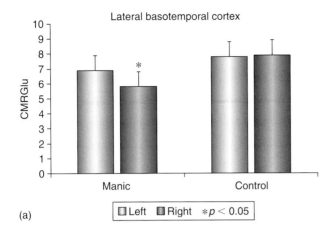

(a)

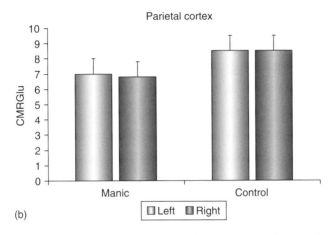

(b)

Figure 27.2 (a) Regional rates of glucose metabolic rates among three patients with mania following subcortical brain lesions and seven age-comparable normal controls. Data are means and standard deviations. Patients with mania had significantly lower metabolic activity in the right basotemporal cortex compared to controls ($p < 0.05$). There was no significant difference in the left temporal cortex of patients and controls. (b) Patients with mania were not significantly different to the controls in terms of metabolic activity in the parietal cortex. CMRGlu: Cerebral glucose metabolic rate in mg of glucose per 100 g tissue per minute.

Assessment of metabolic activity for these three patients compared to seven normal controls between the ages of 35 and 45 who were taking no medication showed that there was a significant asymmetry. The metabolic activity results are shown in Fig. 27.2. Patients one and three had decreased metabolic activity only in the lateral basotemporal region while patient two showed significant metabolic asymmetries in the lateral basotemporal cortex, superior frontal, and parietal cortex.

Although each of these patients had a lesion involving subcortical nuclei or white matter in the right hemisphere, the basotemporal cortex was found to be significantly hypometabolic. The magnitude of the hypometabolic effect in the basotemporal cortex was more than two standard deviations below the overall mean brain metabolic activity in 10 standardized brain regions for patients one and three and more than one standard deviation below for patient two. This study suggests that the right basotemporal region may play an important role in secondary mania through remote hypometabolic effects (diaschises). In the discussion of mechanisms of poststroke depression in Chapter 22, FDG PET studies found *bilateral* hypometabolic activity in both basotemporal and frontal cortices. Thus, mania may involve a specific neurophysiological effect in the right basotemporal cortex while depression involves bilateral basotemporal and frontal dysfunction. This is, however, purely speculative and basotemporal hypometabolism may only play a secondary role in the mechanism of mania.

In another of our studies of secondary mania (this one following traumatic brain injury (TBI)) (Jorge *et al.* 1993), we also found that injury involving the basotemporal cortex was significantly associated with post-TBI mania. There was not, however,

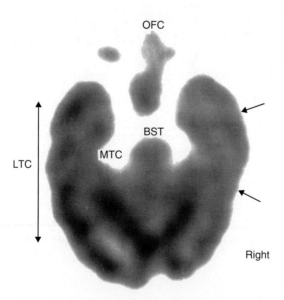

Figure 27.3 Axial slice through the basal temporal lobes following administration of FDG in a 57-year-old man who developed the acute onset of mania within 2 weeks following a stroke involving the right caudate and internal capsule. OFC: orbitofrontal cortex; LTC: laterotemporal cortex; MTC: mediotemporal cortex; BST: brain stem. Arrows indicate the areas of hypometabolic activity in the right temporal cortex (reprinted from Starkstein *et al.* 1990 with permission).

a laterality effect indicating that both right and left hemisphere basotemporal lesions are significantly associated with mania. This lack of a lateralized effect in TBI may have been the result of a high frequency of bilateral injury, which tends to occur in trauma cases, leading to an insufficient number of cases with unilateral injury to reveal any association with right hemisphere injury. It might also suggest that dysfunction of another area of the right hemisphere, in addition to the right basotemporal cortex, plays an important role in the production of secondary mania. Similarly, a study of five patients with primary mania (i.e., mania without a demonstrable brain lesion) using single photon emission computed tomography (SPECT) found significantly lower blood flow in the basal portion of the right temporal lobe compared to seven age-comparable normal controls (Starkstein *et al.* 1990) (Fig. 27.3).

Another case study of a patient with mania provides some further insight into the possible mechanisms of this disorder (Starkstein *et al.* 1989).

CASE STUDY

The patient was a 25-year-old right-handed man who was found to have a vascular malformation involving the right basotemporal lobe with frequent headaches. The patient was referred for embolization of the malformation following a small bleed. Within minutes following the embolization the patient's mood became euphoric and he was very talkative, stating that he was "a new person and this was the best moment of his life." A follow-up CT scan showed partial infarction of the malformation. There was no personal history of prior psychiatric disorder but the patient's mother and twin sister had bipolar disorder.

Because the embolization procedure only partially occluded the vascular formation, the patient underwent a WADA (i.e., injection of Amytal (amylobarbitone) into specific unilateral arterial branches) to determine the pattern of hemispheric dominance. Through a transfemoral selective catheterization, small doses of amylobarbitone were injected into specific branches of the middle cerebral artery. Following injection of 30 mg amylobarbitone into the M1 segment of the left middle cerebral artery, the patient became globally aphasic with a right hemiplegia. Normal verbal comprehension returned in 3 min and 40 s. The patient said that he was feeling fine and responded with laughter. At 6 min and 54 s following the injection, the patient stated that this was one of the happiness moments of his life.

Following similar injection into the right frontal polar artery, the patient continued to make grandiose statements, saying that this was the happiest he has been in his life and that he was enormously happy.

This case demonstrated that after an amylobarbitone injection into the left middle cerebral artery, the patient continued to show symptoms of mania within a few minutes after the return of language function. He was elated and irritable, laughed inappropriately, and showed pressured thoughts and speech. Previous studies have demonstrated that following injections of amylobarbitone into the left internal carotid artery mood changes persist even after recovery from aphasia (Terzian 1965). It has been suggested that a possible mechanism for the production of mood disorders after brain lesions is the "release" of the contralateral hemisphere caused by destruction of inhibitory neural fibers projecting from the ipsilateral to the contralateral cortex (Flor-Henry 1979). In other words, a stroke removes the neurons which normally inhibit the opposite hemisphere, thus allowing it to over-express its normal function. According to this hypothesis, the amylobarbitone injection in the left hemisphere should have at least briefly abolished the manic symptoms. Although it is possible that amylobarbitone injection within another region of the middle cerebral artery (i.e., anterior or posterior branches) might have abolished the manic symptoms, this finding suggests that secondary mania may not be mediated by release from transcallosal inhibitory pathways. This hypothesis, that is mania is mediated primarily by mechanisms within the right hemisphere, is also consistent with the findings in studies of poststroke depression (see Chapters 12 and 21), namely that bilateral stroke lesions do not modify the association between left anterior lesion location and depression, and that severity of depression is correlated only with the proximity of the left hemisphere lesion to the frontal pole.

In summary, studies of patients with poststroke mania have identified risk factors as follows: family history of mood disorder, a right hemisphere lesion involving the orbitofrontal cortex, basotemporal cortex, basal ganglia, or thalamus, and distant effects of injury in the basotemporal cortex. Injury to any one of these structures may lead to dysfunction of the ventral lateral limbic circuit involving the (i.e., orbitofrontal cortex, basotemporal cortex, caudate nucleus, and dorsomedial thalamic nucleus). In addition, the vegetative symptoms associated with mania may be mediated through frontal projections to the septum and hypothalamus. Furthermore, the mechanisms appeared to be predominantly mediated within the right hemisphere and do not involve release of the left hemisphere.

It is interesting that the lesions associated with the production of secondary mania were not simply mirror reflections of the left hemisphere lesions associated with depression. The lesions associated with depression were found to involve the left lateral frontal convexity rather than basotemporal cortex. Furthermore, thalamic lesions have not been found to be associated with depressive disorder. This may indicate that there are different mechanisms for mania and depression which are separate from the lateralized hemispheric effects. Mania may be rare because involvement of more than one area of dysfunction (i.e., a limbic lesion and subcortical atrophy) is required or a genetic vulnerability may be necessary if dysfunction of two separate areas of right hemisphere does not occur. Further work is needed to identify the mechanisms of this interesting clinical phenomenon but several clinical correlates have emerged from anecdotal cases and systematic studies. These clinical correlates have suggested the importance of right limbic system dysfunction in the production of poststroke mania.

REFERENCES

Alexander, G. E., DeLong, M. R., and Strick, P. L. Parallel organization of functionally segregated circuits linking basal ganglia and cortex. *Annu Rev Neurosci* (1986) 9:357–381.

Alexander, G. E., Crutcher, M. D., and DeLong, M. R. Basal ganglia-thalamocortical circuits: parallel substrates for motor, oculomotor, "prefrontal" and "limbic" functions. *Prog Brain Res* (1990) 85:119–146.

Bech, P., Kastrup, M., and Rafaelsen, O. J. Mini-compendium of rating scales for states of anxiety, depression, mania, schizophrenia with corresponding DSM-III syndromes. *Acta Psychiatr Scand* (1986) 73(Suppl 236):29–31.

Blumer, D., and Benson, D. F. Personality changes with frontal and temporal lobe lesions. In D. F. Benson and D. Blumer, eds., *Psychiatric Aspects of Neurologic Diseases*. Grune & Stratton, New York, 1975.

Flor-Henry, P. Uncertain aspects of the localization of the cerebral symptoms relating and determining emotion. *Biol Psychiatr* (1979) 14:677–698.

Jastrowitz, M. Beitrage zur localisation in grosshirn und über deren praktische verwerthung. *Deuts Med Wochenschr* (1888) 14:81–83.

Jorge, R. E., Robinson, R. G., Starkstein, S. E., *et al.* Secondary mania following traumatic brain injury. *Am J Psychiatr* (1993) 150:916–921.

Kleist, K. Die storungen der ichleistungen und ihre lokalisation in orbital-, innen und swischenhirn. *Monatsschr Psychiatr Neurol* (1931) 79:338–350.

Nauta, W. J. H. The problem of the frontal lobe: a reinterpretation. *J Psychol Res* (1971) 8:167–187.

Oppenheim, H. Zur pathologie der grosshirngeschwulse. *Arch Psychiatr Nervenkr* (1890) 21:560–587.

Rylander, G. *Personality Changes after Operations on the Frontal Lobes*. Oxford University Press, London, 1939.

Starkstein, S. E., Berthier, P. L., Lylyk, A., *et al.* Emotional behavior after a WADA test in a patient with secondary mania. *J Neuropsychiatr Clin Neurosci* (1989) 1:408–412.

Starkstein, S. E., Mayberg, H. S., Berthier, M. L., *et al.* Mania after brain injury: neuroradiological and metabolic findings. *Ann Neurol* (1990) 27:652–659.

Terzian, H. Behavioural and EEG effects of intracarotid sodium amytal injection. *Acta Neurochir* (1965) 12:230–239.

Welt, L. Ueber charakterveranderungen des Menschen infolge von lasionen des stirnhirns. *Dtsch Arch Klin Med* (1888) 42:339–390.

28

Treatment of mania following stroke

A controlled double-blind treatment trial of secondary mania has not been conducted. Based on small series and anecdotal case reports, however, lithium has been the most commonly used treatment for secondary mania. There are reports, however, indicating that some cases have not responded to treatment with lithium. Some of these patients had a better response to carbamazepine or valproate and some did not respond to treatment. The treatment responses for the 19 patients in our study of bipolar disorder and mania only are shown in Fig. 28.1. Although there are clearly some patients who did not respond following treatment, most of the episodes of mania improved with treatment using lithium.

Of the total of 27 patients taken from all our studies of secondary mania, 10 of them clearly improved following treatment with lithium and only three clearly did not. In addition, three patients responded to a combination of carbamazepine and lithium, and two patients failed to respond to this treatment combination. The remaining patients were either not treated or treated with a tricyclic antidepressant which would not be expected to improve the manic symptoms.

In spite of the finding that most patients with secondary mania whom we studied responded to lithium treatment, there has been a general consensus in the anecdotal case literature that secondary mania tends to be more difficult to treat than primary mania (Shukla *et al.* 1987; Evans *et al.* 1995). One of the reasons why secondary mania may have been more difficult to treat is that some secondary mania patients had seizure disorders following brain injury. The use of antipsychotic medications in this condition has never been studied. Elderly patients are known to be more vulnerable than younger patients to neuroleptic-associated dyskinesias including tardive dyskinesia (Dubovsky 1994). Thus, neuroleptics should be used with caution and in lower doses than usual in this elderly population.

The doses of other medications used for the treatment of secondary mania in the elderly, such as lithium, carbamazepine, and valproate, should, in many cases, be lower than those used in the treatment of a younger adult and increased slowly. Blood levels, however, should be monitored to determine adequate dosage since

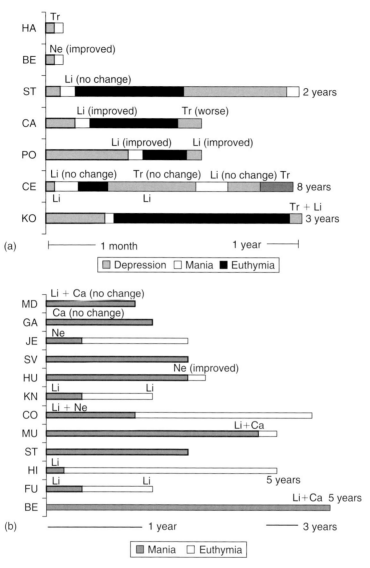

Figure 28.1 (a) Bipolar group: schematic templates of computed tomography scan slices showing largest cross-sectional area of lesion for manic-depressive patients. Lesions mainly involved the right head of the caudate and right thalamus. Longitudinal evolution of mood disorder for individual patients with bipolar disorder. (b) Mania-only group: schematic templates of computed tomography scan slices showing largest cross-sectional area of lesion for mania-only patients. Lesions mainly involved the orbitofrontal cortex and the right basotemporal cortex. Longitudinal evolution of mood disorder for individual patients with mania only (Starkstein and Robinson 1992, reprinted with permission). Tr: tricyclic antidepressant; Ne: nortriptyline; Li: lithium; Ca: carbamazepine.

several of our studies using nortriptyline for depression (Lipsey *et al.* 1984) and pathological crying (Robinson *et al.* 1993) found that the therapeutic range that produces the desired serum concentration was the same for elderly stroke patients and younger adults. The therapeutic range for poststroke mania has not been established for lithium, carbamazepine, or valproate. However, the anecdotal cases would suggest that the blood levels established for treatment of primary mania were effective in the treatment of secondary mania.

Bakchine *et al.* (1989) reported on the double-blind crossover treatment of a single patient with mania following brain injury. In this case, clonidine 600 μg per day, an adrenergic agonist, rapidly reversed the manic symptoms while carbamazepine 1200 mg/day had no effect and levodopa (L-Dopa) 375 mg/day resulted in increased manic symptoms. These findings indicate that clonidine may represent an alternative treatment for patients with secondary mania who fail to respond to the usual treatment and that decreased availability of norepinephrine may play a role in the mechanism of some secondary manias.

In summary, although lithium treatment sometimes clearly fails, until a controlled treatment trial is conducted, the evidence available in the literature suggests that lithium remains the first line of treatment for poststroke mania as it is for primary (i.e., no known brain lesion) mania. Alternative treatments including carbamazepine or valproate, clonidine, benzodiazepines or antipsychotic medications approved for use in primary mania, such as ziprasidone and aripiprazole, need to be evaluated in controlled double-blind treatment trials for their efficacy in poststroke mania.

REFERENCES

Bakchine, S., Lacomblez, L., Benoit, N., *et al.* Manic-like state after orbitofrontal and right temporoparietal injury: efficacy of clonidine. *Neurology* (1989) 39:778–781.

Dubovsky, S. L. Geriatric neuropsychopharmacology. In C. E. Coffey and J. F. Cummings, eds., *Textbook of Geriatric Neuropsychiatry.* American Psychiatric Press, Inc., Washington DC, 1994.

Evans, D. L., Byerly, M., and Greer, R. Secondary mania: diagnosis and treatment. *J Clin Psychiatr* (1995) 53(Suppl 3):31–37.

Lipsey, J. R., Robinson, R. G., Pearlson, G. D., *et al.* Nortriptyline treatment of post-stroke depression: a double-blind study. *Lancet* (1984) i(8372):297–300.

Robinson, R. G., Parikh, R. M., Lipsey, J. R., *et al.* Pathological laughing and crying following stroke: validation of measurement scale and double-blind treatment study. *Am J Psychiatr* (1993) 150:286–293.

Shukla, S., Cook, B. L., Mukherjee, S., *et al.* Mania following head trauma. *Am J Psychiatr* (1987) 144:93–96.

Starkstein, S. E., and Robinson, R. G. Neuropsychiatric aspects of cerebral vascular disorders. In R. C. Yudofsky and R. H. Hales, eds., *Textbook of Neuropsychiatry.* American Psychiatric Press, Washington DC, 1992.

Part IV

Poststroke anxiety disorders

29

Prevalence and specificity of clinical symptoms

Specificity of anxiety symptoms

In order to examine the frequency of anxiety symptoms and their specificity for anxiety disorder, patients with acute stroke were grouped according to whether they did or did not express anxiety or worry. As I discussed in Chapter 7 entitled, "Phenomenology and the specificity of depressive symptoms," among patients with acute stroke, it is not obvious how one should assess the specificity of symptoms used for the diagnosis of anxiety disorder. If one uses the diagnostic criteria to define the study group, it becomes circular reasoning since the anxious patients are defined by the very criteria that are being assessed for specificity. On the other hand, if one groups patients based on the presence of anxiety or any other single symptom, the group would include patients who do not have the full syndrome of generalized anxiety disorder (GAD) but merely one or two symptoms.

The criteria we have chosen is the second method which includes all patients who acknowledge the presence of anxiety or worry. By dividing patients based on the presence or absence of a single symptom (i.e., anxiety or worry) our studies include some patients without the full syndrome of GAD which, therefore, decreases the likelihood of finding symptoms that are specific for anxiety disorders. In other words, if feelings of impending doom or sleep disturbance occur in patients with GAD, comparing the frequency of these symptoms in patients with or without feelings of anxiety would be less likely to show a significant difference than if patients with and without GAD were compared. This method, however, does not prejudice the findings since the anxiety disorder group is not defined by having the symptoms that are being examined.

The frequencies of anxiety symptoms used for the DSM-IV diagnosis of GAD throughout the first 2 years after stroke are shown in Fig. 29.1. During the initial in-hospital evaluation, all symptoms were significantly more frequent among patients with anxiety compared to those without anxiety. Throughout the remainder of the follow-up evaluations at 3, 6, 12 and 24 months, almost all symptoms are

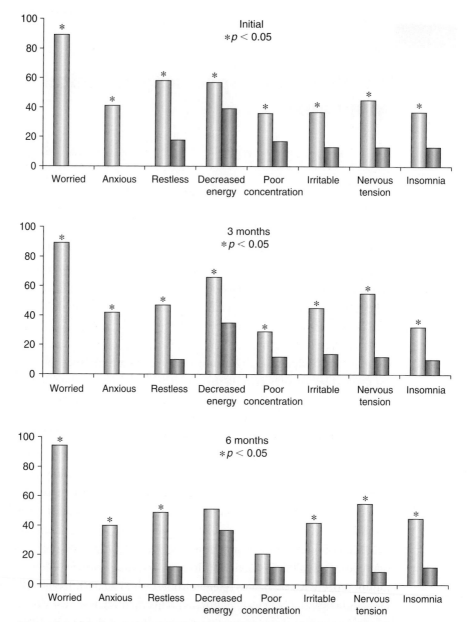

Figure 29.1 The frequency of DSM-IV symptoms for the diagnosis of GAD comparing patients who acknowledged worry or anxious foreboding and those who did not. The goal was to examine the relative specificity of each symptom for anxiety in a physically ill stroke population. During the initial evaluation, all symptoms were significantly more common in those who were worried/anxious compared to those who were not. Over the 2 years of follow-up, restlessness and nervous tension were most consistently associated with anxiety. Only decreased energy was a symptom found with almost the same frequency in non-anxious and anxious patients. Overall, these findings support

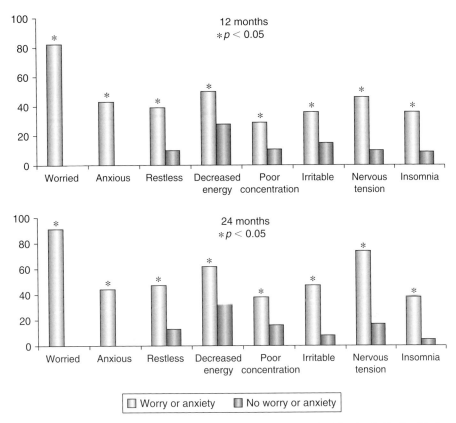

Figure 29.1 (*Cont.*) the specificity of these GAD symptoms to anxiety even in this physically ill, elderly population.

significantly more common in patients with anxiety or worry compared to those without. Decreased energy was the only symptom, which seemed to have a relatively high prevalence even among patients without anxiety. These findings suggest that the symptoms of anxiety are not rampant in a population of patients with an acute medical illness. The symptoms associated with GAD occurred significantly more frequently among patients who had anxiety and, therefore, possible confounds such as hospital nursing night checks leading to insomnia, did not overwhelm the effect of anxiety on any of the symptoms of GAD. The DSM-IV symptoms of GAD should, therefore, be considered to be specific for anxiety disorder.

Prevalence of GAD

The prevalence of GAD in our overall population of 357 patients with acute stroke was 22%. Approximately half (46%) of the patients with GAD also had major depression. Of the overall group of 357 patients with acute stroke, 10% had GAD without associated major depression.

If minor depression is included along with major depression, the association of depression with GAD is even more prominent. In our overall population of 357 patients with acute stroke, major or minor depression was found in 80% of patients with GAD. At 3 months follow-up, 86% of the patients with anxiety disorder had comorbid major or minor depression. At 6 months, the percentage was 90%, at 1 year 67%, and 2 years 84%. Thus, anxiety disorder was associated with major or minor depression in the vast majority of cases.

The prevalence of anxiety disorder reported by all investigators is shown in Table 29.1. Compared with poststroke depression, poststroke anxiety disorders have not received nearly as much attention. Some investigators who examined the frequency of anxiety disorders in patients with stroke did not include anxiety disorders that were comorbid with depression. Across all studies, including follow-up data as well as data from the initial evaluation, the mean pooled data prevalence of anxiety disorder was 14.4%. This number is presumably lower than the number of patients who would have met criteria for GAD with or without comorbid depression. If only studies that identified anxiety with or without depression were included, the mean prevalence of GAD both in hospital and at follow-up was 21%. Thus, anxiety disorders are very common emotional disorders in patients with stroke, both during the acute poststroke period and at follow-up.

Diagnosis of anxiety disorders

As with depressive disorders, the gold standard for the diagnosis of anxiety disorders is a structured or semistructured mental status examination which is applied to the diagnostic criteria of DSM-IV or ICD-10. Although cases of phobic disorder, panic disorder, and obsessive compulsive disorder, have been reported following stroke or brain injury (House 1987; Burvill *et al.* 1995; Max *et al.* 2002). The majority of investigators have focused on the more chronic disorder of GAD associated with stroke. As we showed in Section I of this chapter, all of the symptoms of GAD except perhaps decreased energy are significantly more frequent in patients with anxiety compared to those without anxiety.

Several investigators have examined the utility of screening instruments for the identification of GAD. Schramke *et al.* (1998) examined patients with right and left hemisphere stroke for anxiety and depressive symptoms using the Center for Epidemiological studies depression scale (CESD), Beck Anxiety Inventory, and the Hamilton depression scale. They also administered the structured clinical interview (SCID-R) and found that the rating scales were sensitive to psychiatric disorders but lacked specificity in all groups. There were significant correlations between

Table 29.1. The prevalence of anxiety disorder, as reported in different studies

Investigator	Patient population and time since stroke	N	Criteria	%	Anxiety disorder	% Anxiety disorder + depression	Total (%)
Burvill et al. (1995)	Community (4 months)	294	DSM-III	2	GAD	8% GAD + dep agorophobia	11
House et al. (1991)	Community (1 month)	89	DSM-III	1	GAD	NR	
Castillo et al. (1993)	Acute hospital (2 weeks)	309	DSM-IV	5	GAD	17% GAD + dep	22
Astrom et al. (1996)	Acute hospital (2 weeks)	71	DSM-III-R	13	GAD	15% GAD + maj dep	28
Morris et al. (1990)	Rehabilitation hospital (8 weeks)	99	DSM-III	3	GAD	NR	
Castillo et al. (1995)	Outpatient (1 year)	70	DSM-IV	5	GAD	6% GAD + maj dep	11
	Outpatient (2 years)	66	DSM-IV	6	GAD	12% GAD + dep	18
Morris et al. (1990)	Outpatient (1 year)	56	DSM-III	5	GAD	GAD + dep	5
Astrom et al. (1996)	Outpatient (1 year)	66	DSM-III-R	11	GAD	13% GAD + maj dep	24
	Outpatient (3 years)	48	DSM-III-R	4	GAD	15% GAD + maj dep	19
Leppavuori et al. (2003)	Outpatient (4 months)	277	DSM-IV	4	GAD	17% GAD + dep	21
			Pooled data mean	4	GAD	14% GAD + dep	18

GAD: generalized anxiety disorder.

Maj dep: Major depression.

NR: not reported.

scales suggesting the scales measured a common factor in the controls while in the stroke group, associations were weaker and less likely to be significant. They concluded that caution should be used in applying rating scales of depression and anxiety in neurological patients because, in this population, the scales are sensitive to the stress rather than identifying specific depressive and anxiety disorders.

O'Rourke *et al.* (1998) examined 105 outpatients 6 months following acute stroke using the general health questionnaire-30 (GHQ-30) and the Hospital Anxiety and Depression Scale (HADS). Patients were also blindly assessed using the Schedule for Affective Disorders and Schizophrenia (SADS) and DSM-IV diagnoses. No significant differences were found between the GHQ-30 and the HADS in identifying patients with any DSM-IV diagnosis of depression or anxiety disorders. The authors, however, felt that the recommended cutoff points for identifying cases (i.e., four or five on the GHQ and 8–12 on the HADS) were sub-optimal in this population and suggested that, depending upon the population studied, different cutoff points should be used.

Compared with the "gold standard" diagnoses based on the Psychiatric assessment schedule (Dean *et al.* 1983) and DSM-III diagnoses, the 294 patients included in the Perth Community Stroke Study were analyzed for sensitivity and specificity of the HADS, the Geriatric Depression Scale (GDS) and the GHQ-28 as screening instruments in patients 4 months after stroke (Johnson *et al.* 1995). The GHQ-28 and GDS, but not the HADS depression scale, were shown to be satisfactory screening instruments for depression while the GHQ-28 had an overall superiority. The performance of all three scales for screening poststroke anxiety disorders was less satisfactory. The HADS had the best level of sensitivity but the specificity and positive predictive values were low and the misclassification rate high.

Thus, investigators using screening instruments for the diagnosis of anxiety disorders following stroke have not found a screening instrument which has demonstrated utility either for the diagnosis or severity of anxiety disorders following stroke.

In summary, anxiety disorders are common in patients following stroke in both the acute hospital setting and in chronic outpatient settings. The frequency of anxiety disorders including those that are comorbid with depressive disorder during the acute stroke period was 21% and in outpatient settings was about 20%. Approximately half of the patients with anxiety disorder have accompanying major depressive disorder or minor depression. Symptoms associated with anxiety disorder overlapped with depressive symptoms but were significantly more frequent among patients with anxiety compared to those having stroke without feelings of nervousness or anxiety. The diagnosis of anxiety disorders should be based on mental status examination and clearly defined diagnostic criteria such as DSM-IV. The use of screening instruments in poststroke anxiety disorders has not been very successful with false positive cases being a particularly common problem.

REFERENCES

Astrom, M. Generalized anxiety disorder in stroke patients: a 3-year longitudinal study. *Stroke* (1996) 27:270–275.

Burvill, P. W., Johnson, G. A., Jamrozik, K. D., *et al.* Anxiety disorders after stroke: results from the Perth community stroke study. *Br J Psychiatr* (1995) 166(3):328–332.

Castillo, C. S., Schultz, S. K., and Robinson, R. G. Clinical correlates of early-onset and late-onset poststroke generalized anxiety. *Am J Psychiatr* (1995) 152:1174–1179.

Castillo, C. S., Starkstein, S. E., Fedoroff, J. P., *et al.* Generalized anxiety disorder following stroke. *J Nerv Ment Dis* (1993) 181:100–106.

Dean, C., Surtees, P. G., and Sashidharen, S. P. Comparison of research diagnostic systems in an Edinburgh community sample. *Br J Psychiatr* (1983) 142:247–256.

House, A. Mood disorders after stroke. A review of the evidence. *Int J Geriatr Psychiatr* (1987) 2:211–221.

House, A., Dennis, M., Mogridge, L., *et al.* Mood disorders in the year after first stroke. *Br J Psychiatr* (1991) 158:83–92.

Johnson, G., Burvill, P. W., Anderson, C. S., *et al.* Screening instruments for depression and anxiety following stroke: experience in the Perth community stroke study. *Acta Psychiatr Scand* (1995) 91(4):252–257.

Leppavuori, A., Pohjasvaara, T., Vataja, R., *et al.* Generalized anxiety disorders three to four months after ischemic stroke. *Cerebrovasc Dis* (2003) 16(3):257–264.

Max, J. E., Mathews, K., Lansing, A. E., *et al.* Psychiatric disorders after childhood stroke. *J Am Acad Child Adolesc Psychiatr* (2002) 41(5):555–562.

Morris, P. L. P., Robinson, R. G., and Raphael, B. Prevalence and course of depressive disorders in hospitalized stroke patients. *Intl J Psychiatr Med* (1990) 20:349–364.

O'Rourke, S., MacHale, S., Signorini, D., *et al.* Detecting psychiatric morbidity after stroke: comparison of the GHQ and the HAD Scale. *Stroke* (1998) 29(5):980–985.

Schramke, C. J., Stowe, R. M., Ratcliff, G., *et al.* Poststroke depression and anxiety: different assessment methods result in variations in incidence and severity estimates. *J Clin Exp Neuropsychol* (1998) 20(5):723–737.

30

Clinical and lesion correlates

In the previous chapter, "Prevalence and specificity of clinical symptoms," I listed a number of investigators in Table 29.1 who have examined the clinical and lesion correlates of anxiety disorder following stroke. In an effort to reexamine our findings on the clinical and pathological correlates of poststroke anxiety disorder, we recently analyzed data from our largest group of patients which included 396 acute stroke patients. The background characteristics of patients with or without generalized anxiety disorder (GAD), as defined by DSM-IV symptom criteria, are shown in Table 30.1. Patients were also grouped according to the presence or absence of major depression. More than half of the patients with DSM-IV-defined GAD also had associated major depression. There were significant intergroup differences in background characteristics including age, previous personal history of psychiatric disorder, and previous personal history of alcohol abuse. Two-way analysis of variance (ANOVA) examining the effects of depression (Factor 1) and GAD (Factor 2) demonstrated that GAD was associated with younger age ($p = 0.01$) and having a history of alcohol abuse ($p = 0.01$) while having a previous personal history of psychiatric disorder was associated with depression ($p = 0.01$).

The results of assessment of depression, activities of daily living, cognitive function, and social function are shown in Table 30.2. A two-way ANOVA of the present state examination (PSE) scores demonstrated significant effects of depression and anxiety as well as an interaction ($p = 0.001$). Both the depressed and non-depressed GAD groups had higher PSE scores than the control group. A two-way ANOVA of mean Hamilton depression (Ham-D) scores also demonstrated significant effects of both depression and anxiety ($p = 0.001$) but no significant interaction. The depressed group and the GAD group had higher Ham-D scores than the no mood or anxiety disorder group.

Two-way ANOVA of activities of daily living scale (Johns Hopkins Functioning Inventory or JHFI) demonstrated significant effects of anxiety but not of depression. Similarly, two-way ANOVA of social functioning measures (social ties checklist, STC and social functioning examination, SFE) showed that anxiety had an

Table 30.1. Demographic characteristics

	Not GAD or major depression	GAD, not major depression	Major depression, not GAD	Major depression, plus GAD
n	283	34	32	47
Age (mean ± SD)*	62.3 ± 13.1	58.0 ± 14.1	62.2 ± 14.6	55.2 ± 14.8
Sex (% male)	59.7	64.7	59.4	44.7
Race (% black)	51.6	55.8	34.4	46.8
Socioeconomic status (% class IV–V)	55.1	64.7	75.0	74.5
Marital (% married)	44.5	52.9	43.8	46.8
Education (mean ± SD)	10.2 ± 4.0	9.6 ± 3.9	9.8 ± 3.7	10.3 ± 3.0
Alcohol abuse history (% positive)**	7.7	26.5	15.6	17.8
Family psychiatric history (% positive)	9.8	17.7	9.4	17.8
Personal psychiatric history (% positive)**	6.2	18.2	25.0	23.9

*$p < 0.05$; **$p < 0.01$.

Table 30.2. Psychiatric examination scores*

	Not GAD or major depression	GAD not major depression	Major depression not GAD	Major depression plus GAD
n	283	34	32	47
Depression				
PSE *A–C*	6.2 ± 5.4	18.4 ± 9.0	19.8 ± 7.2	27.8 ± 9.1
HDS *A, B*	4.9 ± 4.4	12.3 ± 6.6	13.2 ± 4.9	18.0 ± 4.8
Activities of daily living				
JHFI *B*	5.3 ± 4.7	8.5 ± 6.2	7.4 ± 4.7	7.7 ± 6.0
Cognitive				
MMSE	23.7 ± 5.6	23.3 ± 5.6	22.9 ± 5.5	21.4 ± 6.8
Social functioning				
SFE *B*	0.16 ± 0.14	0.23 ± 0.17	0.19 ± 0.18	0.24 ± 0.15
STC	3.7 ± 2.0	3.6 ± 1.9	4.0 ± 1.9	4.1 ± 2.1

*Data are expressed as mean ± SD. Two-way ANOVA results: *A = significant depression effect; B = Significant GAD effect; C = significant interaction.*

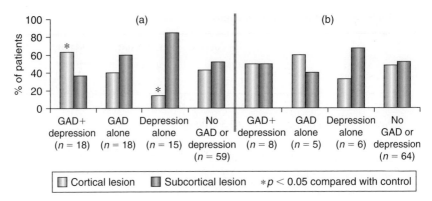

Figure 30.1 The frequency of cortical and subcortical lesions of the left (a) and right (b) hemispheres among patients with depression (major or minor) and GAD. Depression without anxiety was associated with subcortical left hemisphere lesions while the combination of anxiety and depression was associated with left cortical lesions.

effect, whereas depression did not, and there was no interaction. Two-way ANOVA of cognitive examination (mini-mental state examination or MMSE) scores did not demonstrate an effect of depression or anxiety disorder. These findings indicate that patients with anxiety disorders following acute stroke were more impaired in their activities of daily living and social functioning compared with non-anxious non-depressed patients.

Comparison of patients based on the findings of neurological examination demonstrated that there are no significant differences between controls and those with GAD or major depression: motor deficits were found in 77%, 69%, and 66% of the patients, respectively; aphasia was found in 10%, 15%, and 10, respectively.

The lesion correlates of anxiety disorder were examined in 185 patients using either computer tomography (CT) or magnetic resonance imaging (MRI) scan findings. Among patients with left hemisphere lesions, those with GAD plus depression had a significantly higher frequency of cortical lesions than patients with GAD alone or no disorder ($p = 0.04$) (Fig. 30.1). Among patients with right hemisphere lesions, the GAD-only patients had a significantly higher frequency of posterior lesions compared to patients with neither anxiety nor depression ($p = 0.04$) (Fig. 30.2). These findings were identical when we used only major depression suggesting that there is an interaction between the existence of GAD and depression, with depression plus anxiety associated with left cortical lesions and anxiety alone associated with right posterior hemisphere lesions. Since the lesion correlates were found to be dependent upon the presence or absence of depression, this suggests that anxiety disorders occurred with both right and left hemisphere lesions and, if anxiety disorders are the same disorder with and without depression are not lateralized.

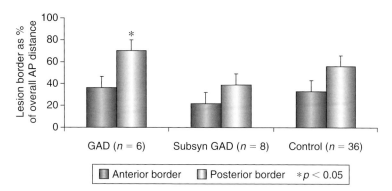

Figure 30.2 The anterior and posterior lesion borders of patients with right hemisphere lesions visualized on CT scan and grouped according to anxiety diagnosis. Patients with GAD had more posterior lesions than the other two groups and the posterior border of the GAD group was significantly more caudal than that of the other two groups (data from Castillo *et al.* 1993).

An earlier study of 98 patients (a subset of the overall group of the 396 acute stroke patients) examined the clinical and lesion correlates of GAD with or without major depression (Starkstein *et al.* 1990). This prior study used DSM-III criteria for GAD and major depression and grouped patients according to whether they had major depression only ($n = 24$), major depression plus GAD ($n = 23$), GAD only ($n = 6$), and or neither depression nor anxiety disorder ($n = 45$). There were no significant differences between groups in age, education, marital status, or frequency of family or previous personal history of psychiatric disorder; however, the patients with anxiety only had a significantly higher frequency of previous history of alcoholism (67% versus 21%, 22%, or 11% respectively, $p < 0.05$).

This study also examined the effect of cortical versus subcortical as well as right versus left lesion location. The effect of cortical versus subcortical lesions among patients with left hemisphere stroke is shown in Fig. 30.3. Among patients with anxiety plus depression there was a significantly higher frequency of cortical lesions compared to patients with depression alone ($p = 0.04$). Among patients with right hemisphere lesions, there was no significant association between the frequency of depression or anxiety and the existence of cortical or subcortical lesions. In contrast, however, depression-only patients had a significantly higher frequency of left subcortical lesions compared to the anxiety plus depression group ($p = 0.04$) (Fig. 30.3). Although there were no associations with cortical or subcortical lesions in the right hemisphere, patients with GAD had significantly more posterior lesions than patients with only anxiety ($p = 0.05$) (Fig. 30.2). Lesion volume, on the other hand, did not correlate significantly with either the presence or absence of depression, anxiety, right or left hemisphere lesions.

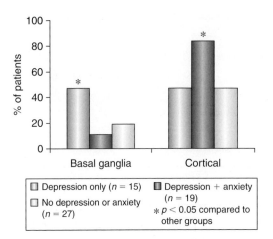

Figure 30.3 Comparison of basal ganglia and cortical lesions among patients with major depression only (depression only), major depression plus GAD (depression + anxiety), and no mood or anxiety disorder (no depression or anxiety). Major depression alone was associated with basal ganglia lesions while major depression plus GAD was associated with cortical lesions (data from Starkstein *et al.* 1990).

Another investigator who has examined the clinical correlate of poststroke anxiety disorder during the acute hospitalization was Astrom (1996). She examined 71 patients with acute stroke and longitudinally followed them over 3 years. During the initial inpatient evaluation, 20 (28%) fulfilled criteria (except for the 6 months duration) for DSM-III-R GAD. Of these patients, 55% had comorbid major depression.

Astrom (1996) found some similar as well as some different clinical correlates of GAD compared with our studies. During the acute poststroke period, GAD was found to be significantly associated with living alone and the existence of dysphasia. In addition, GAD plus major depression was associated with an increased frequency of left hemisphere lesions (i.e. 7 of 17 patients with left hemisphere lesions had major depressive disorder plus GAD compared to only 1 of 17 patients who had GAD alone, $p = 0.002$). On the other hand, GAD alone was associated with right hemisphere lesions (i.e. 5 of 22 patients with right hemisphere lesions had GAD compared to 1 of 17 patients with left hemisphere lesions, $p = 0.04$).

Astrom also examined the clinical correlates of GAD longitudinally. The strongest correlates of GAD were the absence of social contacts outside the family and dependence of patients upon others to perform their primary activities of daily living. These factors were significantly more common in the GAD compared to non-GAD population at 3 months, 1, 2, and 3 years after stroke. However, no other impairment, social, or demographic factors distinguished the GAD from the non-GAD patients throughout the follow-up. In addition, at 3-year follow-up, GAD was associated with both cortical atrophy and subcortical atrophy (as measured by frontal horn ratios on CT scan (i.e. 7 of 7 GAD patients had atrophy versus 19 of 39 non-GAD patients, $p = 0.03$).

Leppavuori *et al.* (2003) examined 277 patients, aged 55–85, between 3 and 4 months following an ischemic stroke (patients with hemorrhagic stroke were not included). GAD due to stroke ($n = 26$) or GAD which preceded the onset of the stroke ($n = 31$) were compared. Combining these two groups, the overall frequency of GAD was 20.6% ($n = 57$). Using a logistic regression, GAD, whether primary or secondary, was associated with a prior history of epilepsy, comorbid depressive disorder, severity of depression, severity of anxiety, and use of anxiolytic drugs. The authors also compared the primary GAD group with the secondary GAD group and found, using a discriminant analysis, that a lower level of psychosocial functioning, history of migraine, and anterior circulation stroke were all associated with GAD secondary to stroke. On the other hand, a history of insomnia was significantly more frequent among patients with primary GAD.

Burvill *et al.* (1995) examined anxiety disorders in 294 patients in the Perth Community Stroke Study at 4 months following stroke. This study found that 49 patients (16.6%) had agoraphobia while 38 (13%) had GAD. The prevalence of anxiety disorder, however, varied by gender occurring in 5% of males and 19% of females. This was compared to the prevalence in community control patients in which 5% of males and 8% of females had GAD. When patients with comorbid depression and GAD were included, the overall prevalence of anxiety disorder increased to 12% in males and 28% in females. Those with onset of GAD and depression following the stroke showed a prevalence of 9% in males and 20% in females. Gender was the only clinical variable that was associated with an increased frequency of anxiety disorder.

As with depressive disorder, it is logical to wonder whether there may be a milder but nonetheless clinically significant form of anxiety disorder. To examine this possibility we compared patients with a subsyndromal form of GAD to patients with GAD (Castillo *et al.* 1993). There were 40 patients who had prominent anxiety or excessive worrying but did not otherwise meet criteria for GAD. Of these patients, 25 (62.5%) had no depression and 15 (37.5%) had major or minor depression. There were no significant differences in their age, gender, or other background characteristics. Perhaps the most surprising finding from this study of subsyndromic GAD, however, was that anxiety appeared in some ways to resemble a continuum rather than a category. For example, the frequency of previous alcohol abuse in patients with subsyndromal GAD was intermediate between the frequency found for patients with GAD and that for patients with no anxiety symptoms. Similarly, in the analysis of lesion location, both subsyndromal GAD and GAD were associated with cortical lesions. On the other hand, we found that intrahemispheric lesion location was significantly different between patients with GAD (who had the most posterior right hemisphere lesions) and patients with subsyndromal GAD (who had the most anterior right hemisphere lesions). Although additional studies of anxiety in patients with stroke need to be conducted, the available data provide some validation for the hypothesis that there may be more than one form of poststroke GAD.

Another major finding from these studies of poststroke GAD was that depression and GAD were closely linked. When considering both major and minor depression, almost all studies found that the vast majority of patients with GAD had comorbid depressive disorder. If only major depression was examined, about one-half of the GAD patients had comorbid major depression (Table 30.1). This finding raises the more fundamental issue of whether GAD is a separate disorder in patients with stroke. Although some anxiety symptoms may be a manifestation of depressive disorder, there were several findings which argue that they are separate disorders. Firstly, anxiety disorder but not depressive disorder was associated with previous alcohol abuse. Secondly, greater impairment in activities of daily living (JHFI), and SFE, were all significantly associated with anxiety disorder. Furthermore, as will be detailed in Chapter 31, the duration of anxiety and depressive disorders were found to be different. Finally, GAD without depression was associated with cortical lesions and posterior right hemisphere injury while depression was associated with left frontal and left basal ganglia lesions suggesting that anxiety may exist independently of depression with its own clinical–pathological correlates.

The frequent occurrence of depression with anxiety disorder in patients without brain lesions has been extensively studied. Roth *et al.* (1972) found depressive symptoms in 65% of anxious patients. Clancy *et al.* (1979) reported that 44% of a series of 112 anxious patients evaluated 6 years after the index episode had secondary depression. Furthermore, patients with comorbid depression and anxiety have been found to be phenomenologically different from patients with either anxiety disorder alone or major depression alone (Fawcet and Kravitz 1983; Paykel *et al.* 1983). In addition, anxious depressed patients have been reported to have increased chronicity of illness, a reduced response to conventional treatments, and a poorer prognosis than patients with major depression alone (Downing and Rickels 1974; Stavrakaki and Vargo 1986). Thus, anxiety, depression, and anxious depression may all be separate disorders.

In summary, the clinical correlates of anxiety disorder during the acute poststroke period include prior history of alcohol abuse, greater impairment in activities of daily living and social functioning, and right hemisphere cortical lesions. Major depression occurred in approximately 50% of patients with GAD and minor depression occurred in another 25–30%. In our studies, prior history of alcohol abuse was associated with anxiety disorder while other investigators have found history of epilepsy and the use of anxiolytic drugs were also characteristic of patients with poststroke anxiety disorders. Although the data suggest that anxiety disorders are distinct from associated depression, further research is needed to determine whether depression, anxiety, and depression plus anxiety all have different etiological mechanisms.

REFERENCES

Astrom, M. Generalized anxiety disorder in stroke patients: a 3-year longitudinal study. *Stroke* (1996) 27:270–275.

Burvill, P. W., Johnson, G. A., Jamrozik, K. D., *et al*. Anxiety disorders after stroke: results from the Perth Community Stroke Study. *Br J Psychiatr* (1995) 166(3):328–332.

Castillo, C. S., Starkstein, S. E., Fedoroff, J. P., *et al*. Generalized anxiety disorder following stroke. *J Nerv Ment Dis* (1993) 181:100–106.

Clancy, J., Noyes, R., Hoenk, P. R., *et al*. Secondary depression in anxiety neurosis. *J Nerv Ment Dis* (1979) 166:846–850.

Downing, R. W., and Rickels, K. Mixed anxiety–depression: fact or myth? *Arch Gen Psychiatr* (1974) 30:312–317.

Fawcet, J., and Kravitz, H. M. Anxiety syndromes and their relationship to depressive illness. *J Clin Psychiatr* (1983) 44:8–11.

Leppavuori, A., Pohjasvaara, T., Vataja, R., *et al*. Generalized anxiety disorders three to four months after ischemic stroke. *Cerebrovasc Dis* (2003) 16(3):257–264.

Paykel, E. S., Parker, R. R., Rowan, P. R., *et al*. Nosology of atypical depression. *Psychol Med* (1983) 13:131–139.

Roth, M., Gurney, C., Garside, R. F., *et al*. The relationship between anxiety states and depressive illness. Part 1. *Br J Psychiatr* (1972) 121:175–181.

Starkstein, S. E., Cohen, B. S., Fedoroff, P., *et al*. Relationship between anxiety disorders and depressive disorders in patients with cerebrovascular injury. *Arch Gen Psychiatr* (1990) 47:785–789.

Stavrakaki, C., and Vargo, B. The relationship of anxiety and depression: a review of the literature. *Br J Psychiatr* (1986) 149:7–16.

31

Longitudinal course

The long-term outcome of anxiety disorders following stroke has been examined by several investigators (Burvill *et al.* 1995; Castillo *et al.* 1995; Astrom 1996; Schultz *et al.* 1997). The first of our two studies compared patients who developed generalized anxiety disorder (GAD) at the time of the acute stroke with patients who developed GAD 3 or more months after their stroke (Castillo *et al.* 1995). In this study we wanted to determine first whether there were significant differences in the clinical correlates of GAD among patients who developed anxiety disorder during the acute poststroke period as compared to anxiety disorder which developed several months after the stroke and, second, the duration of the anxiety disorder. The background characteristics of the patients with GAD (diagnosed using diagnostic and statistical manual of mental disorder-III-revised or DSM-III-R criteria, i.e., 4 of 13 anxiety symptoms, including worry or anxious foreboding had to be present) are shown in Table 31.1. Comparison of the background characteristics of early-onset (i.e., present at the initial in-hospital evaluation) and late-onset (i.e., present for the first time 3 or more months following stroke) GAD groups did not reveal significant differences except that patients with early-onset GAD had a higher frequency of personal history of psychiatric disorder or alcohol abuse compared to the late-onset or the no anxiety disorder (control) patients. The frequency of depression among patients with early- and late-onset GAD is shown in Fig. 31.1. At the initial evaluation, 27% of the 142 acute stroke patients who had at least one follow-up examination had GAD. Among both early- and late-onset cases, the majority of patients had associated major or minor depression (Fig. 31.1). Major depression occurred in 39% of all the early-onset GAD patients and 47% of the late-onset GAD patients. The time of onset of the late-onset cases of GAD with or without depression (major and minor combined) is shown in Fig. 31.1.

We also determined whether the presence of depression may have led to the development of anxiety. Patients with late-onset anxiety disorder were examined for the presence of depression before the onset of GAD. In 10 of 32 patients with late-onset GAD, depression was present before the diagnosis of GAD; however, this was not

Table 31.1. Background characteristics

	No GAD	Early-onset GAD	Late-onset GAD
N	71	39	31
Age (mean ± SD)	50 ± 12	56 ± 13	59 ± 13
Sex (% male)	66	49	47
Race (% African-American)	74	56	56
Socioeconomic status (% Hollingshead IV–V)	79	77	68
Marital status (% married)	44	51	47
Education (mean years ± SD)	9 ± 4	9 ± 4	10 ± 4*
Alcohol abuse history (% positive)	10	13	0
Family psychiatric history (% positive)	6	5	10
Personal psychiatric history or alcohol abuse history (% positive)	18	31	6*
Ischemic stroke, N (%)	43/51 (84.3)	24/26 (92.3)	25/27 (92.6)
Hemorrhagic stroke, N (%)	8 (15.7)	2 (7.7)	2 (7.4)

*$p < 0.05$. Reprinted with permission from Castillo *et al.* 1995.

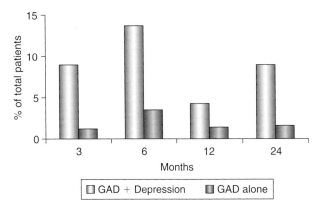

Figure 31.1   The frequency of GAD with or without depression during the acute hospital period (early-onset) and 3–24 months (late-onset) following stroke. Of 142 patients seen acutely and at follow-up, the number of early- and late-onset cases associated with depression was quite similar. The great majority of GAD cases had associated depression (data from Castillo *et al.* 1995).

significantly different from the frequency of depression among patients who did not develop GAD during the same follow-up period (i.e., 10 of 55 patients, $p = 0.16$).

We determined the duration of GAD (with or without depression) using survival analysis. The duration of late-onset GAD was significantly longer (median = 3.0

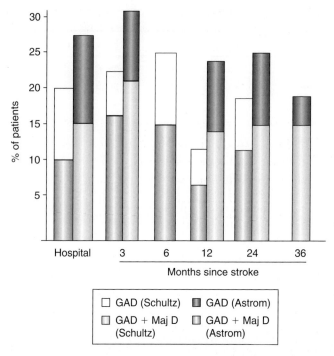

Figure 31.2   The frequency of GAD with and without major depression (Maj D) over 3 years following acute stroke. Results obtained from our study (Schultz *et al.* 1997) using DSM-IV criteria were compared to the results of Astrom (1996) using DSM-III-R criteria. Results indicate a slightly lower frequency of GAD using DSM-IV criteria and emphasize the prominence of major depression in this population of patients with poststroke anxiety disorder.

months, interquartile range = 0.0 month) than that of early-onset GAD (median = 1.5 months, interquartile range = 6.0 months, p = 0.02). This finding held true even when we removed patients with comorbid depression. The median duration for late-onset GAD (without depression) was 3.0 months (interquartile range = 1.5 months) while the duration of early-onset GAD (without depression) was 1.5 months, interquartile range = 0.0 month, p = 0.001). However, because of increased variability in the duration of anxiety disorder among depressed patients, the duration of GAD (associated with depression) was not significantly different for late-onset compared to early-onset disorder (median = 3.0 months versus median = 1.5 months, p = 0.58).

     Astrom (1996) examined 71 acute stroke patients for anxiety disorder and re-examined 70 of these patients at 3 months: 66 at 1 year, 57 at 2 years, and 48 at 3 years. The decreasing number was primarily due to mortality. The prevalence of GAD at each time point is shown in Fig. 31.2. Astrom (1996) found that GAD was more persistent in her population of stroke patients than we had found in our population. Of 21 patients with GAD diagnosed in hospital or at 3-month follow-up, only five patients (23%) had recovered from GAD by the 1-year follow-up. At 3-year follow-up, only 5 of 13 patients (38%) had recovered – four within the first year and only one more by the 3-year follow-up. This appeared to be due to comorbid major depression and GAD as 11 of these 13 patients seen at 3 years had this comorbid condition.

Burvill *et al.* (1995) also examined the longitudinal course of poststroke anxiety disorders. Of 294 total patients, 71 were diagnosed with anxiety disorder. Among the 71 patients with anxiety disorders, 49 had agoraphobia and 51% had recovered by 12-month follow-up. Furthermore, when patients with anxiety disorder alone were compared to patients with anxiety plus comorbid depression, there was a significantly increased mortality among the patients with comorbid anxiety and depression. Thus, Burvill *et al.* like Astrom found that many poststroke anxiety disorders lasted for more than a year following stroke.

In our study of early- versus late-onset GAD (Castillo *et al.* 1995), analysis of impairment in activities of daily living (Johns Hopkins functioning inventory or JHFI) or cognitive impairment (mini-mental state examination or MMSE), or social functioning examination (SFE) did not show significant intergroup differences across the control, early- and late-onset GAD groups. Similarly, on neurological examination there were no significant intergroup differences found in the frequency of motor or sensory deficits, aphasia, or visual field disturbances. Finally, analysis of lesion location or lesion volume revealed no significant differences between the early- and late-onset GAD groups in the frequency of right versus left hemisphere lesions, cortical versus subcortical lesion location, or the mean distance of the anterior or posterior lesion border from the frontal pole or lesion volume.

The finding that early-onset but not late-onset GAD was associated with a premorbid history of psychiatric disorder or alcohol abuse suggests that early-onset GAD may be an exacerbation or recurrence of a prestroke disorder. The second finding was that early-onset disorder had a significantly shorter duration than late-onset disorder as determined by survival analysis. Both of these findings suggest that the pathophysiological mechanisms of early- versus late-onset disorder may be different.

Our finding that the median duration of poststroke GAD was between 1.5 and 3 months, indicates that most of these disorders would not fulfill the DSM-IV duration criteria for GAD, which requires the continuous presence of symptoms for 6 months or more. It also raises the question of whether these disorders should be called GAD. An argument can be made, however, that the anxiety disorders following stroke meet the symptom criteria for GAD that is similar to the presentation of GAD without brain injury. Astrom (1996) found that 62% of her patients with poststroke GAD did not recover over 3 years. Perhaps referring to these disorders as poststroke anxiety disorders might avoid the question of whether the 6-month duration of symptoms is essential for a diagnosis of GAD. Clearly additional research is needed to determine which patients develop transient rather than chronic anxiety disorders.

Another interesting finding (Castillo *et al.* 1995) was that both early- and late-onset anxiety disorders were associated with depression. In the majority of cases, depression and poststroke anxiety disorder seemed to start concurrently. There were a few cases in which depression preceded late-onset anxiety but these were no more common in the anxious compared with the non-anxious patients.

Although the mechanism of poststroke anxiety disorder will be discussed in more detail in Chapter 33, the finding that early- and late-onset anxiety disorders have different durations and clinical correlates with premorbid conditions is consistent with the hypothesis that early- and late-onset poststroke anxiety disorders may have different etiologies.

Our second study (Schultz *et al.* 1997) which examined the longitudinal course of anxiety disorder following stroke, looked cross-sectionally at associations between anxiety disorder and depressive disorder in-hospital at 3, 6, 12, and 24 months following stroke (Schultz *et al.* 1997). In contrast to the first study (Castillo *et al.* 1995), the diagnosis of GAD was based on DSM-IV criteria excluding the 6-month duration. The DSM-IV criteria require that anxiety and worry be exhibited as well as three of six additional symptoms. These symptoms, which include restlessness, fatigue, poor concentration due to anxiety, irritability, sleep disturbance, and nervous tension, are less dependent on somatic symptoms than DSM-III-R criteria and, therefore, may enable better separation of these patients from those with depressive disorders than was achieved by DSM-III-R. The overall prevalence of GAD was 19% at initial evaluation, 22% at 3 months, 25% at 6 months, 11% at 1 year, and 18% at 2 years (Fig. 31.2). The duration of GAD without depression was 4.5 months (interquartile range = 0.0 month) while the duration of GAD cormorbid with depression was 1.5 months (interquartile range = 4.5) $p = 0.3792$. The prevalence of comorbid anxiety and major depression at each visit was 10% at intake, 16% at 3 months, 15% at 6 months, 6% at 1 year, and 12% at 2 years (Fig. 31.3).

Analysis of Hamilton depression scores demonstrated significantly higher depression scores among the anxious depressive disorder patients compared to the depression-only group or the control groups at both the in-hospital and 3-month follow-up evaluations. At the 6-, 12-, and 24-month follow-ups, there were no significant differences between the group with depression and that with anxious depression. This finding suggests that the nature of anxious depression and/or depression alone may be changing over time.

There was also an interesting effect of gender on the prevalence and course of anxiety disorder. Significantly more women than men had a diagnosis of either DSM-IV GAD disorder or DSM-IV major depression compared to the control

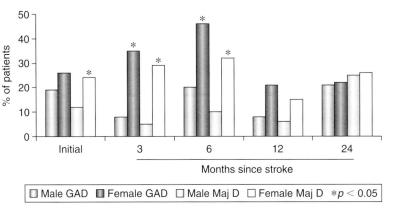

Figure 31.3   The frequency of DSM-IV defined major depression (Maj D) and GAD grouped according to gender over the first 2 years following acute stroke. Both GAD and major depression were significantly more common in females than males during the 3- and 6-month follow-up but, by 1 and 2 years poststroke, there were no gender-related differences in the frequency of these disorders (data from Schultz et al. 1997).

group at 3 months, 6 months, and a trend difference at 12 months (Fig. 31.3) ($p = 0.007$, 0.04, and 0.06, respectively). Consistent with this finding, Hamilton depression scores were significantly higher in females than males (for the entire group of patients) during the first 6 months of follow-up (intake $p = 0.002$, 3 months $p = 0.003$, and 6 months $p = 0.002$).

The finding that depression and anxiety were more common in women confirmed the phenomenon that women without brain injury have roughly twice the likelihood that men have of developing depressive or anxiety disorders over the course of their lifetimes (Weissman and Klerman 1977; Kessler et al. 1994). It is interesting that a physical injury such as stroke might be associated with different frequencies of psychiatric manifestations in men and women. This suggests that the cause of depression is not strictly the lesion, rather, the lesion may trigger some premorbid vulnerability, such as a genetic predisposition. Alternative explanations may include cultural influences, hormonal influences, or differences in psychological response to impairment. This gender-related difference in vulnerability to mood disorder is another fruitful area for further research.

In summary, the natural course of anxiety disorder appears to depend upon whether the disorder develops acutely after stroke or during the chronic poststroke period. The mean duration of anxiety disorder which developed after 3 or more months poststroke was 3.0 months compared to acute onset GAD which had a mean duration of 1.5 months. Astrom, however, found that 62 of her patients with GAD following acute stroke continued to have GAD and comorbid major depression at 3 years. Burvill et al. similarly found that 49% of patients with agoraphobic anxiety disorder continued to have this disorder at 12-month follow-up. The natural course of poststroke anxiety disorders clearly deserves further investigation.

REFERENCES

Astrom, M. Generalized anxiety disorder in stroke patients: a 3-year longitudinal study. *Stroke* (1996) 27:270–275.

Burvill, P. W., Johnson, G. A., Jamrozik, K. D., *et al.* Anxiety disorders after stroke: results from the Perth Community Stroke Study. *Br J Psychiatr* (1995) 166(3):328–332.

Castillo, C. S., Schultz, S. K., and Robinson, R. G. Clinical correlates of early-onset and late-onset poststroke generalized anxiety. *Am J Psychiatr* (1995) 152:1174–1179.

Kessler, R. C., McGonagle, K. A., Zaho, S., *et al.* Lifetime and 12-month prevalence of DSM-III-R psychiatric disorders in the United States. *Arch Gen Psychiatr* (1994) 51:8–19.

Schultz, S. K., Castillo, C. S., Kosier, J. T., *et al.* Generalized anxiety and depression following stroke. *Am J Geriatr Psychiatr* (1997) 5:229–237.

Weissman, M. M., and Klerman, G. L. Sex differences in the epidemiology of depression. *Arch Gen Psychiatr* (1977) 34:98–111.

32

Relationship of anxiety to outcome

For many years clinicians have recognized the importance of anxiety disorder as well as depression in patients following stroke (Schwartzman 1976). The spectrum of anxiety disorders includes panic disorder, generalized anxiety disorder (GAD), obsessive compulsive disorder (OCD) and phobic disorders. There have been anecdotal reports of panic disorder (Maricle *et al.* 1991) and OCD occurring in patients with stroke. These are relatively rare conditions arising from ischemic brain injury. Our research investigations have not systematically examined patients for panic disorder or OCD. We have, however, systematically examined patients for GAD. Although this has not been a major area of investigation for other researchers, there are a number of reports of the presentation, diagnosis, and clinical and pathological correlates of poststroke anxiety disorder (Burvill *et al.* 1995; Astrom 1996).

In contrast to the relatively large number of studies which have examined the relationship between the existence of poststroke depression and physical and cognitive recovery following stroke, relatively few studies have examined the effect of anxiety disorder on physical and cognitive recovery from stroke. We examined 142 consecutive patients who were evaluated following acute stroke and followed-up at either 3 or 6 months ($n = 110$) or 12 or 24 months follow-up ($n = 103$) (Shimoda and Robinson 1998). The patients lost to follow-up were due to mortality (15%) or failure to show for appointments (10%). The patient characteristics are shown in Table 32.1. The only significant difference in background characteristics was a greater number of females in the major depressive disorder (MDD) and the MDD plus GAD groups than in the no disorder group ($p = 0.049$).

Using a two-way repeated measures ANOVA (factor 1, presence or absence of in-hospital GAD; factor 2 presence or absence of in-hospital MDD), we analyzed the independent and interactive effects of GAD and MDD. Non-MDD patients tended to be older than patients with MDD, non-MDD 59.2 ± 12.4 versus MDD 54.0 ± 13.0, $p = 0.056$ and the non-GAD patients tended to have large lesion volumes than patients with GAD, non-GAD 7.4 ± 7.3 versus GAD 3.4 ± 2.8, $p = 0.054$). Due to these group differences, the analyses of the effect of in-hospital

Table 32.1. Demographic characteristics

Patients' Characteristics	Not MDD		MDD	
	Control ($n = 100$)	GAD only ($n = 15$)	MDD only ($n = 9$)	MDD + GAD ($n = 18$)
Age (years ± SD)	59.5 ± 12.2	56.9 ± 14.0	53.6 ± 12.7	54.2 ± 14.2
Education (years ± SD)	9.3 ± 4.1	9.6 ± 4.7	7.8 ± 3.8	9.4 ± 3.2
Sex (% female)*	37.0	33.3	77.8	72.2
Race (% black)	67.0	60.0	77.8	55.6
Marital (% married)	49.0	60.0	11.1	50.0
Alcohol abuse (% positive)	6.0	13.3	11.1	50.0
Socioeconomic status (% class IV–V)	26.0	26.7	88.9	83.3
Family psychiatric history (% positive)	6.0	0	11.1	11.1
Past psychiatric history (% positive)	11.0	20.0	44.4	22.2
Medication				
Antidepressants (% positive)	5.0	0	22.2	11.1
Other psychotropics (% positive)	0	0	0	0

*$p < 0.05$ control and GAD only compared with other groups.
Reprinted from Shimoda and Robinson 1998 with permission.

GAD on recovery were done using patients matched for age (±2 years), education (±2 years), and lesion volume (±2% of total brain volume). The group sizes were 100 no mood or anxiety disorder, 15 GAD, 9 MDD, 18 GAD and MDD. At short-term follow-up, mini-mental state examination (MMSE) scores showed a significant effect of in-hospital MDD and time but no significant effect of GAD or coexistence of both GAD and MDD. At long-term follow-up, there was a significant effect on MMSE scores of the existence of in-hospital MDD ($p < 0.01$) but no effect of GAD and no effect of having both GAD and MDD.

Repeated measures ANOVA of JHFI scores for patients at 3- to 6-month follow-up showed a significant effect of in-hospital MDD ($p = 0.004$) and time but no significant effect of GAD or the coexistence of in-hospital MDD and GAD. At 12 to 24 month follow-up, however, there were significant effects of MDD ($p = 0.04$) and the coexistence of MDD and GAD ($p = 0.02$), but no effect for GAD alone or other interactions (Fig. 32.1) (Shimoda and Robinson 1998). Thus, patients who had both MDD and GAD in-hospital were more impaired in their activities of daily living (ADL) at 1 or 2 years follow-up than were control patients, patients with GAD alone, or patients with MDD alone.

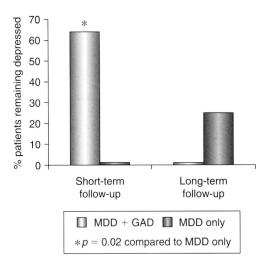

Figure 32.1 The percent of patients with MDD at the time of the initial in-hospital evaluation with or without anxiety disorder who remained depressed at 3 6 months (short-term) follow-up and 12–24 months (long-term) follow-up. Patients with MDD plus GAD were significantly more likely to remain depressed at 3–6 months follow-up than MDD patients without GAD. There were no significant effects of in-hospital anxiety disorder on depression at long-term follow-up (data from Shimoda and Robinson 1998).

Finally, we examined the effect of in-hospital GAD or MDD on social functioning at short- and long-term follow-up. At 3 to 6 months follow-up, there were significant interactions of in-hospital MDD or GAD by time ($p = 0.03$) as well as the coexistence of both MDD and GAD by time ($p < 0.01$) (Fig. 32.3). Repeated measures ANOVA of in-hospital social functioning examination scores at 1 or 2 years follow-up showed significant interactions for MDD or GAD by time and the coexistence of MDD and GAD by time. These results indicate that in contrast to the major role that poststroke depression plays on both cognitive and functional physical recovery from stroke, anxiety disorder by itself does not influence recovery but the combination of MDD and GAD in-hospital significantly limits recovery in ADL at 1–2 years follow-up. In contrast, however, GAD does influence social functioning after stroke and in combination with MDD plays a significant role in the quality of patients' social lives over the first 2 years following stroke. The social functioning of patients with in-hospital GAD consistently deteriorated over 2 years compared to patients without GAD, while patients with GAD plus MDD had the greatest amount of social deterioration over 2 years.

Perhaps the most significant finding from this study was that the coexistence of MDD and GAD diagnosed at the time of the initial in-hospital evaluation had a

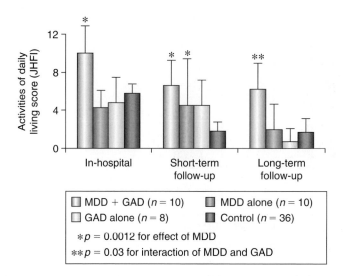

Figure 32.2 ADL scores (mean ± SEM) in patients with MDD and/or GAD in-hospital. Patients with MD
had significantly more impaired ADL scores at short-term follow-up (3–6 months). At
long-term follow-up (1–2 years), there was an effect of MDD ($p = 0.02$) and a significant
interaction of MDD and GAD ($p = 0.03$). Thus, the long-term recovery in ADLs was
significantly worse in patients with MD and GAD in-hospital than patients without this
combination of disorders (data from Shimoda and Robinson 1998).

greater impairment in ADL at 1 to 2 years follow-up than MDD alone, anxiety disorder alone, or no mood or anxiety disturbance (Fig. 32.2). Although it is possible
that a more sensitive measure of cognitive impairment than the MMSE might have
demonstrated subtle effects of anxiety, the effect of anxiety on cognitive function
was not nearly as great as the effect of depression.

Although the explanation for these findings is uncertain, the most straightfor-
ward explanation may be related to our finding described in Chapter 8 on the
course of poststroke depression that MDD associated with anxiety disorder lasts
longer than MDD alone (Fig. 32.1). A more prolonged depression may lead to
worse physical and social functioning outcomes. The ultimate way to examine this
hypothesis would be to compare recovery in ADL and social functioning in patients
with anxiety plus depressive disorder compared to patients with depressive disorder
alone who are matched for the duration of depression. In this study, we unfortu-
nately did not have sufficient numbers of patients with prolonged depression but
no anxiety disorder to examine this issue.

Astrom (1996) also reported that MDD associated with GAD had a longer duration
than MDD alone. In Chapter 30, we reported that MDD plus GAD was associated

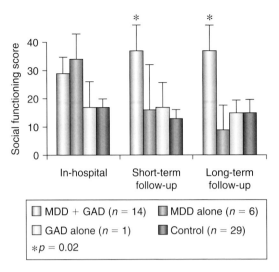

Figure 32.3 Social functioning outcome in patients with MDD or GAD in-hospital. Patients with both
MDD and GAD in-hospital had significantly worse social functioning at both short-term
(3–6 months) follow-up and long-term (1–2 years) follow-up than patients with these
disorders alone or no mood disorder. At both short- and long-term follow-up, there was a
significant MDD by GAD by time interaction ($p = 0.03$) indicating that the combination of
anxiety and depression was associated with the worst social outcome at 1–2 years
poststroke (data from Shimoda and Robinson 1998).

with a higher frequency of cortical lesions than MDD alone. Feeney and Baron
(1986) reported that cortical lesions in rats produced long-lasting hypometabolic
effects on the brain at sites distant from that of the lesion. These distant effects may
be more extensive and persistent after cortical lesions as compared to subcortical
lesions and thus lead to longer lasting depressions.

To my knowledge, this is the first time that an important role of anxiety disorder
in recovery from stroke has been demonstrated. The duration of depression, the
degree of impairment in ADL, and social functioning were all found to be influenced
by the combination of MDD and anxiety disorder. Although these effects may be
mediated primarily by the duration of depression, it is an intriguing therapeutic possibility that treatment of anxiety disorder during the acute poststroke period might
improve physical recovery as well as and social adjustment following stroke.

In summary, although the role of anxiety disorders in recovery from stroke has
rarely been examined, this study demonstrated that there are not only effects of the
interaction between depression and anxiety disorder but also anxiety disorder
alone in social functioning following a stroke. This suggests that treatment of anxiety disorder during acute stroke period might improve physical recovery as well as
social adjustment following stroke.

REFERENCES

Astrom, M. Generalized anxiety disorder in stroke patients: a 3-year longitudinal study. *Stroke* (1996) 27:270–275.

Burvill, P. W., Johnson, G. A., Jamrozik, K. D., *et al.* Anxiety disorders after stroke: results from the Perth Community Stroke Study. *Br J Psychiatr* (1995) 166(3):328–332.

Feeney, D. M., and Baron, J.-C. Diaschisis. *Stroke* (1986) 17:817–830.

Maricle, R. A., Sennhauser, S., and Burry, M. Panic disorder associated with right parahippocampal infarction. *J Nerv Ment Dis* (1991) 179(6):374–375.

Schwartzman, S. T. Anxiety and depression in the stroke patient: a nursing challenge. *J Psychiatr Nurs Ment Health Serv* (1976) 14(7):13–18.

Shimoda, K., and Robinson, R. G. Effect of anxiety disorder in impairment and recovery from stroke. *J. Neuropsychiatr Clin. Neurosci* (1998) 10:34–40.

33

Mechanism and treatment of poststroke anxiety disorder

Background

Several clinical studies have reported (Starkstein *et al*. 1990; Castillo *et al*. 1993; Astrom 1996), findings which must be explained by any hypothesis about the mechanism of poststroke anxiety. The major clinical finding is the frequent co-occurrence of anxiety disorder with depression. Approximately half of the patients with poststroke anxiety disorder were found to have major depression and about one-third minor depression. The second clinical finding is that the clinical and pathological correlates of anxiety disorder and depressive disorder are different. For example, the duration of anxiety disorder and depression are different. Anxiety but not depression is associated with prior alcohol abuse, acute onset anxiety but not acute onset depression is associated with right hemisphere lesion location, and anxiety and depression have independent or sometimes additive effects on recovery of activities of daily living (ADL), cognitive functioning, and social functioning.

Numerous hypotheses have been proposed to explain the neurobiological basis of anxiety disorders (Gorman *et al*. 1989) as well as the comorbidity of anxiety and depression. Paul (1988), for example, hypothesized that depression and anxiety may both be triggered by changes in the balance between inhibitory γ-aminobutyric acid (GABA) systems and excitatory noradrenergic systems. According to this theory, excessive arousal (perhaps created by the stress of stroke or other medical illness) may lead to decreased GABAergic inhibition, which could then lead to increased noradrenergic activity which produces the clinical manifestations of anxiety. Increased norepinephrine (NE) turnover could then result in a depletion of intracellular NE stores, which coupled with a continued depletion of GABA could lead to anxiety and depression. However, when we examined the temporal sequence in the relationship between anxiety and depressive disorder, as described in Chapter 31, we did not find that anxiety disorder preceded depressive disorder.

An alternative hypothesis has been proposed by Stahl (1997). According to this hypothesis, the abnormality arises in the somatodendritic serotonin 1A (5-HT-1a) receptor. Prior to an anxiety disorder, the autoreceptor becomes downregulated. This allows an excess of serotonin to be released, leading to anxiety. On the other hand, the release of 5-HT produces 5-HT-1a activation, which leads to a decrease in serotonin release and ultimately to depression. Pharmacological agents which are partial agonists in the downregulated state and partial antagonists in the upregulated state are effective in treating both anxiety and depression.

In the case of poststroke anxiety and depressive disorders, there is some evidence for serotonergic depletion (in left temporal cortex) as well as serotonin receptor upregulation, in right temporoparietal cortex, in response to right hemisphere stroke (Mayberg et al. 1988)(see Chapter 21 on the mechanism of depression). If stroke leads to a rapid release of serotonin and downregulation of 5-HT-1A receptors, anxiety could result. A failure to replace the released serotonin (while the neuron begins to repair injured axons) would then lead to an upregulation of the 5-HT-1A receptor and ultimately depression. The duration of anxiety and depression might reflect the period of time necessary for receptor changes to take place.

Gainotti (1972) found a significantly higher frequency of anxiety reactions in patients with Broca's aphasia (i.e., impaired ability to initiate speech associated with lesions of the left inferior-posterior frontal cortex) and suggested that this may be the psychological response of the patient to repeated failure in verbal communications. Not all anxious-depressed patients in our studies, however, had non-fluent aphasia or left frontal lesions, suggesting that other mechanisms are also involved. Gur et al. (1987) showed that a linear decrease in the ratio of cortical metabolic rate to overall brain metabolic rate (i.e., lower cortical metabolism) is associated with an increasing severity of anxiety. This study indicates that disruption of cortical function may play a role in the production of primary anxiety disorders (i.e., anxiety without brain injury).

These hypotheses obviously do not answer all the questions or explain the clinical observations but they do provide some testable ideas for further exploration of the mechanism of poststroke anxiety disorder.

Treatment of poststroke anxiety disorder

The first treatment study of generalized anxiety disorder (GAD) following stroke was based on a merged analysis of results from previous treatment studies conducted by our research group (Kimura and Robinson 2003). These previous treatment studies included poststroke depression (Lipsey et al. 1984), pathological laughing and crying (Robinson et al. 1993) and a comparison of nortriptyline and fluoxetine for poststroke depression (Robinson et al. 2000). From the total of 106 patients in these three double-blind studies, 27 patients had a diagnosis of GAD as well as poststroke depression (i.e., 17 major and 10 minor depressions). Patients with GAD had to acknowledge the presence of worry or anxious foreboding as well as three out of six additional symptoms (excluding the 6-month duration criteria). These symptoms included restlessness, fatigue, poor concentration, irritability, nervous tension, and sleep disturbance. There was only one patient who dropped out during the course of the treatment trial (one patient from the Iowa study with major depression dropped out while receiving a dose of 100 mg/day of nortriptyline). We analyzed the 27 GAD patients with comorbid depression using an intention to treat analysis.

The studies were merged by equalizing approximately the duration of exposure to nortriptyline. The patients from both the Lipsey (1984) and the Robinson *et al.* (1993) studies were given 20 mg of nortriptyline for 1 week, 50 mg for 2 weeks, 70 mg for 1 week and 100 mg for 2 weeks. The patients from the Robinson *et al.* (2000) study were given 25 mg for 1 week, 50 mg for 2 weeks, 75 mg for 3 weeks and 100 mg for 6 weeks. For the merged analysis, evaluations completed at the beginning of the study (0 mg), 2 weeks (50 mg), 4 weeks (70 mg), and 6 weeks (100 mg) were considered approximately equivalent to those at weeks 0, 3 (50 mg), 6 (75 mg), and 9 (100 mg) in the Robinson *et al.* 2000 study.

Among the 27 patients with GAD, 13 patients were assigned nortriptyline and 14 patients were assigned to placebo. Analysis of variance (ANOVA) of baseline Hamilton anxiety (Ham-A) and Hamilton depression (Ham-D) scores with two factors (factor one, treatment versus placebo, factor two, study population) showed no significant active versus placebo effects or treatment by study population effects. There were no significant differences between the nortriptyline and placebo groups in demographic characteristics (Table 33.1). There were also no significant differences in stroke type, lesion location, and neurological deficits between the nortriptyline and placebo groups. Baseline Ham-A scores were not significantly different between the nortriptyline and the placebo groups (15.8 ± 4.3 SD nortriptyline versus 15.9 ± 5.1 SD placebo).

Repeated measures ANOVA of Ham-A scores using intention to treat analysis demonstrated a significant treatment by time interaction ($p = 0.002$) (Kimura and Robinson 2003)(Fig. 33.1). Planned comparisons revealed that the nortriptyline group was significantly more improved than the placebo at doses of 50 mg ($p < 0.05$); 75 mg ($p < 0.01$) and 100 mg/day ($p = 0.02$). The response rate for the nortriptyline group based on having a greater than 50% reduction in Ham-A score was 69.2% (9 of 13 patients) while the placebo response rate was 21.4% (3 of 14 patients) (Fisher exact $p = 0.02$).

We also compared the efficacy of nortriptyline between GAD comorbid with major depression and GAD with minor depression. Among patients with GAD and comorbid major depression, there was no significant pretreatment difference

Table 33.1. Demographic characteristics in 27 stroke patients with GAD

Characteristic	Nortriptyline (n = 13)	Placebo (n = 14)	p-value
Diagnosis (N)			
Major depression	6	11	0.1201
Minor depression	7	3	
	Mean ± SD	Mean ± SD	
Demographics			
Age (years)	64.8 ± 11.3	55 ± 15.2	0.07
Education (years)	11.4 ± 4.1	11.6 ± 2.8	0.91
Time since stroke (days)	73 ± 101	117 ± 159	0.44
Nortriptyline concentration at 100 mg (range)	83.4 ± 44.9 (16–152)		
Male sex	6 (46.2)	7 (50.0)	0.84
White	10 (76.9)	12 (85.7)	0.65
Right-handed	11 (84.6)	13 (92.9)	0.60
Married	6 (46.2)	10 (71.4)	0.25
Hollingshead social class IV or V	8 (57.1)	6 (42.9)	0.33
Family psychiatric history	4 (30.8)	2 (14.3)	0.38
Personal psychiatric history	2 (15.4)	3 (21.4)	1.00
Personal alcohol abuse history	3 (23.1)	6 (42.9)	0.42

Note: Values are number (percentage) unless otherwise indicated.

in Ham-A scores between the nortriptyline group (n = 6, mean Ham-A score 17.5 ± 4.5 SD) and the placebo group (n = 11, mean Ham-A 16.2 ± 5.5 SD). Repeated measures ANOVA of Ham-A scores showed a significant time by treatment interaction ($p = 0.02$). Among patients with GAD and comorbid minor depression, there were too few patients in the placebo group (n = 3) to analyze the data.

In addition, the nortriptyline group showed significant greater improvement in ADL Johns Hopkins functioning inventory (JHFI) scores than the placebo group ($p = 0.048$, effect size 1.24) (Table 33.2). There were no significant differences in mini-mental scores between the groups.

In an effort to determine whether there was a significant difference in the rate of response of anxiety symptoms compared to depressive symptoms, we compared the magnitude of change in Z score for both Ham-A and Ham-D scores for each

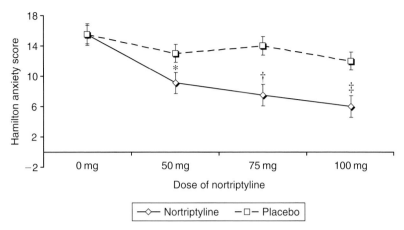

Figure 33.1 Mean Ham-A scores among patients with GAD and comorbid depression following stroke at increasing doses of nortriptyline. The nortriptyline group ($n = 13$) showed significantly greater improvement in anxiety symptoms than the placebo group ($n = 14$) ($p = 0.002$). Error bars represent standard errors of the mean (SE). (reprinted from Kimura and Robinson (2003) with permission) [*]$p < 0.05$, [†]$p < 0.01$, [‡]$p < 0.02$.

Table 33.2. Scores on neuropsychiatric measures for 27 stroke patients with GAD in a double-blind trial of nortriptyline or placebo

	Nortriptyline ($n = 13$)		Placebo ($n = 14$)	
	Baseline	End of treatment	Baseline	End of treatment
Measure	Mean $\pm$ SD	Mean $\pm$ SD	Mean $\pm$ SD	Mean $\pm$ SD
Present state examination[*]	24.1 $\pm$ 14.2	6.3 $\pm$ 6.7	24.4 $\pm$ 5.2	15.1 $\pm$ 9.1
17-item Ham-D[†]	17.0 $\pm$ 4.8	6.8 $\pm$ 7.0	17.4 $\pm$ 4.0	14.6 $\pm$ 7.9
Mini-mental state examination	23.8 $\pm$ 6.1	25.9 $\pm$ 4.0	25.8 $\pm$ 4.7	26.4 $\pm$ 6.9
Johns Hopkins functioning inventory[‡]	8.6 $\pm$ 6.4	5.5 $\pm$ 3.4	7.8 $\pm$ 5.3	7.4 $\pm$ 5.5

[*] Significantly greater improvement in the nortriptyline group ($F = 4.50$, d.f. $= 1, 25$; $p = 0.04$).
[†]Significantly greater improvement in the nortriptyline group ($F = 6.17$, d.f. $= 1, 25$; $p = 0.02$).
[‡]Significantly greater improvement in the nortriptyline group ($F = 4.37$, d.f. $= 1, 22$; $p = 0.048$).

dose of nortriptyline (Fig. 33.2). The change in Z score was significantly greater in Ham-A scores than Ham-D scores at a nortriptyline dose of 50 mg ($p = 0.035$, effect size $= 1.50$) (Kimura and Robinson 2003). This suggests that anxiety symptoms responded more rapidly than depressive symptoms to nortriptyline therapy.

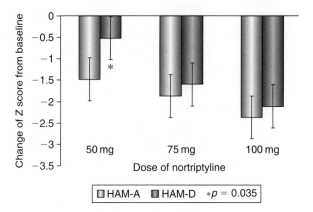

Figure 33.2 Change of Z score from baseline (pretreatment) scores for both Ham-A and Ham-D scales among patients treated with nortriptyline (n = 13). At a dose of 50 mg which represents 2–3 weeks of treatment, Ham-A scores had dropped significantly more than Ham-D scores from the baseline values (*p = 0.035). This suggests a more rapid response of anxiety symptoms than depressive symptoms to nortriptyline treatment [data from Kimura and Robinson (2003)].

To our knowledge, this was the first study which examined the use of nortriptyline or any other antidepressant–anti-anxiety agent in a double-blind randomized trial of poststroke GAD comparing placebo with active treatment. Patients who were given nortriptyline demonstrated significantly greater improvement in anxiety symptoms than patients who were given placebo. In addition, active treatment also led to significantly greater improvement in ADL compared with placebo as well as more rapid improvement of anxiety symptoms than depressive symptoms.

Although this study combined two groups of patients with different durations of treatment, we tried to combine them in a way that made them comparable in the duration of time that they received each dose of nortriptyline. We also had to examine the treatment of comorbid GAD and depression rather than GAD alone because all of our study patients had comorbid depression. Finally, after 2 or more weeks of 100 mg of nortriptyline, all patients had blood levels of nortriptyline that were in the therapeutic range for treatment of depression (Table 33.1).

Besides the finding that nortriptyline effectively treated anxiety disorder in patients with stroke, this study also found that nortriptyline was superior to placebo in improving ADL. In Chapter 32, we showed that there was an interactive effect of poststroke major depression and GAD on long-term recovery in ADLs. The additive effect may have enabled us to demonstrate the effect of treatment with a relatively small group of patients. The effect size for treatment on ADLs was 1.24 indicating a large effect.

Finally, this study demonstrated that the time (dose) at which significant changes occurred in anxiety symptoms was earlier than the time course of response to depression. This is consistent with our suggestion that GAD after stroke is etiologically different than poststroke depression. Elucidation of the mechanisms of these disorders, however, will require further investigation.

In summary, for the first time, a double-blind randomized treatment study using a merged analysis of prior treatment studies has demonstrated that GAD may be effectively treated with nortriptyline. Presumably the new generation anti-anxiety and antidepressant medications may also demonstrate significant anti-anxiety effects. Our findings also suggest that the impairments in ADL associated with stroke, depression, and anxiety disorder can be significantly improved by treatment of poststroke anxiety and depression. Additional treatment trials focused specifically on patients with poststroke anxiety disorders who do not have comorbid depression or other disorders in a randomized double-blind placebo controlled study are needed.

REFERENCES

Astrom, M. Generalized anxiety disorder in stroke patients: a 3-year longitudinal study. *Stroke* (1996) 27:270–275.

Castillo, C. S., Starkstein, S. E., Fedoroff, J. P., *et al.* Generalized anxiety disorder following stroke. *J Nerv Ment Dis* (1993) 181:100–106.

Gainotti, G. Emotional behavior and hemispheric side of the brain. *Cortex* (1972) 8:41–55.

Gorman, J. M., Liebowitz, M. R., Fyer, A. J., *et al.* A neuroanatomical hypothesis for panic disorder. *Am J Psychiatr* (1989) 146(2):148–161.

Gur, R. C., Gur, R. E., Resnick, S. M., *et al.* The effect of anxiety on cortical crebral blood flow and metabolism. *J Cereb Blood Flow Metab* (1987) 7:173–177.

Kimura, M., and Robinson, R. G. Treatment of poststroke generalized anxiety disorder comorbid with poststroke depression. Merged analysis of nortriptyline trials. *Am J Geriatr Psychiatr* (2003) 11(3):320–327.

Kimura, M., Robinson, R. G., and Kosier, T. Treatment of cognitive impairment after poststroke depression. *Stroke* (2000) 31(7):1482–1486.

Lipsey, J. R., Robinson, R. G., Pearlson, G. D., *et al.* Nortriptyline treatment of post-stroke depression: a double-blind study. *Lancet* (1984) i(8372):297–300.

Mayberg, H. S., Robinson, R. G., Wong, D. F., *et al.* PET imaging of cortical S_2-scrotonin receptors after stroke: lateralized changes and relationship to depression. *Am J Psychiatr* (1988) 145:937–943.

Paul, S. M. Anxiety and depression: A common neurobiological substrate? *J Clin Psychiatry* (1988) 49(Suppl 10):13–16.

Robinson, R. G., Parikh, R. M., Lipsey, J. R., *et al.* Pathological laughing and crying following stroke: validation of measurement scale and double-blind treatment study. *Am J Psychiatr* (1993) 150:286–293.

Robinson, R. G., Schultz, S. K., Castillo, C., *et al.* Nortriptyline versus fluoxetine in the treatment of depression and in short term recovery after stroke: a placebo controlled, double-blind study. *Am J Psychiatr* (2000) 157:351–359.

Stahl, S. M. Mixed depression and anxiety: serotonin1A receptors as a common pharmacologic link. *J Clin Psychiatr* (1997) 58(Suppl 8):20–26.

Starkstein, S. E., Cohen, B. S., Fedoroff, P., *et al.* Relationship between anxiety disorders and depressive disorders in patients with cerebrovascular injury. *Arch Gen Psychiatr* (1990) 47:785–789.

Part V

Other poststroke disorders

34

Psychosis

Although the literature contains many reports of psychotic syndromes associated with brain lesions, there are relatively few systematic studies of patients with psychosis following stroke. Davison and Bagley (1968) reviewed 50 reports of schizophrenia-like syndromes associated with disruption of normal brain anatomy or physiology. They concluded that no single type of brain injury or location was causally associated with these syndromes. Levine and Finkelstein (1982) and Price and Mesulam (1985) reported, however, that schizophrenia-like symptoms were strongly associated with right hemisphere infarctions as well as seizure disorders. Levine and Finkelstein (1982) reported on eight patients who developed hallucinations between 1 month and 11 years after a cerebrovascular infarction or traumatic brain injury. None of them had a previous personal history of psychiatric disorder and all of them were right handed. All of the patients had right hemisphere lesions with partial or complete involvement of the temporoparietal-occipital junction. The hallucinations and delusions developed acutely and lasted a period of days to months. In addition to the association with right hemisphere lesions, seven of the eight patients had seizures that developed after the brain injury: six of them had focal seizures while the remaining patient had generalized seizures. The seizures had preceded the onset of psychosis in five patients and followed the onset in the remaining two. In most patients, the hallucinations occurred in close temporal proximity (hours to days) to the occurrence of seizures.

Another series of cases was reported by Price and Mesulam (1985). Five right-handed patients aged 45–78 years developed delusions and/or hallucinations following infarcts in the right hemisphere. Only one patient had hallucinations and two patients had epileptiform activity on electroencephalogram (EEG). Thus, seizures may be sufficient in combination with a right hemisphere lesion but are not necessary to produce hallucinations and delusions.

Levine and Grek (1984) reported nine cases of delusions following right hemisphere infarction. They found that delusions were associated with pre-morbid brain atrophy more than with the exact location or size of the brain infarct.

There are several types of hallucinations that can occur in patients with brain injury. These have been termed atypical psychosis, peduncular hallucinosis, release hallucinations, organic psychosis, and agitated delirium. The term "agitated delirium" was used by Hornstein (1967) to describe nine patients who immediately after unilateral or bilateral infarctions of the calcarine cortex or the fusiform gyrus developed auditory or visual hallucinations accompanied by agitation, restlessness, memory disturbances, distractibility, unawareness of their behavioral disorder and visual loss. It is unclear, however, whether these disorders represented true delirium with decreased level of consciousness, slowing on the EEG, and fluctuating levels of symptomatology or were manifestations of an agitated psychotic state.

The term "peduncular hallucinosis" was used first by L'Hermitte (1922) to describe a patient with visual hallucinations and neurological findings compatible with a lesion in the midbrain and pons. The term hallucinosis was used to differentiate these visual hallucinations from a hallucination in which the patient believed that the sensory perception was real. Hallucinosis involves a perception without a stimulus but the patient does not believe the sensory perception is real. This ego-dystonic perception with preserved insight of the nonreality of the perception constitutes a hallucinosis.

Patients with peduncular hallucinosis may have perceptions of visual or auditory stimuli such as sounds of machines or visions of objects or animals. The lesions usually involve visual or auditory pathways within the brain stem, although some patients with peduncular hallucinosis have lesions of the brain stem, substantia nigra, or dorsal tegmentum (Geller and Bellur 1987) (Feinberg and Rapcsak 1989).

We have identified five patients hospitalized with schizophrenia-like symptoms which began following an identifiable stroke (Rabins *et al.* 1991). The clinical characteristics of these five patients are shown in Table 34.1. I have also compared these patients with our overall acute stroke population (Table 34.2). Patients who developed a schizophrenia-like syndrome were older and had a significantly higher frequency of family history of psychiatric disorder. Of the two patients with a positive family history, one had a son with schizophrenia and one patient had one sister with hallucinations and another sister with Parkinson's disease who was given electroconvulsive therapy (ECT). One patient with post-stroke psychosis was adopted and therefore their family history was uncertain. All patients had hallucinations and delusions. One patient had mild depressive symptoms but the other patients had no evidence of depression. The onset of symptoms occurred within hours following the stroke in two cases and within several days in another two cases. In only one case was the onset 2 months after the stroke lesion.

These five patients with schizophreniform psychosis were compared with five matched patients who were within ±2 years of the patient's age and whose stroke was in the same brain region, as defined according to the brain regions described by

Table 34.1. Descriptive characteristics of five patients who developed atypical schizophreniform psychosis after a right hemisphere stroke

Characteristic	Patient				
	A	B	C	D	E
Age	70	85	68	72	63
Sex	M	F	M	F	M
Family history	Son had schizophrenia	Sister received ECT and had Parkinson's; Brother had alcoholism; Sister had hallucinations	None	Adopted	None
Past psychiatric history	None	None; Mild Parkinson's tremor in hand	Alcohol abuse	None	None
Hearing	L hearing aid	Inconsistent responses; mod bilateral loss	Normal	Normal	Not tested
Time after lesion symptoms started	Within hours	2 months	Within days	2 days	1 day
Hallucinations	Yes	Yes	Yes	Visual, auditory	1 day
Delusions	Yes	Yes	Yes	Yes	Yes
Depression	Mild	No	No	No	No
Neurologic symptoms	L hemineglect; L hemiplegia arm > leg; L hemianopsia seizures	L ext plantar; L tone	L hemiparesis; L hemianopsia; seizures	Seizure at onset	L hemiparesis; L hemianopsia
Treatment	Thiothixene 8 mg	Pimozide 3 mg; perphenazine 8 mg; haloperidol 12 mg; thioridazine 400 mg; trifluoperazine; lithium 450 mg; ECT	Phenytoin; thiothixene	Haloperidol 10 mg	None
Response to treatment	Less delusional	No improvement	Released off medication; hallucinations and delusions resolved; still suspicious	Full resolution by 5 years	Slow incomplete resolution

Note: L = left; ECT = electroconvulsive therapy.
From Rabins *et al.* 1991 reprinted with permission.

Table 34.2. Background characteristics

	Psychosis ($n = 5$)	All stroke ($n = 301$)
Age (mean year ± SD)	72 ± 13*	61 ± 17
Education (mean year ± SD)	11 ± 15	9 ± 6
Sex (% male)	60	57
Family history (% positive)	50*	9
Personal history (% positive)	20	10

*$p < 0.05$

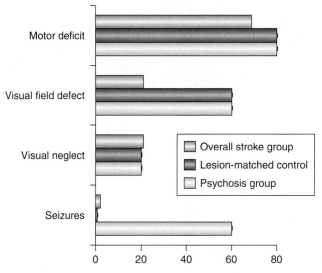

Figure 34.1 The frequency of several neurological symptoms in patients with schizophreniform disorders ($n = 5$), lesion- and age-matched controls ($n = 5$), and overall acute stroke population ($n = 301$). There were no differences in the frequency of motor deficit or visual neglect but the psychosis patients had a significantly greater frequency of seizures and visual field defects than the overall stroke population.

Levine and Grek (1984), and whose lesion volume was classified in the same category: small (1–5% of brain area), medium (6–15%), or large (>15%). The neurological findings are shown in Fig. 34.1. The psychotic patients and the lesion-matched controls were not significantly different in any of their neurological findings except for the frequency of seizures. Three of the five patients who developed hallucinations had seizures: one patient's seizures began immediately after the stroke, while for two patients the onset of seizures began more than 3 months after the stroke. The onset of seizures and the onset of hallucinations were not identical. The frequency of visual field defects was also higher in patients with hallucinations than in the overall

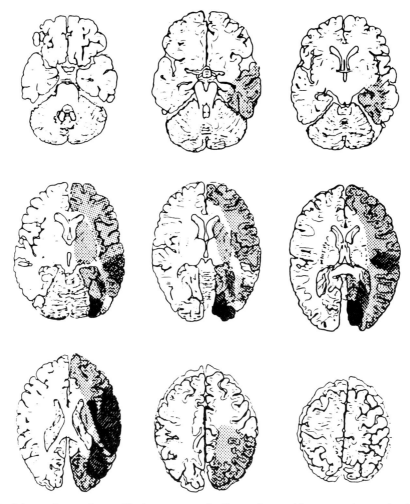

Figure 34.2 Schematic templates of lesions among the five patients with post-stroke psychosis. Note that the lesions are exclusively in the right hemisphere and are predominantly cortical in their location. Only one patient had a subcortical infarct.

group of acute stroke patients. The lesion locations of the five patients with hallucinations are shown in Fig. 34.2. The lesion locations and a comparison with the overall stroke population are shown in Table 34.3. All of the patients with delusions and hallucinations had a right hemisphere lesion, compared to 45% in the overall stroke group. In addition, four out of the five (80%) had cortical lesions, compared to 42% in our unselected stroke patients. There were no differences in lesion volume between the psychotic patients, the lesion-matched controls, or the overall stroke population.

In addition to the assessment of lesion hemisphere and intrahemispheric lesion location, a number of other measurements of subcortical and cortical structures in

Table 34.3. Lesion measurements

	Psychosis ($n = 5$)	Control ($n = 5$)	All stroke (%) ($n = 301$)
Right	5*	5	45
Left	0	0	36
Bilateral/basal	0	0	18
Cortical	4	4	42
Subcortical	1	1	45
Combined	0	0	12
Volume	5.4 ± 1.5	7.4 ± 1.3	6.2 ± 6.5

*$p = 0.02$

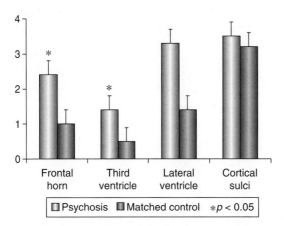

Figure 34.3   Measurements of cortical sulci and ventricular to brain ratios in patients who developed delusions and hallucinations following stroke and lesion and age-matched controls who were non-psychotic. Although the psychotic patients had higher mean ± SEM ratios on all measures, the significant differences were found in the frontal horn ratio (distance between the frontal horns of the lateral ventricles divided by the width of the brain at that level) and the third ventricle ratio (area of the third ventricle divided by the transpineal width). These findings indicate that the psychotic patients had greater subcortical atrophy than non-psychotic patients. This atrophy probably preceded the stroke, suggesting that these patients may have had a pre-morbid vulnerability that was brought out by the right hemisphere stroke.

the brain were made, the results of which are shown in Fig. 34.3. Patients with schizophreniform disorder were not significantly different than the lesion-matched control patients in the extent of cortical atrophy, as measured by the width of four cortical sulci. On the other hand, the subcortical measures of ventricular to brain ratios were all higher in the patients with hallucinations compared to the lesion-matched controls (Fig. 34.3). After a Z score transformation of the CT data (i.e., a statistical transformation so that scores may be compared across scales) so that all measures could be compared in one analysis, two-way analysis of variance (ANOVA) (factor one group: schizophrenic versus controls; factor two, all CT measures) demonstrated a significant group effect ($p < 0.05$). This indicates that, across all measures, the psychotic patients had more brain atrophy than the lesion-matched controls. A comparison of individual measures showed that the psychotic patients had significantly larger frontal horn and third ventricle to brain ratios, indicating prominent subcortical atrophy.

Although the number of cases was quite limited, this study found some interesting clinical correlations. First, the patients who developed delusions and hallucinations following stroke were older than the overall population of acute stroke patients and they were more likely to have a family history of psychiatric disorder. In addition, these patients were more likely to have seizures, visual field defects, right hemisphere lesions, and subcortical atrophy. These findings also suggest that the reason why hallucinations and delusions are uncommon following stroke is that more than one factor is needed. Data from lesion-matched control patients demonstrated that the existence of a right hemisphere lesion is not sufficient to produce this syndrome, but that a right hemisphere lesion, particularly of the posterior temporoparieto-occipital junction, is necessary. This right hemisphere lesion may act in combination with one or more additional factors such as seizures, genetic vulnerability, or subcortical atrophy. A combination of two or more factors appears to be necessary for the production of this unusual but dramatic manifestation of brain injury.

Recently, Tonkonogy and Geller (1999) reported on 13 patients with late onset paranoid psychosis compared with 35 elderly patients with early onset paranoid psychosis. The mean age of the late onset patients was 66.3 and the present age of the early onset patients was 63.9. Magnetic resonance imaging revealed that late onset patients had white matter hyperintensities in 69.2% of the cases compared with the 22.9% of the early onset cases ($p = 0.0055$, 2-tailed Fisher's exact test). Ventricular enlargement and cortical atrophy, however, were more frequent in the early onset group. Ventricular enlargement occurred in 28.6% of the early onset patients, cortical atrophy in 22.9%, while none of the patients with late onset psychosis had ventricular enlargement or cortical atrophy ($p = 0.0007$, 2-tailed Fisher's exact test). Thus, the patients with late onset psychosis appeared to have vascular disorder involving small vessel pathology leading to white matter hyperintensities. These vascular lesions may have played a role in the onset of schizophrenic disorders. In contrast, however, Howard *et al.* (1995) did not find a significant difference in the number of white matter hyperintensities visualized by magnetic resonance imaging among 38 patients with late onset paranoid schizophrenia compared with 31 healthy age comparable community volunteers. Periventricular white matter and subcortical gray matter hyperintensities, however, were associated with elevated blood pressure and older age in both control and psychotic patients.

A clinical history can be illustrative of the variety of psychotic phenomena which may occur following stroke. The first case is one of the patients reported by L'Hermitte (1922). The patient was a 72-year-old woman with no personal history of psychiatric disorder. The patient suffered the acute onset of vertigo and several days later exhibited a palsy of the left sixth cranial nerve as well as an intention tremor of the right arm. She also developed paralysis of the third and fourth cranial nerves, a right hemiparesis, and a Babinski sign. Two weeks later she reported seeing animals of bizarre appearance but as soon as she tried to touch them they disappeared through the floor. The patient never thought that these perceptions were real and reported that the animals sometimes turned into human figures, such as children playing with dolls.

The second patient presents a case of auditory and visual hallucinations. The patient was a 72-year-old right-handed, widowed African–American woman with a high school education and no previous psychiatric history. She had been married for 24 years and worked as a housekeeper until her retirement 3 years prior to admission. She lived alone and 15 days prior to admission experienced the sudden onset of severe right occipital headache. The following day the patient noted numbness of her left arm, slurring of speech, and left facial droop. She had focal seizure activity involving her left arm. Two days later the patient heard a loud buzzing noise while dressing. The patient interpreted this noise as being due to a large bee and she began shedding her clothing "in order to get rid of the bee." The patient then had numerous visual and auditory hallucinations including seeing a fire in the street and hearing the voice of a relative who said that he was coming to kill her. The patient hid in the bedroom closet, hearing someone coming up the stairs. The patient reported seeing people of normal size sitting at her kitchen table and discussing her among themselves. They made derogatory and vulgar comments about her and on one occasion suggested that she should jump out the window. She also experienced occasional tactile hallucinations, such as having her hair pulled by her "visitors." On examination, the patient was alert, cooperative, and oriented. She had a score of 29 out of 30 on the mini-mental state examination. On EEG there was no evidence of seizure activity. The hallucinations gradually declined in frequency following treatment with haloperidol (Haldol). Four weeks later the patient discontinued the haloperidol. She had no further auditory hallucinations or visual hallucinations.

In summary, psychosis following stroke involves a variety of presentations ranging from patients who have no insight about the non-reality of their hallucinations and delusions to patients who retain their awareness of reality in spite of the existence of hallucinations. Psychotic disorders have generally been associated with right hemisphere lesions although not exclusively (Low *et al.* 1999). In many cases, the psychosis was associated with stroke lesions affecting the parietal temporo-occipital junction. Although some lesions that produced hallucinations were subcortical, most were cortical. Both seizures and subcortical brain atrophy have been associated with hallucinations. Small vessel disease has also been associated with the development of psychosis. Generally, patients have responded to treatment with neuroleptic medication although in some treatment resistant cases, anticonvulsant medications have been reported to be useful (Levine and Grek 1984). This phenomenon of hallucinations and delusions associated with focal brain injury may reveal insights into the mechanisms of psychosis. Although they are rare following stroke, post-stroke psychosis deserves further investigation.

REFERENCES

Davison, K., and Bagley, C. R. Schizophrenia-like psychoses associated with organic disorder of the central nervous system: a review of the literature. In R. Herrington, ed., *Current Problems in Neuropsychiatry: Schizophrenia, Epilepsy, the Temporal Lobe*. Headley Ashford, Kent, England, 1968.

Feinberg, W. M., and Rapcsak, S. Z. Peduncular hallucinosis following paramedian thalamic infarction. *Neurology* (1989) 39:1535–1536.

Geller, T. J., and Bellur, S. W. Peduncular hallucinosis: magnetic resonance imaging confirmation of mesencephalic infarction during life. *Ann Neurol* (1987) 21:602–604.

Hornstein, S., Chamberlin, W., and Conomy, J. Infarction of the fusiform and calcarine regions: agitated delirium and hemianopia. *Trans Am Neurol Assn* (1967) 92:85–89.

Howard, R., Cox, T., Almeida, O., *et al*. White matter signal hyperintensities in the brains of patients with late paraphrenia and the normal, community-living elderly. *Biol Psychiatr* (1995) 38(2):86–91.

L'Hermitte, J. Syndrom de la callotte du pédoncle cérébral. Les troubles psycho-sensorieles dans les lésions du mesencéphale. *Rev Neurol* (1922) 38:1359–1365.

Levin, D. N., and Finkelstein, S. Delayed psychosis after right temporoparietal stroke or trauma: relation to epilepsy. *Neurology* (1982) 32:267–273.

Levine, D. N., and Grek, A. The anatomic basis of delusions after right cerebral infarction. *Neurology* (1984) 34:577–582.

Low, J. A., Yap, K. B., and Chan, K. M. Posterior cerebral artery territory infarct presenting as acute psychosis. *Singapore Med J* (1999) 40(11):702–703.

Price, B. H., and Mesulam, M. Psychiatric manifestations of right hemisphere infarctions. *J Nerv Ment Dis* (1985) 173:610–614.

Rabins, P. V., Starkstein, S. E., and Robinson, R. G. Risk factors for developing atypical (schizophreniform) psychosis following stroke. *J Neuropsychiatr Clin Neurosci* (1991) 3:6–9.

Tonkonogy, J. M., and Geller, J. L. Late-onset paranoid psychosis as a distinct clinicopathologic entity: magnetic resonance imaging data in elderly patients with paranoid psychosis of late onset and schizophrenia of early onset. *Neuropsychiatry Neuropsychol Behav Neurol* (1999) 12(4):230–235.

35

Anosognosia and denial of illness

In 1914, Babinski (1914) reported that some patients with severe hemiplegia appeared to be unaware of their deficit. He called this absence of awareness "anosognosia," a term derived from the Greek words "gnosis" (knowledge), "a" (without), and "noso" (disease). The medical literature of the late 19th and 20th centuries reported a variety of failures of awareness of one's own deficits or diseases including Anton's syndrome of cortical blindness (Anton 1896), unawareness of hemianopsia, amnesia, dementia, aphasia (particularly fluent aphasia), and mental illnesses like schizophrenia or dementia.

As they are unaware of their illness, patients with anosognosia may be less likely to seek treatment and remain compliant with prescribed medications. They may also engage in potentially dangerous activities based on their belief that they are able to do things that they are not, such as believing themselves capable of driving an automobile when they are not (Heilman and Valenstein 1993). Clinicians, therefore, should monitor their patients' awareness of their limitations.

Denial of illness is similar to anosognosia because patients fail to acknowledge their illness or deficits associated with it. Denial of illness has been reported among patients with brain injury as well as patients without brain injury (Weinstein and Kahn 1955). When stroke patients deny hemiplegia or sensory deficit, the distinction between denial and anosognosia is negligible. The two conditions may, in fact, be manifestations of the same underlying mechanism. On the other hand, when patients who do not have brain injury deny an obvious impairment or even the existence of a major medical condition like myocardial infarction (Hackett and Cassem 1974), this appears to be a different process than the one associated with brain injury. The nature of brain injury may create cognitive or sensory impairments which contribute to a deficit in awareness of impairment, while unawareness in patients who have not sustained brain injury probably represents a psychological response to impairment.

Another phenomenon related to anosognosia is the indifference reaction. First described by Hecaen *et al.* (1951) and Denny-Brown *et al.* (1952), patients with the indifference reaction do not deny the existence of impairment, but their unconcern seems clearly inappropriate to (or perhaps unaware of) the severity or implications of the illness or impairment. This phenomenon, therefore, appears to share some features with anosognosia such as unawareness of the severity of illness as well as a lack of empathic understanding of the patient's mental state.

The "alien hand syndrome" is a similar and potentially related condition characterized by the patient's inability to recognize that his hand, usually the left, is his own. Patients may try to throw the hand out of the bed or strike it with the right hand as though it was an interloper invading their personal space. The alien hand behavior may include buttoning a shirt with their right hand while the left hand follows undoing the work of the right hand. Although relatively unusual, this is among the most striking examples of failed awareness of some part or deficit of one's own body. When they appear as manifestations of brain injury, it is usually but not exclusively the right hemisphere that has sustained the insult (Starkstein *et al.* 1992; Heilman and Valenstein 1993).

There have been many attempts to explain these multiple variations of failed awareness. Weinstein and Kahn (1955) proposed psychological etiologies suggesting that denial is a psychological defense mechanism which attenuates the emotional impact of a catastrophic event such as hemiplegia. Alternatively, it has also been proposed that anosognosia is a confusional state induced by the medical illness or its treatment (Hecaen *et al.* 1951). Others (Levine *et al.* 1991) suggested that anosognosia may occur when patients do not receive sufficient sensory feedback to their brains that their limb is weak or that their proprioceptive system is impaired and consequently, they do not sense an absence of motor activity. Hemispatial neglect has also been proposed as a contributory mechanism. If patients neglect their left visual field, they may be unaware that there is no movement of their left arm. Still others have hypothesized a phantom limb phenomenon where the patient senses his arm has moved when it has not. Disconnection between the right and left hemisphere has also been proposed to explain anosognosia (Geschwind 1965a, b) with areas in the right hemisphere disconnected from language centers in the left hemisphere leading to a consequent language-mediated unawareness of impairment. None of these hypotheses, however, has been shown to explain all or even the majority of the cases of anosognosia or denial of illness.

We examined 80 patients for the presence of anosognosia and looked for clinical correlates of this disorder (Starkstein *et al.* 1992). The background characteristics of the patients are shown in Table 35.1. Patients were enrolled if they had no previous history of stroke and no evidence of moderate or severe comprehension deficits as determined by passing part 1 of the token test (DeRenzi and Faglioni 1978). The patients were predominantly African–American from lower socioeconomic classes in their late 50s or 60s and were examined within the first 2 weeks following acute stroke. There were no significant differences between patients with

Table 35.1. Stroke patients with anosognosia (*n* = 80)

	None (*n* = 53)	Mild (*n* = 8)	Moderate (*n* = 9)	Severe (*n* = 10)
Age	56 ± 11	62 ± 11	69 ± 13	62 ± 11
Education	11 ± 4	9 ± 3	11 ± 4	10 ± 3
Gender (*n*, male)	29	5	5	6
Race (*n*, black)	33	6	6	6
Left handedness	3	0	2	1
Number of married	16	2	5	2
Hollingshead class IV–V	30	7	3	8
Fam hx psych disorder	9	0	2	1
Personal hx psych disorder	8	0	1	1
Past hx psych disorder	13	0	2	1
Days since stroke	5.7 ± 3.9	7.1 ± 4.9	6.7 ± 4.8	5.6 ± 3.5

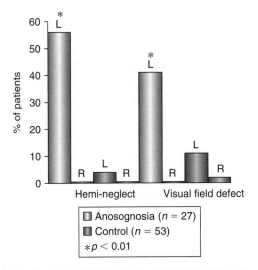

Figure 35.1 The association of anosognosia with left-sided (L) neglect to double simultaneous stimulation and visual field defect. More than half of the patients with anosognosia showed L hemi-neglect and L visual field defect significantly more frequently than stroke patients without anosognosia.

severe anosognosia and those with no anosognosia in terms of any of their background characteristics.

Neurological examination revealed no significant differences between groups in the frequency of motor or sensory deficits, cerebellar or brain stem neurological findings, or frequency or type of aphasia. The patients with anosognosia, however, had a significantly higher frequency of left-sided hemi-neglect (Fig. 35.1) which was

Table 35.2. Frequency of motor and visual anosognosia in patients with mild, moderate, and severe disorders

	Motor impairment anosognosia/total with impairment	Visual field impairment anosognosia/total with impairment
Mild	8/8	0/3
Moderate	9/9	0/4
Severe	10/10	2/5

determined by the presence of extinction (i.e., being unaware of a stimulus when two or more stimuli are given simultaneously) on double simultaneous stimulation for auditory, visual, or tactile stimulation. Subjects were asked to point with one finger to the side stimulated. Out of 10 double simultaneous stimulations, neglect was determined by failure to identify bilateral stimulation on five or more of the trials. Hemi-spatial neglect was assessed by asking the patient to copy a complex figure which included 10 lines to the left of the midline and 10 lines to the right and draw five figures from memory (i.e., flower, cube, star, clock, and house). The complex figure was scored as the total number of lines omitted on each side of the midline and the other figures were scored as the number of omissions from each lateralized component. Patients with motor deficits in their dominant hand were not given this test.

Patients with anosognosia were also found to have a significantly greater frequency of visual field deficits than controls (Fig. 35.1). Of 27 patients with anosognosia, 11 had a left-sided hemianopia, which was significantly greater than the 6 hemianopias among 53 patients without anosognosia.

The presence of anosognosia was determined for motor and visual deficits by asking the patient if there was anything wrong with their motor movement or their eyesight. Patients were considered to have mild anosognosia if they acknowledged their disorder only after the examiner stated that they had an impairment of their motor or visual function (Bisiach *et al.* 1986). Moderate anosognosia was defined by the patient's acknowledgment of impairment only after it was identified in a neurological examination. Severe anosognosia was demonstrated by the patient's failure to acknowledge the disorder even after the existence of a motor or visual field deficit was demonstrated to them. Table 35.2 shows the frequency of motor and visual anosognosia found in patients with mild, moderate, and severe disorders. All 25 patients with hemiparesis and anosognosia had a failure to recognize their motor deficits while only 2 of 12 patients with visual field defects and anosognosia failed to recognize this impairment ($p < 0.001$). This finding demonstrates that anosognosia of motor impairment is significantly more frequent than anosognosia

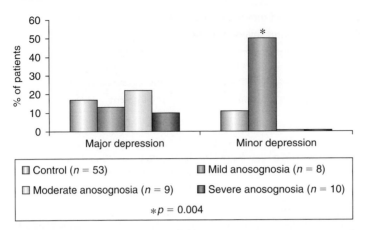

Figure 35.2 The frequency of major and minor depression by severity of anosognosia. Major depression was equally common in stroke patients with anosognosia as stroke patients without anosognosia. This indicates that unawareness of physical impairment does not lead to unawareness of mood disorder.

of visual field impairment and that someone may have anosognosia for motor impairment but not of visual field deficits.

There were no significant differences between groups in terms of their total score on the present state examination (PSE), the Hamilton depression scale, or the Hamilton anxiety scale (Fig. 35.2). This finding does not support the idea that anosognosia of motor impairment might extend to unawareness of an emotional disorder. Patients who had mild or moderate anosognosia had slightly higher depression scores than those with no anosognosia (Fig. 35.2). Similarly, frequencies of major depression were not significantly different across groups (Fig. 35.3). The only significant difference in the frequency of depression was that patients with mild anosognosia had more cases of minor depression compared to patients with no anosognosia ($p = 0.004$). If anosognosia is hypothesized to prevent patients from recognizing their own depression, one would expect significantly lower frequencies of depression among the group with anosognosia as compared to that without.

It might be argued that patients with anosognosia would have more severe depression if it were not for the existence of anosognosia. In order to examine this issue, we matched 6 patients with anosognosia (one with mild, one with moderate, four with severe) and 6 patients without anosognosia for lesion side (four pairs with right hemisphere lesions and two pairs with left hemisphere lesions) and location (two pairs with temporo-occipital lesions, one pair with fronto-dorsolateral lesions, and three pairs with basal ganglia lesions). The groups were also comparable in terms of age (62.1 ± 13.8 years anosognosia versus 58.5 ± 10.4 years no anosognosia), years of education (8.6 ± 3.2 versus $11.9 \pm 2.6, p = $ NS). There were

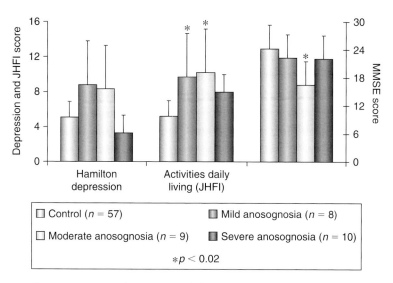

Figure 35.3   Impairment scores on the MMSE and the JHFI as well as severity of depression scores on the Hamilton depression scale. Note that patients with anosognosia had greater severity of impairment than patients without anosognosia.

no significant differences between these lesion-matched patients in their total PSE score (14.8 ± 16.5 anosognosia versus 8.1 ± 10.4 control). In addition, three of the 6 patients with anosognosia were depressed (two with major depression and one with minor depression) compared with two of the 6 patients without anosognosia (one had major and one had minor depression). Thus, even after controlling for demographic and lesion location variables, depression was no less common in the anosognosic compared to the control population.

Scores on the activities of daily living (Johns Hopkins functioning inventory or JHFI) scale demonstrated that patients with mild or moderate anosognosia had a significantly greater degree of impairment than control patients (Fig. 35.3). Similarly, upon cognitive examination, patients with moderate anosognosia were significantly more impaired as assessed by the mini-mental state examination (MMSE), than the control group (Fig. 35.3). There were no significant differences between groups in the numbers of social ties.

These findings suggest that the degree of physical and cognitive impairment is more related to the existence of anosognosia than is the presence or absence of depression. Patients with anosognosia were more impaired physically and cognitively than patients without anosognosia.

Results of neuropsychological testing revealed that patients with anosognosia had a significantly higher frequency of ignoring one stimulus during double simultaneous tactile, visual, or auditory stimulation (i.e., unilateral extinction or neglect)

(Fig. 35.4). Patients were given 10 double simultaneous stimulations intermixed with 20 single stimulations. The number of errors in pointing to the correct side or sides of stimulation was significantly higher in patients with mild, moderate, or severe anosognosia compared with controls. In addition to this unilateral extinction on double simultaneous tactile, visual or auditory stimulation, patients with anosognosia also showed evidence of hemi-spatial neglect (Fig. 35.4). When asked to copy a complex figure with 10 lines to the left of the midline and 10 lines to the right, patients with anosognosia omitted a significantly larger number of the lines on the left side compared to patients without anosognosia (Fig. 35.4). Similarly, when asked to point to the side of the body contralateral to the brain lesion using the hand on the ipsilateral side of the body, significantly more patients showed no movement to the target or delayed movement compared to the control patients without anosognosia (Fig. 35.4). These neuropsychological test findings demonstrate that patients with anosognosia have both sensory extinction and left-sided neglect compared to patients without anosognosia.

In addition to the neuropsychological impairments, patients also had deficits in their ability to recognize facial emotion, emotional intonation in voice. Patients were shown 20 photographs of Ekman and Friesen faces (i.e., facial pictures of actors and actresses) trying to facially display sad, happy, or angry emotions (Ekman and

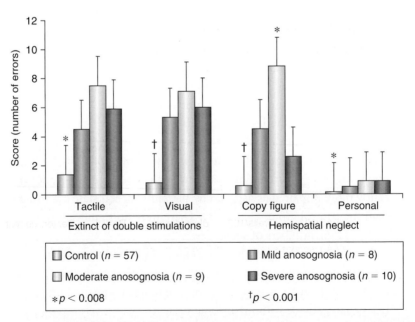

Figure 35.4 Tactile, visual, and spatial neglect in patients with anosognosia and controls. Patients with all severities of anosognosia had significantly more severe neglect in all modalities tested than stroke patients without anosognosia.

Friesen 1975). Patients with anosognosia made significantly more errors in this task than control patients without anosognosia. In addition, patients listened to 13 different sentences spoken in a happy, sad, or angry intonation. All sentences were simple, declarative statements such as "the lamp is on the table." Although all patients were able to hear the auditory stimulation, patients with anosognosia made significantly more errors (i.e., receptive or sensory aprosody) than control patients without anosognosia ($p < 0.05$). These findings suggest that the impairment in patients with anosognosia is not simply an unawareness of one side of their body in space but also an inability to recognize the emotional meaning of sensory input.

In order to control for the effect of lesion location on neuropsychological test performance, we matched another set of 8 patients with anosognosia and 8 control patients who had received detailed neuropsychological assessment for both hemisphere and location of brain injury (Starkstein *et al.* 1993a). Patients were given tests of comprehension (token test, DeRenzi and Faglioni 1978), frontal lobe function (Trail making test and controlled word association Test (FAS), Reitan 1971), as well as visual construction (block design, Wechsler and Wechsler 1955), attention (digit span) and learning/memory (Benton visual retention test and Rey auditory verbal learning test (RAVLT); Spreen and Strauss 1991). Patients with anosognosia were significantly more impaired than those without anosognosia in the frontal lobe tests including the controlled word association test (FAS, Benton 1968) ($p < 0.02$), and the Trails A and B tests ($p < 0.001$) (Fig. 35.5). The groups did not perform significantly differently on the construction, attention, or memory tasks, suggesting that anosognosia was associated with cognitive impairment in frontal lobe function and not a general cognitive dysfunction.

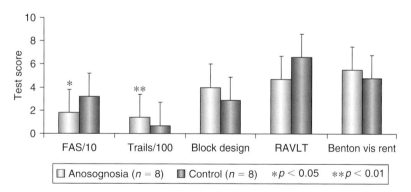

Figure 35.5 Performance of patients with and without anosognosia who were matched for lesion location on several neuropsychological examinations. Patients with anosognosia were significantly more impaired than controls on verbal fluency (FAS) and Trails A and B but not on any of the other construction, attention, learning, or memory tasks. These findings suggest that anosognosia is associated with frontal lobe dysfunction (data taken from Starkstein *et al.* 1993a). Benton vis rent: Benton visual retention test.

In light of the findings that patients with anosognosia tend not to recognize one side of their body or space, have frontal lobe dysfunction and are unable to recognize the meaning of emotional sensory stimulation, the finding that severity of depressive symptoms or frequency of depressive disorder was not significantly different between patients with and without anosognosia is even more interesting. This finding suggests that the patient's inability to recognize their own impairment as well as an unawareness of one side of their body and space does not necessarily imply an inability to recognize their own inner feelings of sadness, hopelessness, loss of pleasure, or self-blame.

As one might expect, lesion location also plays an important role in the existence of anosognosia. There were 66 patients who had a lesion demonstrable on CT scan, and patients with anosognosia had a significantly higher frequency of right hemisphere lesions than patients without anosognosia (Fig. 35.6). Analysis of intrahemispheric lesion location revealed that patients with mild or severe anosognosia had an increased frequency of temporoparietal lesions or thalamic lesions than patients without anosognosia, and patients with moderate anosognosia had a significantly higher frequency of basal ganglia strokes than patients without anosognosia (Fig. 35.6). There were no significant intergroup differences in other lesion locations and there were no significant differences in the frequency of hemorrhagic infarcts.

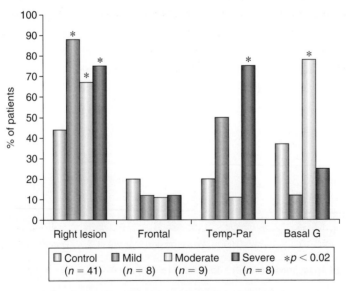

Figure 35.6 The frequency of lesion locations in patients with and without anosognosia. The strongest association was between anosognosia and right hemisphere lesions. Patients with severe anosognosia were more likely to have temporoparietal (Temp-Par) lesions than any other group while moderate severe anosognosia was associated with basal ganglia (Basal G) lesions. Note that frontal lesions were not associated with the existence of anosognosia in this population.

Brain atrophy was measured on CT scan in 51 of these patients (patients who were excluded had cerebellar or brain stem lesions or multiple lesions or tilted images). Patients with anosognosia ($n = 18$) were compared to controls ($n = 33$) without anosognosia. The group with anosognosia had significantly greater frontal horn to brain size ratios, third ventricular to brain size, and lateral ventricular to brain size ratios (Fig. 35.7). These findings indicate that subcortical atrophy is associated with anosognosia.

In an effort to examine the independent effects of all of these factors that were shown to be associated with anosognosia, a stepwise regression analysis was performed in which the presence or absence of anosognosia was examined in relation to extinction, neglect, facial emotion recognition, receptive aprosody, subcortical atrophy, lesion location, and impairments in activities of daily living. The two significant variables (which accounted for 57% of the variance) were the frontal horn to brain size ratio ($r = 0.69$) and a right temporoparietal or thalamic lesion location ($r = 0.75$).

Following our first study of 80 acute stroke patients for clinical correlates of anosognosia, we have recently examined the effect of antidepressant (i.e., fluoxetine or nortriptyline) treatment on anosognosia among 44 patients who completed 12 weeks of treatment and were seen 21 months later for follow-up. This was a secondary analysis of our depression treatment study (Robinson *et al.* 2000). In this study, all patients were administered the denial of illness scale (DIS). Based on our first 80 patients, all patients with a score of 5 or more on the DIS had at least mild anosognosia. Thus, in the treatment study, patients with scores of 5 or greater on the DIS were considered to have anosognosia/denial. Background characteristics of 9 patients who

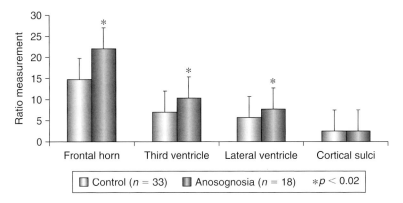

Figure 35.7 Ventricle to brain size ratios for patients with anosognosia were significantly larger than those for patients without anosognosia. The cortical measures were not different between groups indicating that patients with unawareness of their physical impairment following a stroke have more subcortical brain atrophy (which probably preceded the stroke). Compromised subcortical function in the right hemisphere may mediate this phenomenon of anosognosia.

Table 35.3. Demographic characteristics

Characteristic	Non-denial ($n = 35$)		Denial ($n = 9$)	
	Mean	*SD*	*Mean*	*SD*
Age (years)	69.6	10.3	65.3	14.3
Education (years)	11.9	2.3	12.2	2.5
	n	*%*	*n*	*%*
Male	19	54.3	5	55.6
Caucasian	33	94.3	9	100.0
Married	16	47.7	7	77.8
Socioeconomic status (%)	12	34.3	5	55.6
(Hollingshead class IV or V)				
Right handedness	35	100.0	9	100.0
Prior psychiatric history	4	11.4	1	11.1
Family psychiatric history	4	11.4	2	22.2

fulfilled the DIS criteria were compared with 35 patients who did not (Table 35.3). There were no significant differences between the patient groups in background characteristics including prior personal or family history of psychiatric disorder. The mean age of the patients with denial was 65.3 ± 14.3 years and the non-denial patients 69.6 ± 10.3 years. They were also comparable in years of education, 12.2 ± 2.5 for the patients with denial versus 11.9 ± 2.3 non-denial. Fifty-six percent of the denial patients and 54% of the non-denial patients were males and all patients were right handed. The severity of impairment measures did not reveal any significant differences between the denial and non-denial groups including the mini-mental examination score (24.6 ± 5.5 denial versus 26.2 ± 5.1 non-denial), activities of daily living score or social functioning score (Table 35.4). On neurological examination 91% of the controls and 78% of the denial patients had ischemic infarcts. The volume of all visible lesions in the control group was 6.5 ± 8.7 SD% of whole brain volume while the lesion volume was 3.5 ± 3.6 SD% of whole brain volume in the denial patients. These lesion volumes were not significantly different ($p = 0.43$). On the other hand, lesion location was significantly different between the two groups. Eighty-eight percent of the denial patients had a right hemisphere lesion compared with only 45% of the control patients (Fisher's exact $p = 0.05$) (Fig. 35.8). When intrahemispheric lesion location was determined, 50% of the patients with denial had a basal ganglia lesion in the right hemisphere compared with 8% of the controls. Similarly, patients with denial tended to have a greater frequency of insular lesions in the right hemisphere than control patients.

Relationships of denial of illness and Diagnostic and Statistical Manual, 4th ed. (DSM-IV) diagnoses of major depression, minor depression, or generalized anxiety disorder are shown in Fig. 35.9. There were no significant differences in the

Table 35.4. Psychiatric variables

Characteristic	Non-denial ($n = 35$)		Denial ($n = 9$)		Significance
	Mean	SD	Mean	SD	
MMSE	26.2	5.1	24.6	5.5	0.3939
JHFI	6.5	3.3	8.0	5.4	0.3140
FIM	48.6	9.7	46.5	12.4	0.5818
SFE	0.12	0.15	0.14	0.25	0.7427
STC	3.5	1.9	2.4	1.3	0.1249

FIM: functional independence measure; SFE: social functioning examination; STC: social ties checklist.

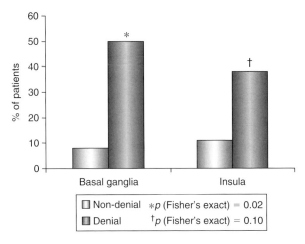

Figure 35.8 Intra hemispheric lesion location and denial of illness. Both basal ganglia and insular lesions of the right hemisphere were associated with denial of illness (anosognosia) (reprinted from Robinson 2004 with permission). From Self-Awareness Deficits in Psychiatric Patients, edited by Bernard D. Beitman and Jyotsna Nair, Copyright © 2004 by Bernard D. Beitman and Jyotsna Nair. Used by permission of W.W. Norton & Company Inc.

frequency of major depression, minor depression or generalized anxiety disorder between patients with or without denial.

Hamilton depression and Hamilton anxiety scores were negatively correlated with scores on the denial of illness scale. The correlation with the Hamilton depression score was $r = -0.35$, $p = 0.02$ and the correlation with the Hamilton anxiety score was $r = -0.33$, $p = 0.01$. The strength of the correlations, however, was only moderate and severity of denial would explain only about 10% of the variance in Hamilton depression scores or Hamilton anxiety scores. These findings suggest, nevertheless, that denial may impair recognition of some anxiety and depressive symptoms or minimize the self-report of such symptoms.

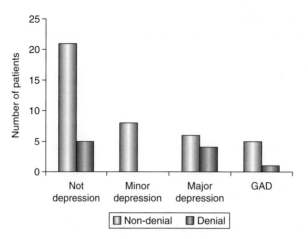

Number of patients

Figure 35.9 Relationship between denial of illness (anosognosia) and diagnosis of major or minor
depression, or GAD using DSM-IV diagnostic criteria. Note that depression and GAD were
just as common in the denial compared with the non-denial stroke patients (reprinted
from Robinson 2004 with permission). From Self-Awareness Deficits in Psychiatric
Patients, edited by Bernard D. Beitman and Jyotsna Nair, Copyright © 2004 by Bernard D.
Beitman and Jyotsna Nair. Used by permission of W.W. Norton & Company Inc.

We also evaluated differences in denial scores among patients with DIS scores
of 2 or higher who received nortriptyline, fluoxetine or placebo. Using double-
blind methodology and random assignment to treatment, there were 12 patients who
received nortriptyline or fluoxetine for 12 weeks and 12 patients who received placebo.
Although there were not enough patients with denial scores over 5 to analyze only
patients with denial of illness, we used only patients with some degree of denial
and we matched patients for severity of denial score. The placebo group initially
had a mean score of 3.83 ± 1.8 SD compared to the nortriptyline and fluoxetine
group with a mean score of 3.83 ± 1.64 SD. The results of the trial are shown in
Fig. 35.10. Repeated measures analysis of variance comparing the active and placebo
group revealed a significant time by treatment interaction ($p = 0.049$). Based on *post
hoc* comparisons, patients who received placebo had significantly higher denial
scores at the end of the treatment trial than patients who received active medication.
The patients who received placebo over the 12-week course of treatment increased
their denial score while there was no significant change in denial scores among
patients treated with active medication.

Since the patients were, on average, 2–3 months poststroke at the beginning of
the treatment trial, these findings suggest that there may be an increased severity of
unawareness of illness among some patients over the course of the first 5–6 months
following stroke. Although treatment with antidepressants did not eliminate or
decrease the severity of unawareness of illness, patients receiving active medication
did not increase their severity of denial. This treatment trial could not be called a

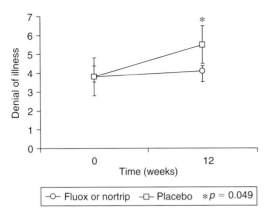

Figure 35.10 Denial of illness scores (DIS) before and after 12 weeks of double-blind treatment with nortriptyline, fluoxetine or placebo. There was a statistically significant time by treatment interaction (F1, 22–4.35, $p = 0.049$) showing that active treatment was superior to placebo in preventing DIS from increasing over the 3 months of treatment (reprinted from Robinson 2004 with permission). From Self-Awareness Deficits in Psychiatric Patients, edited by Bernard D. Beitman and Jyotsna Nair, Copyright © 2004 by Bernard D. Beitman and Jyotsna Nair. Used by permission of W.W. Norton & Company Inc.

successful therapeutic intervention, but it does suggest that intervention may be possible. Stimulants or new generation atypical antipsychotic mediations might decrease the severity of anosognosia during the first few months following stroke.

In summary, we were able to identify several consistent findings across both of the studies which we have conducted of anosognosia/denial following stroke. Anosognosia and denial of illness, for example, were not associated with prior history of psychiatric disorder but were strongly associated with right hemisphere lesions, particularly in the basal ganglia and temporal parietal regions. Our first study found frontal executive dysfunction and left-sided neglect were strongly associated with anosognosia. Furthermore, both studies found that anosognosia and denial were not associated with major or minor depression or generalized anxiety disorder.

Based on the findings from these studies, how might the mechanism of anosognosia be appreciated? In the first study 28% of patients screened following stroke had at least a mild degree of anosognosia. In our treatment study, 20% of patients denied illness. If the overall prevalence is approximately 20–25% for anosognosia, this represents a substantial portion of the stroke population. The predominance in the right hemisphere, particularly temporal parietal and basal ganglia suggests there is a functional hemispheric asymmetry which allows dysfunction of the right hemisphere to mediate this phenomenon. It should be noted, however, that three patients in the first study and two patients in the treatment study had anosognosia following left hemisphere lesions. Thus, the mechanisms leading to anosognosia can occur in patients with left as well as right hemisphere lesions. Based on the cortical–basal ganglia–thalamic loops identified by Delong and Alexander, the neurocircuitry mediating

anosognosia may involve dysfunction in the pathways extending from the right parietal or right temporal lobes to the basal ganglia to thalamus and oribotofrontal cortex. Interruption of the right parietal–thalamic–cortical pathway could impede
integration of sensory input as well as higher level association. The third finding
shared by both studies was that denial of physical impairment does not imply denial
of emotional disorder. Patients with and without unawareness of paralysis have the
same frequency of major depression, minor depression, and general anxiety disorder.
Thus, the mechanisms for recognition of emotional disorders may be independent
of the circuitry which mediates awareness of physical illnesses.

Our studies made two additional findings. The first study identified impairment
in frontal lobe function reflected in significantly impaired performance on verbal
fluency and trails b. There were no differences, however, between patients with
anosognosia on block design, RAVLT, or verbal retention tasks. In addition, the
larger frontal horn, third ventricle, and lateral ventricle to brain ratios were significantly increased in patients with anosognosia compared to those without this condition. This finding suggests that subcortical atrophy may play a role in the mediation
of this process. Thus, lesions involving the right temporal parietal cortex or basal ganglia may interrupt normal cortical–basal ganglia–thalamic frontal circuitry in the
right hemisphere. When accompanied by subcortical atrophy, these physiological
insults may cause even greater dysfunction of the subcortical pathways in the basal
ganglia and thalamus. The disruption of sensory projections from the thalamus to
the sensory and association cortex of the right hemisphere may precipitate neglect
and sensory extinction of input from the left side of the body. Unawareness of hemiplegia could result from an impairment of integrative functions mediated by dysfunction of the right frontal lobe and compromised appreciation of sensory input
following subcortical afferent disconnection from cortex or remote effects (diachesis)
responsible for establishing associations. The characteristic nonchalance and inappropriate affect of the indifference reaction could reflect disruption of negative
emotion associated with right hemisphere lesions or dysfunction (Davidson *et al.*
1999). Thus, emotional dysfunction of the right hemisphere could lead to predominance of the left hemisphere in mediating positive emotion with cheerfulness
and indifference. Other explanations might be proposed for anosognosia and emotional indifference. The treatment study, however, suggests that pharmacological
intervention may be useful in preventing either the progression of anosognosia or
its amelioration. Certainly further studies of intervention for this common and
disruptive syndrome associated with stroke are clearly needed.

Gianotti (1989) suggested that the diagnosis of depression in patients with
right hemisphere lesions might be hampered by the inability of these patients to
express affect or describe their mood and by their tendency to deny depression and
related behavioral vegetative symptoms. He also suggested that anosognosia and
depression may not co-exist except in the chronic stage when anosognosic patients

are much more aware of their impairment. A case history of a patient with anosognosia and major depression will illustrate both the clinical features of this condition as well as the fact that anosognosia and depressive disorder may co-exist.

CASE STUDY

The patient, a 71-year-old right-handed man, suffered the sudden onset of weakness on his left side. On neurological examination, the patient had severe paresis of his left leg but only a mild deficit in the left arm. The patient, however, did not use his left arm. There were no sensory deficits. Although the patient was able to localize a unilateral stimuli in the visual, tactile, or auditory modality, bilateral stimuli were only reported on the right side in 5 of 10 tactile, 4 of 10 visual, and 3 of 10 auditory stimulations. On the line-crossing task, the patient only crossed lines on the right side of the paper. The patient was able to recognize the appropriate facial emotion of happy, sad, or angry expressions in only 10 of 20 photographs. A CT examination showed a lesion in the anterior cerebral artery territory in the right hemisphere involving the cingulate gyrus, part of the supplementary motor area, and the outflow of the genu of the corpus callosum.

On clinical interview, the patient said that he was in the hospital because of a carpal tunnel syndrome in his right hand, which he did have although this was not the reason for his admission to hospital, and he denied any motor deficit on his left side. He stated that he could not control his left side, that his left arm and leg were "disjointed and separated from the rest of his body." He said that he hated his left arm and called it a "jerk." He also reported that the left arm moved without his moving it and he felt that a strange limb was lying beside him. Involuntary and antagonistic movements of his left hand were so frequent that the nurses had to secure his left hand to the bed. On the present state examination, the patient reported that he was worried about his wife's health (his wife was actually in good health) and felt restless, tense, and very anxious. He also reported feeling depressed most of the day and especially during the morning hours. He felt hopeless about the future and did not want to see friends. He also felt that he was to blame for everything that had gone wrong with him and his family.

The patient met DSM-III-R criteria for major depressive disorder. There was no personal or family history of previous depressive or other psychiatric disorder. Both the anosognosia and left-sided neglect resolved by 1 month following stroke. Although the patient was started on antidepressant treatment 3 weeks after the stroke, the major depression did not resolve until the third month following stroke.

REFERENCES

Babinski, J. Contribution a l'etude des troubles mentaux dans l'hemiplegie organique cerebrale (anosognosie). *Rev Neurol (Paris)* (1914) 27:845–848.

Benton, A. L. Differential behavioral effects in frontal lobe disease. *Neuropsychology* (1968) 6:53–60.

Bisiach, E., Vallar, G., Perani, D., *et al.* Unawareness of disease following lesions of the right hemisphere: Anosognosia for hemiplegia and anosognosia for hemianopia. *Neuropsychologia* (1986) 24:471–482.

Davidson, R. J., Abercrombie, H., Nitschke, J. B., *et al.* Regional brain function, emotion and disorders of emotion. *Curr Opin Neurobiol* (1999) 9(2):228–234.

Davidson, R.J., and Irwin, W. The functional neuroanatomy of emotion and affective style. *Trends Cog Sci* (1999) 3(1):11–21.

Denny-Brown, D., Meyer, J. S., and Horenstein, S. The significance of perceptual rivalry resulting from parietal lesions. *Brain* (1952) 75:434–471.

DeRenzi, E., and Faglioni, P. Development of a shortened version of the token test. *Cortex* (1978) 14:41–49.

Ekman, P., and Friesen, W. V. *Unmasking the Face: a Guide to Recognizing Emotions from Facial Clues.* Prentice Hall, New Jersey, 1975.

Gainotti, G. Disorders of emotions and affect in patients with unilateral brain damage. In F. Boller and J. Graffman, eds., *Handbook of Neuropsychology.* Elsevier, Amsterdam, 1989.

Geschwind, N. Disconnexion syndromes in animals and man – I. *Brain* (1965a) 88(2):237–294.

Geschwind, N. Disconnexion syndromes in animals and man – II. *Brain* (1965b) 88(3):585–644.

Hackett, T. P., and Cassem, N. H. Development of a quantitative rating scale to assess denial. *J Psychosom Res* (1974) 18:93–100.

Hecaen, H., deAjuriaguerra, J., and Massonet, J. Les troubles visoconstructifs para lesion parieto occipitale droit. *Encephale* (1951) 40:122–179.

Heilman, K. M., and Valenstein, E. *Clinical Neuropsychology.* Oxford University Press, Oxford, 1993.

Levine, D. N., Calvanio, R., and Rinn, W. E. The pathogenesis of anosognosia for hemiplegia. *Neurology* (1991) 41(11):1770–1781.

Reitan, R. M. Trail making test results for normal and brain-damaged children. *Percept Mot Skills* (1971) 33(2):575–581.

Robinson, R. G., Schultz, S. K., Castillo, C., *et al.* Nortriptyline versus fluoxetine in the treatment of depression and in short term recovery after stroke: a placebo controlled, double-blind study. *Am J Psychiatry* (2000) 157:351–359.

Robinson, R.G. Anosognosia and denial of illness following stroke. In B.D. Beitman and J. Nair, eds., *Self-Awareness Deficits in Psychiatric Patients. Neurobiology, Assessment, and Treatment.* WW Norton & Co, New York, 2004.

Spreen, O., and Strauss, E. *A Compendium of Neuropsychological Tests.* Oxford University Press, New York, 1991.

Starkstein, S. E., Fedoroff, J. P., Price, T. R., *et al.* Anosognosia in patients with cerebrovascular lesions. A study of causative factors. *Stroke* (1992) 23:1446–1453.

Starkstein, S. E., Fedoroff, J. P., Price, T. R., *et al.* Neuropsychological deficits in patients with anosognosia. *Neuropsychiatry Neuropsychol Behav Neurol* (1993a) 6:43–48.

Starkstein, S. E., Fedoroff, J. P., Price, T. R., *et al.* Denial of illness scale. A reliability and validity study. *Neuropsychiatry Neuropsychol Behav Neurol* (1993b) 6(2):93–97.

Wechsler, D., and Wechsler, M. *Adult Intelligence Scale Manual.* Psychological Corp., New York, 1955.

Weinstein, E. A., and Kahn, R. L. *Denial of Illness: Symbolic and Psychological Aspects.* C.C. Thomas Publishing, Springfield IL, 1955.

36

Catastrophic reaction

The sudden onset of anxiety, tears, aggressive behavior, swearing, displacement, refusal, denouncement, and compensatory boasting constitute a syndrome referred to by Goldstein (1948) as a catastrophic reaction (CR). Goldstein believed that this syndrome represented a response to the inability of an organism to cope when faced with a serious defect in their physical or cognitive function. These emotional outbursts would generally last only a few seconds and were usually associated with a stressor, such as a demanding, cognitive examination or a request to perform a task. Gainotti (1972) was the first investigator, to my knowledge, who systematically studied CRs in patients with stroke or other causes of brain damage. Gainotti examined 160 patients with brain injury due to stroke, traumatic brain injury or other causes. Eighty patients had left-sided lesions and 80 patients had right-sided lesions. Of those, 53 had vascular lesions of the left hemisphere and 58 vascular lesions of the right hemisphere. When the presence of CRs was compared between patients with left and right hemisphere lesions, patients with left hemisphere lesions had significantly greater frequency of anxiety reactions, tears, swearing, refusal, and renouncement. He noted that patients with Broca's aphasia were particularly prone to developing CRs with 68% of these patients showing outbursts of tears during the examination. Gainotti believed that both psychological and physiological factors played a role in the development of the depressive/CRs. In patients with Broca's aphasia, he believed that inactivation of a physiological mechanism such as cortical control of emotional discharge was the main determinant of a CR. On the other hand, among patients with anomic aphasia, tears appeared long after the patient showed increased anxiety and failure at verbal communication which Gainotti hypothesized led to a psychological cause for the CR and response to disability. It should be remembered that in this Gainotti study, the nature of the brain injury ranged from neoplastic to traumatic and there was great variability in the time since injury to examination. Thus, these mechanistic hypotheses are, at best, highly speculative.

Subsequently, Gainotti (1989) suggested that patients diagnosed with poststroke depression were actually having CRs. According to this hypothesis, the CR had been triggered by the stress of the examination, leading the patient to report more depressive symptomatology than they actually experienced and subsequently an inappropriate diagnosis of poststroke depression when the underlying disorder was a CR.

In an effort to examine the frequency of CR and its relationship with depression, we developed a CR scale (Starkstein *et al.* 1993) which is shown in Table 36.1. Patients who were assessed using the anosognosia and denial of illness scales were also assessed by the CR scale. A total of 70 patients were investigated in this way, but 8 of them were excluded because of a prior history of cerebrovascular lesion ($n = 5$) or comprehension deficits on the token test ($n = 3$). Most of the items on the CR scale were selected from Gainotti's and Goldstein's reports on the CR. The neurologist who administered the CR scale was blind to the findings of the psychiatrist who conducted the present state examination for assessment of depression or anxiety disorders.

The internal consistency of the CR scale was determined by Cronbach's α, which calculates a mean correlation coefficient between each individual item in the scale

Table 36.1. CR scale

Key 0 = None
   1 = Slight (once during the interview)
   2 = Moderate (several times during the interview)
   3 = Extreme (most of the interview)

1. Patient appeared to be anxious (i.e., patient showed an apprehensive attitude or expressed fears).
2. Patient complained of feeling anxious or afraid (i.e., patient referred to feeling tense or having psychological concomitants of anxiety).
3. Patient became tearful (i.e., patient cried at some point during the evaluation).
4. Patient complained of feeling sad or depression (i.e., patient spontaneously reported sad feelings during the evaluation).
5. Patient behaved in angry manner (i.e., patient shouted, contradicted the examiner, performed tasks in a careless way).
6. Patient complained of feeling angry (i.e., patient reported being upset with the evaluation and/or the examiner).
7. Patient swore (i.e., patient swore at some point during the evaluation).
8. Patient expressed displaced anger (i.e., patient complained about the hospital, doctors, and fellow patients).
9. Patient refused to do something (i.e., patient stopped doing a task or refused to answer some questions).
10. Patient described a feeling of suddenly become depressed or hopeless (i.e., patient reported feeling worthless, sad, and lacking in confidence).

From Starkstein *et al.* (1993) reprinted with permission.

and all the other items. The CR scale showed a high degree of internal consistency ($\alpha = 0.85$). Interrater reliability was determined by having a second interviewer present for 10 interviews in order to provide a second rating of the CR scale. The correlation between the raters' total scores on the CR scale was $r = 0.91$ ($p < 0.01$).

The background characteristics of the patients included in the study are shown in Table 36.2. CRs occurred in 12 of 62 patients studied (i.e., 19%) based on having a score of 8 or greater on the CR scale. Although there were no significant differences in age, gender, or education, patients with a CR had a significantly higher frequency of familial and personal history of psychiatric disorder than patients without a CR.

A plot of CR scores for all 62 patients showed a bimodal distribution with a cutoff score of 8 separating the two modes. Based on this frequency distribution, patients with CR scores of less than 8 were considered not to have a CR while patients with CR scores $\geqslant 8$ were considered to have CR. Using a step-wise multiple regression analysis to determine which items on the CR scale were most frequently associated with the diagnosis of CR, the CR items which accounted for most of the variance in total CR score were suddenly becoming depressed or hopeless ($p < 0.01$), expressing displaced anger ($p < 0.01$), and feeling anxious or afraid ($p < 0.01$).

There were no significant between-group differences in the neurological findings: motor impairment was found in 92% of the 12 patients with CR and 78% of the 50 patients without CR; sensory deficits were found in 42% of the CR patients and 30% of those without CR; aphasia was found in 25% of the CR patients and 12% of those without CR ($p = $ NS).

Table 36.2. Demographic findings

Variable	CR ($n = 12$)	No CR ($n = 50$)
Age (years)	57.6 ± 15.4	58.7 ± 13.2
Education (years)	10.7 ± 4.0	10.0 ± 3.1
Gender (% female)	45	37
Race (% black)	64	69
Alcoholism (% positive)	33 ± 4	18 ± 9
Personal history of psychiatric disorder (% positive)*	33 ± 4	10 ± 5
Family history of psychiatric disorder (% positive)**	25 ± 3	4 ± 2
% right-handed	83 ± 10	92 ± 46
Time since stroke (days)	6.3 ± 3.3	6.1 ± 2.9

Note: Values are mean $\pm$ SD.
*$p < 0.05$; **$p < 0.05$.
From Starkstein *et al.* (1993) reprinted with permission.

The frequency of depression in the CR and non-CR patients is shown in Fig. 36.1. The frequency of major depression was significantly greater in patients with CR compared to those without CR ($p < 0.0001$). In addition to the increased frequency of major depression, patients with CR had significantly higher Hamilton anxiety (Ham-A) scale scores and greater impairment in activities of daily living as measured by the Johns Hopkins functioning inventory (JHFI) than patients without CR (Fig. 36.2). Patients with CR, however, were not significantly more cognitively impaired than those without CR (Fig. 36.2).

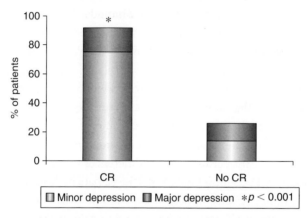

Figure 36.1   The percentage of patients with and without CRs who also have a depressive disorder. There was a significantly greater frequency of major depression but not minor depression, among patients with CRs (data from Starkstein *et al.* 1993).

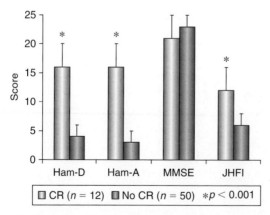

Figure 36.2   The impairment scores of patients with and without CRs following acute stroke. The patients with CR had more severe depression (Ham-D) and anxiety (Ham-A) symptoms and greater impairment in activities of daily living (JHFI) than patients who did not have CR. Patients with CR, however, were not more cognitively impaired than patients without CR (data from Starkstein *et al.* 1993). MMSE: mini-mental state examination.

Since there was a significant association between CR and the existence of major depression, we matched patients in the CR and non-CR groups for depression diagnosis to determine whether there were other factors which may be associated with the existence of CR. In each group, there were 10 patients (7 with major, 2 with minor depression, and 1 non-depressed patient). There were no significant between-group differences in age, education, gender, family, or personal history of psychiatric disorder [family history of psychiatric disorder in the CR group 30% versus 0% for the non-CR group ($p = $ NS), prior psychiatric history 20% in the CR group versus 40% in the non-CR group ($p = $ NS)]. There were no differences in neurological findings and there were no significant between-group differences in Hamilton depression (Ham-D) score, Ham-A score, activities of daily living, or mini-mental state examination (MMSE) score.

Of the 51 patients whose brain imaging scans showed a single stroke lesion, patients with CR ($n = 9$) had a significantly higher frequency of lesions involving the basal ganglia compared to patients without CR ($n = 42$) (Fig. 36.3). There was no significant association, however, between lesion volume and the existence of CR (CR group 3.1 ± 3.6 SD versus non-CR 8.1 ± 9.4% of brain volume SD, $p = $ NS). The CR group tended to have smaller lesions because they had a significantly higher frequency of subcortical lesions than the non-CR group (i.e., 8 of 9 versus 20 of 42).

Structural brain imaging examination indicated that patients with CR had significantly more anterior lesions (i.e., the distance of the anterior border of the lesion from the frontal pole as a percentage of the total anterior–posterior distance) than their matched pair without CR. The distance from the frontal pole in patients with CR was 28.4 ± 6.0, SD versus 42.0 ± 5.9 ($p < 0.01$) in those

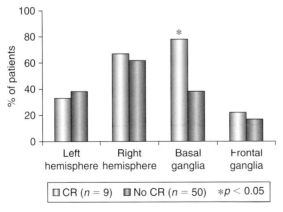

Figure 36.3   The lesion locations found on computerized tomographic (CT) scan in 51 patients with or without CRs. The only lesion site which was significantly associated with the existence of CR was the basal ganglia. There was no association found with laterality of lesion (data from Starkstein *et al.* 1993).

without. In addition to the association of CR and more anterior lesions, the CR group also had a higher frequency of subcortical lesions: 8 of 9 (89%) in the CR group had subcortical lesions as compared to 4 of 9 (33%) in the non-CR group ($p = 0.01$). Thus, even when we controlled for the difference in frequency of depression (which has been discussed in Chapter 10 to be strongly associated with left basal ganglia lesions), the CR continued to be associated with the existence of subcortical (primarily basal ganglia) lesions. In addition, the association with a more anterior lesion location suggests that lesions involving the head of the caudate may be the most likely to produce CR.

Although Gainotti (1989) speculated that poststroke depression is no more than a CR, our findings indicate that depression is strongly associated with the CR but the prolonged nature of depression along with the fact that depression and not CR is associated with left frontal and left basal ganglia lesions during the acute poststroke period. In addition, there were 9 patients with CR who had major depression but there were 7 patients without CR who had major depression. Thus, CR is not an explanation for all poststroke depressions. Similarly, although 11 of the 12 patients with CR had major or minor depression, there was a patient who had CR without depressive disorder.

The issue that is more difficult to answer is whether the CR could, in some patients, represent a variant or "form fruste" of major depression. In support of this suggestion (Starkstein *et al.* 1993), we found that patients with CR were more likely to have a personal and family history of depression. On the other hand, when we controlled for the frequency of depression in CR and non-CR groups, there was no significant difference between the groups in the frequency of family or personal history of psychiatric disorder. Furthermore, when we controlled for depression, the patients with CR had more anterior and subcortical lesions than the non-CR patients. These findings, however, do not rule out the possibility that the CR could characterize a subgroup of poststroke major depression.

It was suggested by Goldstein (1948) that the CR represents a response of patients confronted with their limitations. Patients with CR were found to be more impaired in their activities of daily living than non-CR patients (Fig. 36.2); however, two findings in this study argue against this interpretation. First, the CR patients were not more significantly impaired in terms of neurological deficits than the patients without CR. Secondly, there was no significant difference between the CR and non-CR patients in the severity of their cognitive impairment. If the CR was a response to impairment, one would expect that cognitive impairment would have at least as much effect on psychological response as physical impairment, but it was only the physical impairment that was associated with the existence of CR.

Another possible explanation for the association between CR and depression is lesion location. Patients with CR had significantly more anterior and subcortical lesions than patients without CR, a finding which held true even when the increased frequency of depression was controlled. House *et al.* (1989) has also reported that patients with poststroke "emotionalism" (defined as increased tearfulness with episodes of crying that were sudden and not under normal social control) had higher depression scores than patients without emotionalism, as well as a significantly higher frequency of left frontal lesions.

Another possible explanation of the association between CR and depression is that CR represents an emotional release from a tonic, emotional inhibition similar to emotional lability or a pseudobulbar affect (see Chapter 40, "Pathological laughing and crying"). Many features of the CR, such as anger, affective changes, and swearing, have been reported to occur in patients with neurological diseases affecting the basal ganglia such as Huntington's disease, Wilson's disease, and focal ischemic lesions (Caine and Shoulson 1983; Richfield *et al.* 1987; Dening and Berrios 1989). Thus, the CR may represent the effect of subcortical basal ganglia lesions interrupting the cortical-basal ganglia-thalamic loops (Alexander *et al.* 1990) resulting in the release of the emotion-generating areas of orbital and prefrontal cortices. This might lead to disinhibited behavior related to the release of tonic inhibition of the frontal cortex. This same lesion could lead to the production of depression by disruption of the ventral lateral limbic circuit (i.e., orbital frontal-amygdala, basal ganglia, thalamus) in the left hemisphere. Finally, the CR may not represent a unique clinical syndrome but may constitute a behavioral aggression found in some depressed patients related to disconnection and disinhibition of specific areas of the frontal cortex. Whatever the cause, however, this is an interesting behavioral phenomenon associated with stroke as well as other neuropsychiatric disorders such as Alzheimer's and Huntington's diseases and one that can lead to significant disruption of the care and rehabilitation of poststroke patients. Additional research is needed to determine the cause and natural course as well as effective treatments for this disorder.

The only other systematic study of CRs was conducted by Carota *et al.* (2001). Twelve patients with CRs, as defined as an outburst of frustration, depression, and anger when confronted with a task, were identified in a prospective population of 326 patients with first ever stroke, hospitalized and examined within 48 hours of stroke. CRs were found to be rare in this population but associated with nonfluent aphasia and left opercular lesions. The authors concluded that CRs, poststroke depression and emotionalism were distinct but related disorders.

As discussed in Chapter 6, Gainotti *et al.* developed a poststroke depression rating scale (PSDRS) to identify depression in patients with stroke and differentiate it from primary depression (Gainotti *et al.* 1997). In this study, 124 patients admitted to hospital with acute stroke who were between 2 weeks and 6 months poststroke were examined for 10 areas of psychopathology as assessed by the PSDRS including

CRs. CRs were scored as: well controlled reaction = 0, rather controlled reaction = 1, more evident anxious or aggressive manifestations = 2, clear manifestations or anxiety = 3, clear signs of anxiety with sporadic fits of crying = 4, test practically impossible to carry out due to fits of anxiety and crying = 5. Patients with endogenous depression, no depression, or minor poststroke depression all scored a mean of 0.5 on the CR scale. Patients with major poststroke depression, however, had a mean score of 1.5 on the catastrophic scale. This was significantly higher than the non-depressed or minor depressed patients ($p < 0.001$).

Gainotti repeated this finding in another study in which 58 patients <2 months poststroke were compared with 52 patients between 2 and 4 months poststroke and 43 patients who were >4 months poststroke and 30 patients without brain injury who had been hospitalized for major depression (Gainotti *et al.* 1999). Patients who were <2 months, 2–4 months, or >4 months poststroke had mean scores on the CR scale of 2.0 compared to 0.5 among the patients with primary depression. Consistent with his 1972 hypothesis, Gainotti *et al.* concluded that the symptom profiles and the temporal evolution of poststroke depression suggest that psychological rather than neurological factors mostly account for this important consequence of stroke.

In summary, CRs occur in a significant number of patients following stroke. Prevalence estimates have ranged from 4% to 19%. The clinical correlates have included impairment severity, poststroke major depression, and basal ganglia lesions. These reactions can be very disruptive to families and social functioning. No controlled treatment studies have been conducted to determine whether these reactions can be controlled. As with other disorders following stroke, there are both psychological as well as neurophysiological hypotheses to explain these socially devastating disorders.

REFERENCES

Alexander, G. E., Crutcher, M. D., and DeLong, M. R. Basal ganglia-thalamocortical circuits: parallel substrates for motor, oculomotor, "prefrontal" and "limbic" functions. *Prog Brain Res* (1990) 85:119–146.

Caine, E. D., and Shoulson, I. Psychiatric syndromes in Huntington's disease. *Am J Psychiatr* (1983) 140:728–733.

Carota, A., Rossetti, A. O., Karapanayiotides, T., *et al.* Catastrophic reaction in acute stroke: a reflex behavior in aphasic patients. *Neurology* (2001) 57(10):1902–1905.

Dening, T. R., and Berrios, G. E. Wilson's disease: psychiatric symptoms in 195 cases. *Arch Gen Psychiatr* (1989) 46:1126–1134.

Gainotti, G. Emotional behavior and hemispheric side of the brain. *Cortex* (1972) 8:41–55.

Gainotti, G. Disorders of emotions and affect in patients with unilateral brain damage. In F. Boller and J. Graffman, eds., *Handbook of Neuropsychology*. Elsevier, Amsterdam, 1989.

Gainotti, G., Azzoni, A., Razzano, C., *et al.* The Post-Stroke Depression Rating Scale: a test specifically devised to investigate affective disorders of stroke patients. *J Clin Exp Neuropsychol* (1997) 19(3):340–356.

Gainotti, G., Azzoni, A., and Marra, C. Frequency, phenomenology and anatomical–clinical correlates of major post-stroke depression. *Br J Psychiatr* (1999) 175:163–167.

Goldstein, K. *Language and Language Disturbances.* Grune and Stratton, New York, 1948.

House, A., Dennis, M., Molyneau, A., *et al.* Emotionalism after stroke. *Br Med J* (1989) 298(6679):991–994.

Richfield, E. K., Twyman, R., and Berent, S. Neurological syndrome following bilateral damage to the head of the caudate nuclei. *Ann Neurol* (1987) 22:768–771.

Starkstein, S. E., Fedoroff, J. P., Price, T. R., *et al.* Catastrophic reaction after cerebrovascular lesions: frequency, correlates, and validation of a scale. *J Neurol Neurosurg Psychiatr* (1993) 5:189–194.

37

Apathy

The definition of apathy in the dictionary is described as "a lack of feeling or emotion or a lack of interest or concern." In a study of 124 poststroke patients who were examined at either 2, 6, or 12 months following stroke, apathy was reported in 27% of the patients while depression was reported in 61% and irritability in 33% (Angelelli *et al.* 2004). Apathy has been associated with bilateral paramedian, or interior thalamic infarctions (Ghika-Schmid and Bogousslavsky 2000; Krolak-Salmon *et al.* 2000), or frontal lobe lesions (Daffner *et al.* 2000). Helgason *et al.* (1988) has also reported that apathy was associated with the medial temporal and lateral diencephalic lesions associated with anterior choroidal artery infarction.

Although there are relatively few publications examining apathy in patients with stroke, it constitutes an important neuropsychiatric syndrome because of its effects on rehabilitation, social interaction, and return to work. Apathetic patients may refuse to participate in rehabilitation exercises, feed, dress, and care for themselves or to interact with others. Thus, the importance of apathy in patients with stroke is highly significant.

Utilizing the same group of patients that we used for studies of anosognosia and catastrophic reactions, 80 patients were also assessed for apathy using a modified version of the "apathy scale" developed by Marin (1991) and Starkstein *et al.* (1992). The apathy scale is shown in Table 37.1: apathy scores range from 0 to 42, with higher scores indicating more severe apathy. Interrater reliability for the apathy scale, based on two independent evaluations during the same interview, showed good interrater agreement ($r = 0.81, p < 0.01$). Using the Cronbach alpha assessment of internal consistency, the mean correlation of each item with the other items in the scale showed that the apathy scale has good internal consistency (Cronbach alpha $= 0.76$). Based on a previous assessment of the apathy scale (i.e., a study of 50 patients with Parkinson's disease; Starkstein *et al.* 1992), a cut-off score of 14 points separated a bimodal distribution, in which patients with apathy scored 14 points or greater on the apathy scale.

Table 37.1. Apathy scale

| Date: | Patient initials: |
| Rater | Patient No.: |

A STRUCTURED INTERVIEW GUIDE TO THE APATHY SCALE

I'd like to ask you some questions about how you have been feeling the past 2 weeks or since your stroke (if less than 2 weeks)

1. Learning

Are you interested in learning new things?	0 = a lot
Does learning new activities interest you as much as in the past?	1 = some
Do you have a desire to learn anything new?	2 = slightly
	3 = not at all

2. Interest

Do you have anything that interests you?	0 = a lot
Do you have interest in your usual activities?	1 = some
Do activities interest you as much as in the past?	2 = slightly
	3 = not at all

3. Insight

Are you concerned about your condition?	0 = a lot
Do you think anything is wrong with you?	1 = some
Does your condition worry you?	2 = slightly
	3 = not at all

4. Energy

Do you put much effort into things?	0 = a lot
Do you have the energy to do things like you did in the past?	1 = some
Do you feel the desire to put a lot of effort into your work?	2 = slightly
	3 = not at all

5. Initiative

Are you always looking for something to do?	0 = a lot
Do you feel like doing projects?	1 = some
Do you have the desire to start a new project?	2 = slightly
	3 = not at all

6. Future goals

Do you have plans and goals for the future?	0 = a lot
Do you think and plan for the future?	1 = some
Is achieving your goals an important factor in your life?	2 = slightly
	3 = not at all

Table 37.1. (*Continued*)

7. Motivation

Do you have motivation?	0 = a lot
Do you feel inspired to accomplish tasks?	1 = some
Does the desire to accomplish something give you energy?	2 = slightly
	3 = not at all

8. Energy

Do you have the energy to do your daily activities?	0 = a lot
Do you rarely feel too tired to do daily chores?	1 = some
Do you have the energy to take care of yourself?	2 = slightly
	3 = not at all

9. Initiative

Does someone have to tell you what to do each day?	0 = not at all
If someone doesn't ask you to do things, do you just sit?	1 = slightly
Do you need prodding to get going?	2 = some
	3 = a lot

10. Pleasure

Are you indifferent to things?	0 = not at all
Do you lack pleasure in anything?	1 = slightly
Does doing something leave you feeling, so what?	2 = some
	3 = a lot

11. Caring

Are you unconcerned with many things?	0 = not at all
Do you feel like you don't care about things?	1 = slightly
Have you stopped caring about what happens?	2 = some
	3 = a lot

12. Motivation

Do you need a push to get started on things?	0 = not at all
Do you need someone to bug you before you can do things?	1 = slightly
Does someone else have to help you to begin tasks?	2 = some
	3 = a lot

13. Emotion

Are you neither happy nor sad, just in-between, no matter what happens?	0 = not at all
Do you feel your emotions are gone?	1 = slightly
Do you feel "blah" about everything that happens?	2 = some
	3 = a lot

14. Insight

Would you consider yourself apathetic?	0 = not at all
Have you lost your interest and motivation?	1 = slightly
Compared to the past, are you more apathetic now?	2 = some
	3 = a lot

Table 37.2. Diagnostic criteria for apathy[a]

Lack of motivation relative to the patient's previous level of functioning or the standards of his or her age and culture, as indicated either by subjective account or observation by others.

Presence, with lack of motivation, of at least one symptom belonging to at least two of the following three domains:
- Diminished goal-directed behavior
  – Lack of effort
  – Dependency on others to structure activity
- Diminished goal-directed cognition
  – Lack of interest in learning new things or in new experiences
  – Lack of concern about one's personal problems
- Diminished emotion
  – Unchanging affect
  – Lack of emotional responsivity to positive or negative events

The symptoms cause clinically significant distress or impairment in social, occupational, or other important areas of functioning.

The symptoms are not due to a diminished level of consciousness or the direct physiological effects of a substance (e.g., a drug of abuse, a medication).

[a] Adapted from Starkstein (2001) and reprinted with permission.

The validity of the assessment measure was examined by asking a neurologist who was blind to the score on the apathy scale to rate 12 consecutive patients for the presence or absence of apathy. Six patients were rated as apathetic, the remaining six non-apathetic. Clinically diagnosed apathetic patients had a mean apathy scale score of 14.8 ± 5.7 compared to the mean score of 5.5 ± 2.2 ($p < 0.001$) for non-apathetic patients. Formal diagnostic criteria for apathy have been proposed by Starkstein *et al.* (2001) (Table 37.2).

The background characteristics of the patients in this study grouped according to their depression diagnosis and their apathy scale score are shown in Table 37.3 (Starkstein *et al.* 1993). Differences in background characteristics were examined using a two-way analysis of variance (ANOVA) (factor 1, presence or absence of apathy; factor 2, presence or absence of depression). Two-way ANOVA for age showed that it has a significant effect on apathy (i.e., patients with apathy, with or without depression, were significantly older than patients without apathy). Depressed patients had a significantly higher frequency of personal history of psychiatric disorder but there was no difference in the frequency of personal history of psychiatric disorder between apathetic and non-apathetic patients. No other significant between-group differences in the remaining demographic characteristics were found.

The neurological findings are shown in Table 37.4: there were no between-group differences in motor, sensory, visual, or language disturbances.

Table 37.3. Demographic findings

	Control	Depressed	Apathetic	Apathetic + depressed
Number of patients	44	18	9	9
Age (mean ± SD in years)*	61.1 ± 12.9	52.0 ± 15.7	64.0 ± 12.4	63.8 ± 12.6
Education (mean number of years ± SD)	9.5 ± 3.1	9.9 ± 2.9	11.0 ± 2.7	9.8 ± 4.5
Race (% black)	66	66	78	33
Gender (% female)	39	55	44	67
Alcoholism (% positive)	14	6	0	22
Personal history of psychiatric disorder (% positive)**	16	33	11	56
Family history of psychiatric disorder (% positive)	20	17	11	11
Handedness (% right, handers)	90	94	89	75
Time since stroke (mean ± SD)	6.1 ± 3.8	5.9 ± 4.1	6.9 ± 4.7	6.6 ± 4.2

*$p < 0.05$, **$p < 0.05$; reprinted with permission Starkstein *et al.* (1993).

Table 37.4. Neurological and neuroanatomic findings

	Normal	Depressed	Apathetic	Apathetic + depressed
Number of patients	44	18	9	9
Motor deficits				
Mild	27	33	33	11
Moderate	7	11	22	0
Severe	23	17	22	56
Sensory deficits	39	28	56	33
Aphasia	11	22	33	22
Dysarthria	43	44	33	33
Left hemisphere (% positive)[a]	22	25	33	50
Right hemisphere (% positive)[a]	66	67	50	38
Bilateral lesions (% positive)[a]	3	8	17	13
Posterior fossa (% positive)[a]	9	0	0	0
Ischemic lesions (% positive)[a]	78	75	67	63
Posterior internal cap (% positive)*,[a]	9	17	67	13
Lesion area (% mean ± SD)	3.7 ± 5.0	11.4 ± 14.0	8.9 ± 12.0	4.2 ± 4.0

*$p < 0.05$.
[a]Lesion localization could be determined in 32 normals, 12 depressed, 6 apathetic, and 8 apathetic and depressed. Reprinted with permission Starkstein *et al.* (1993).

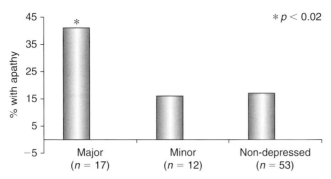

Figure 37.1   The frequency of apathy (i.e., score of 14 or more on the apathy scale) among patients with major or minor depression, or no depression. Patients with major depression were significantly more likely to have apathy than patients with minor depression or no depression ($p < 0.02$) (data from Starkstein *et al.* 1993).

The frequency of apathy among patients with major, minor, or no depression is shown in Fig. 37.1. There was a significantly increased frequency of apathy among the patients with major depression. However, 9 of 53 non-depressed patients (17%) had apathy. Among the overall group of 80 patients, 11% had both apathy and depression, 22% had depression but no apathy, and 55% had neither apathy nor depression. When patients with major depressions were examined separately from those with minor depression, it was found that apathy was significantly more prevalent in patients with major depression (Fig. 37.1) than in those with minor or no depression, of whom only eight (16%) had apathy ($p < 0.02$). Moreover, one-way ANOVA for apathy scores between those with major, minor, and no depressions showed that patients with major depression had significantly higher scores than those with either minor or no depression ($p = 0.01$). These findings indicate that although major depression and apathy occurred independently, apathy was significantly associated with major but not minor depression.

Using two-way ANOVA (factor 1, presence or absence of depression; factor 2, presence or absence of apathy) revealed that there was a significant effect of apathy on mini-mental state examination scores, and a significant interaction between apathy and depression. Patients with apathy and depression had significantly greater cognitive impairment than patients without apathy. In addition, using activities of daily living as the outcome measure, it was shown that there were significant effects of both depression ($p = 0.002$) and apathy ($p = 0.0001$), as well as a significant interaction between apathy and depression ($p = 0.05$) (Fig. 37.2). The depressed group included patients with either major or minor depression.

Examination of the CT and MR scans found lesions in 32 control patients, 12 depressed patients, six apathetic patients, and eight apathetic patients with depression.

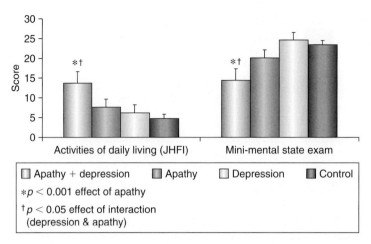

Figure 37.2 Impairment in activities of daily living and cognitive function related to the presence of apathy and/or depression (major or minor). Patients with apathy and depression were significantly more impaired than patients with depression or apathy alone or no emotional disturbance. This suggests that these two disorders may be additive in their effects on performance in these examinations (data from Starkstein *et al.* 1993).

There were no significant differences between groups in either the volume of the infarction or the frequency of right or left hemisphere involvement. Patients with apathy only had a significantly higher frequency of lesions involving the posterior limb of the internal capsule compared with the other three groups (Fig. 37.3). There were no other significant between-group differences in terms of lesion location.

In summary, this study found that a significant number (23%) of patients with stroke had a significant degree of apathy. The apathetic patients were characterized by being older, having a higher frequency of major but not minor depression, having a greater degree of physical and cognitive impairment, and having lesions involving the posterior limb of the internal capsule.

Okada *et al.* (1997) examined 40 patients with stroke, 20 of whom were judged to have apathy based on the apathy scale (Table 37.1). Patients with apathy were found to have significantly lower scores on verbal intelligence and frontal lobe function tasks and significantly higher depression scores than non-apathetic patients. Using the [133]Xe (Xenon) inhalation method, regional blood flow in patients with apathy was significantly reduced in the right dorsolateral frontal and left frontotemporal regions compared with the non-apathetic patients (Okada *et al.* 1997). Furthermore, apathy scores for all patients were significantly negatively correlated with regional cerebral blood flow in the right dorsolateral frontal and the left frontotemporal region. This same group reported that a new group of 29 patients with subcortical stroke showed significantly lower scores of verbal fluency

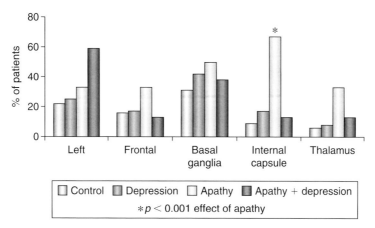

Figure 37.3   The frequency of specific lesion locations in patients with apathy and/or depression. The only lesion location that was significantly more frequent in patients with apathy compared to the other groups was the posterior arm of the internal capsule. This may reflect the interruption of pallidomcscncephalic fibers from the inner pallidum to the pedunculopontine nucleus which in cats and rodents plays an important role in goal-oriented locomotion (data from Starkstein *et al.* 1993).

and global cognitive function compared with the non-apathetic patients. In addition, apathy scale score was significantly correlated with the novelty p3-evoked potential latency and amplitude at the frontal site. Thus an event-related-evoked potential associated with a novel stimulus demonstrated a decreased response in the frontal lobes on electroencephalogram (EEG) recording among apathetic compared with non-apathetic patients. In summary, both of these studies have suggested that patients with apathy following stroke have decreased activity, particularly in the frontal lobes bilaterally as evidence by decreased blood flow and decreased amplitude and prolonged onset of evoked potentials stimulated by a novel object.

Finset and Andersson also examined apathy in patients with stroke ($n = 30$), traumatic brain injury ($n = 27$), and hypoxic brain injury ($n = 13$). Apathy was associated with subcortical right hemisphere lesions as well as a decreased score on the active approach oriented coping questionnaire (Andersson *et al.* 1999). Ghika-Schmid and Bogousslavsky (2000) examined 12 patients with anterior thalamic infarcts. Although the acute period was characterized by perseverative behavior and anterograde memory retrieval deficit as well as intrusions, naming difficulties and dysarthria within a few months follow-up, the persisting abnormalities included memory dysfunction and apathy. This report as well as other anecdotal reports in the literature suggested that apathy following stroke, particularly associated with bilateral lesions, may persist for many years. Van der Werf reported on a patient with right intralaminar nuclei infarction of the thalamus with apathy and cognitive deficits persisting for more than 17 years (Van der Werf *et al.* 1999).

The association of apathy in some reports with greater physical impairment might suggest that apathy results from more extensive stroke lesions. However, this hypothesis is not supported by the fact that in our study of poststroke apathy there were no significant intergroup differences in lesion volume (Starkstein *et al.* 1993). In addition, the most impaired group with both apathy and depression had smaller lesions than the depressed or apathetic groups. Alternatively the existence of apathy may have worsened performance in cognitive and physical tasks. Our finding that there were no significant differences on neurological examination is consistent with this suggestion. This is another issue that deserves further investigation.

It was interesting that apathy was demonstrated to be associated with major but not minor depression. This finding is consistent with previous findings which have differentiated between major and minor depressions. For example, major but not minor depression was associated with cognitive impairment (see Chapter 14) and major but not minor depression was associated with a failure to suppress serum cortisol after dexamethasone administration (see Chapter 21) (Lipsey *et al.* 1985; Bolla-Wilson *et al.* 1989). This association between apathy and major depression suggests that they might be causative of one another, or that they might share similar mechanisms. Alternatively, the association might be due to some significant overlap in clinical symptomatology. For example, both psychomotor retardation and diminished interests in daily activities (two important symptoms of apathy) are included in the diagnostic criteria for major but not dysthymic depression. This kind of overlap might increase the frequency of association between apathy and major depression.

The studies that have been conducted suggest that lesions of many brain regions, particularly thalamic, frontal, and subcortical, are associated with apathy. These findings suggest that the cortical–basal ganglia–thalamic circuits which have been implicated in the development of depression may also play a role in apathy. The ansa lenticularis, which is the main output of the internal pallidum, occupies part of the posterior limb of the internal capsule (Nauta 1989). This pathway projects to the pedunculopontine nucleus. This structure, located within the mesencephalic locomotor region in cats and rodents, sends monosynaptic projections to motor neurons in the anterior horn and plays a prominent role in goal-oriented locomotor behavior (Bechara and van der Kooy 1989).

Another pallidal projection also goes through the ansa lenticularis and reaches the pedunculopontine nucleus after a synapse in the substantia nigra pars reticulata (Nauta 1989). This pallidonigral projection provides limbic innervation to both a somatic motor mechanism and the dopaminergic nigrostriatal system. Disruption of this circuit may underlie the bradyphrenia demonstrated in apathetic patients.

Thus, apathy may involve biogenic amine dysfunction and interruption of efferent pathways passing through the basal ganglia and the internal capsule. Lesions of the ventral striatum could produce disruption of the ascending biogenic amine pathways and extend into the thalamus, thus producing disruption of both the ascending biogenic amine pathways and the cortical–basal ganglia–thalamic circuit. This anatomic explanation could explain why both major depression and apathy are associated with one another. Although other explanations might be proposed, this is a testable hypothesis and might stimulate further research in this important clinical problem.

REFERENCES

Andersson, S., Krogstad, J., and Finset, A. Apathy and depressed mood in acquired brain damage: relationship to lesion localization and psychophysiological reactivity. *Psychol Med* (1999) 29:447–456.

Angelelli, P., Paolucci, S., Bivona, Y., *et al.* Development of neuropsychiatric symptoms in post-stroke patients: a cross-sectional study. *Acta Psychiatr Scand* (2004) 110(1):55–63.

Bechara, A., and van der Kooy, D. The tegmental pedunculopontine nucleus: a brainstem output of the limbic system critical for the conditioned place preferences produced by morphine and amphetamine. *J Neurosci* (1989) 9:3440–3449.

Bolla-Wilson, K., Robinson, R. G., Starkstein, S. E., *et al.* Lateralization of dementia of depression in stroke patients. *Am J Psychiatr* (1989) 146:627–634.

Daffner, K. R., Mesulam, M. M., Scinto, L. F., *et al.* The central role of the prefrontal cortex in directing attention to novel events. *Brain* (2000) 123(Part 5):927–939.

Ghika-Schmid, F., and Bogousslavsky, J. The acute behavioral syndrome of anterior thalamic infarction: prospective study of 12 cases. *Ann Neurol* (2000) 48(2):220–227.

Helgason, C., Wilbur, A., Weiss, A., *et al.* Acute pseudobulbar mutism due to discrete bilateral capsular infarction in the territory of the anterior choroidal artery. *Brain* (1988) 111:507–519.

Krolak-Salmon, P., Croisile, B., Houzard, C., *et al.* Total recovery after bilateral paramedian thalamic infarct. *Eur Neurol* (2000) 44(4):216–218.

Lipsey, J. R., Robinson, R. G., Pearlson, G. D., *et al.* Dexamethasone suppression test and mood following stroke. *Am J Psychiatr* (1985) 142:318–323.

Marin, R. S. Reliability and validity of the apathy evaluation scale. *Psychiatr Res* (1991) 38:143–162.

Nauta, W. J. H. Reciprocal links of the corpus striatum with the cerebral cortex and the limbic system: a common substrate for movement and thought? In J. Mueller, ed., *Neurology and Psychiatry: A Meeting of Minds.* S. Karger, Basel, Switzerland, 1989, pp. 43–63.

Okada, K., Kobayashi, S., Yamagata, S., *et al.* Post stroke apathy and regional cerebral blood flow. *Stroke* (1997) 28:2437–2441.

Starkstein, S. E., Fedoroff, J. P., Price, T. R., *et al.* Apathy following cerebrovascular lesions. *Stroke* (1993) 24:1625–1630.

Starkstein, S. E., Mayberg, H. S., Preziosi, T. J., *et al.* Reliability, validity and clinical correlates of apathy in Parkinson's disease. *J Neuropsychiatr Clin Neurosci* (1992) 4:134–139.

Starkstein, S. E., Petracca, G., Chemerinski, E., *et al.* Syndromic validity of apathy in Alzheimer's disease. *Am J Psychiatry* (2001) 158(6):872–877.

Van der Werf, Y. D., Weerts, J. G., Jolles, J., *et al.* Neuropsychologial correlates of a right unilateral lacunar thalamic infarction. *J Neurol Neurosurg Psychiatr* (1999) 66(1):36–42.

38

Disturbance of prosody

Monrad-Krohn (1947) described prosody as the melodic line of speech produced by variations of pitch, rhythm, and stress of pronunciation. Heilman and Valenstein (1993) divided prosody into two types: affective aprosody, described as the loss or defect in expression, repetition, or comprehension of emotionally intoned speech and prepositional aprosody, characterized by a loss of or defect in expression, repetition, or comprehension of sentences with prepositional content such as questions, statements, or commands. Heilman *et al.* (1975) reported that patients with right temporoparietal lesions had more deficits in their comprehension of affective prosody than patients with left temporoparietal lesions. Cancelliere and Kertesz (1990) reported an increased frequency of impairment in affective prosody involving comprehension of emotion in speech associated with basal ganglia lesions but failed to find a significantly higher frequency among patients with right hemisphere as compared with left hemisphere lesions. Patients with comprehension aprosody or expressive aprosody may appear to have an emotional disorder because of their inability to either express emotion in the tone, pitch or rhythm of their voice, or comprehend emotional intonation in the voices of others. They appear to be flat or blunted in their facial expression.

Prosody may also be extended in its concept to include the expression or comprehension of not only verbal language but also facial and gestural affective appearance (Ross 1981). Thus, patients with a comprehension affective prosody might be unable to recognize emotional intonation in a person's affective expression. Similarly, patients with an expressive affective aprosody would be unable to show a facial expression consistent with their own mood or a posed mood.

Ross (1981) proposed that the expression and comprehension of emotions are organized in the right hemisphere in an analogous fashion to language in the left hemisphere. Thus, patients with right temporoparietal infarction would have difficulty in the comprehension of prosodic intonation, while patients with lesions of the right posterior-inferior frontal lobe would have abnormalities in the affective prosodic expression of language. Furthermore, it was hypothesized by Ross that patients with impaired affective comprehension prosody would have disturbances in the recognition of their own emotional state which could lead to the denial of depression when in fact a depression was present. Therefore, failure of patients to recognize their own depression, it was argued, could lead to under-diagnosis. The existence of patients with right hemisphere lesions with "masked" depression could also negate or weaken the association of depression with left frontal or left basal ganglia lesions. Thus, although at the time of Ross's study, a systematic study of patients with aprosody had not been undertaken, there were anecdotal reports of patients with prosody impairments which seemed to interfere with their neuropsychiatric evaluation (Ross and Rush 1981) and perhaps ultimately with the previously identified clinical correlates of post-stroke depression.

We undertook a systematic study to examine comprehension prosody including comprehension of both verbal intonation and facial expression (Starkstein *et al.* 1994). We did not examine prepositional prosody, expressive prosody of facial emotion, or expressive verbal intonation of emotion, but we did investigate comprehension prosody. Comprehension prosody is the issue most relevant to our studies since any impairment might interfere with the patient's ability to recognize their own emotional state and, therefore, lead to under recognition of depression or other disorders. Expressive aprosody would not be expected to interfere with a patient's ability to recognize that they were depressed (even though their facial appearance might be flat) and report the associated depressive symptoms.

This study included 65 of the 91 patients who were also examined for apathy, catastrophic reactions, and anosognosia. This represented a consecutive series of patients who were subjected to a battery of assessments of prosody, excluding only three patients who had a prior stroke and three patients who had severe verbal comprehension deficits as determined by their score on the token test ($n = 59$) (De Renzi and Ferrai 1978). All patients were examined within 10 days following acute stroke. In addition to the patients with acute stroke, a control group of 17 normal volunteers, aged from 33 to 62 years, was assessed for performance on the comprehension, verbal prosody, and facial emotion recognition tests.

In order to determine whether prosody is associated with other cognitive impairments, a detailed battery of neuropsychological tests was administered to these patients. This battery included assessment of neglect, as measured by counting the number of extinctions on double simultaneous stimulation in three sensory modalities (auditory, visual, and somesthetic); hemi-spatial neglect, as measured by counting the number of lines missed when copying a complex figure with 10 lines to the left and 10 lines to the right of midline; personal neglect, determined by asking patients to touch the hand ipsilateral to that with clinical signs using the contralateral hand; motor neglect, determined by asking the patients to open and close both hands 20 times and motor impersistence, assessed by asking the patients to keep their eyes closed for up to 30 s.

Recognition of facial emotion was determined by showing the patient 15 faces selected from the Ekman *et al.* (1972) series showing emotions of sadness ($n = 5$), happiness ($n = 5$), or anger ($n = 5$). Patients were asked to identify the emotion expressed in the face by selecting from a multiple choice answer sheet showing schematic drawings of faces with happy, sad, or angry expressions (appropriate labels were written underneath).

Comprehension of verbal emotional prosody was determined by asking 59 patients in this study to listen through head phones to 13 different six- or seven-word sentences that were recorded by a female speaker using a happy (five sentences), sad (five sentences), or angry (three sentences) tone of voice. All sentences were simple declarative sentences such as, "the lamp is on the table." These prosody tests were obtained from Dr. Kenneth Heilman who had standardized these tapes in previous research projects and graciously provided them for us to use in this study. Sentences were presented in random order and patients were asked to repeat the first phrase to ensure that there was no possible contamination by auditory comprehension deficits. Patients indicated the tone of voice by pointing to a line drawing of a figure indicating a sad, happy, or angry face with the corresponding words typed under the face.

A second task of emotional prosody comprehension was assessed by administering to the patients 16 sentences of six or seven words as in task one. Four sentences had both a happy tone of voice and a happy semantic content (e.g., "the children laughed at the clown"). Four sentences had a happy intonation and a sad semantic content (e.g., "the woman lay ill and dying"), four sentences had a sad intonation and a happy semantic content, and four sentences had both a sad intonation and sad semantic content. Thus, for 50% of the stimuli, the emotional prosody and the semantic content of the sentences were congruent while in the remaining 50% they were incongruent. Patients were asked to ignore the semantic content of the message and to indicate only the type of emotional prosody being used. Patients also filled out the anosognosia questionnaire and were assessed by the denial of illness scale as described in Chapter 35.

Based on their scores on the prosody tasks, patients were grouped as having no, mild, or severe prosody. On the first prosody task, the mean number of correct responses out of 13 sentences was 12.9 ± 0.2 for the normal controls. No control subject made more than one error. The mean score for the 16 items with matching or incongruent semantic and emotional content was 15.3 ± 0.9 and no control subject made more than three errors. Patients who correctly identified fewer than 8 emotions on the first task, or fewer than 13 on the second task were considered abnormal. These cutoff scores were based on the observed bimodal distribution among the stroke patients with splits at 9 points for the first task and 13 points for the second task. There were 19 patients (32%) who had abnormal scores on both prosody tasks and

10 patients (17%) who had abnormal scores on only one task (five patients failed task one and five patients failed task two). Patients who failed both tasks were considered to have severe aprosody, those who failed one task were considered to have mild aprosody, and the rest were controls.

The background characteristics and neurological findings of the patients with none, mild, or severe aprosody are shown in Table 38.1. There were no significant differences between groups in terms of background characteristics or neurological findings. The frequency of depression in each group is shown in Fig. 38.1. Although the frequency of major depression in controls was about twice the rate seen in patients with aprosody, there was no significant difference in the frequency of either major or minor depression in patients with or without aprosody. Similarly, there were no significant differences in Hamilton depression (Ham-D) scores or Hamilton anxiety score between the control, mild, or severe aprosody groups.

In Chapter 7, "Phenomenology and specificity of depressive symptoms," I indicated that approximately 5% of patients with acute stroke would have met criteria for major depressive disorder had they acknowledged a depressed mood. These patients might be regarded as "masked depressions." Therefore, we looked at patients with aprosody to see if any of them with mild or severe aprosody would have met criteria for major depression had they not failed to acknowledge a depressed mood. We found that none of the non-depressed patients in either the mild or severe aprosody groups had symptoms otherwise sufficient for a diagnosis of major depression but no depressed mood.

Table 38.1. Demographic and neurological findings

Characteristic	No aprosody	Mild aprosody	Severe aprosody
Number of patients	30	10	19
Age (mean $\pm$ SD in years)	52.3 $\pm$ 15.3	59.9 $\pm$ 7.1	60.9 $\pm$ 15.5
Education (mean no. of years $\pm$ SD)	11.3 $\pm$ 3.1	8.6 $\pm$ 2.6	10.0 $\pm$ 3.3
Gender (% females)	47 (14)	30 (3)	42 (8)
Handedness (% right-handers)	83 (25)	100 (10)	89 (16)
Time since stroke (mean days)	6.1 (2.3)	5.9 (3.0)	7.2 (1.9)
Motor deficits (%)	71 (21)	80 (8)	79 (15)
None (%)	13 (4)	20 (2)	21 (4)
Mild (%)	37 (11)	60 (6)	47 (9)
Moderate (%)	7 (2)	10 (1)	11 (2)
Severe (%)	27 (8)	10 (1)	21 (4)
Visual field deficits (%)	33 (10)	10 (1)	16 (3)
Sensory deficits (%)	13 (4)	30 (3)	26 (5)
Aphasia (%)	20 (6)	20 (2)	11 (2)
Dysarthria (%)	47 (14)	30 (3)	11 (2)

Modified from Starkstein *et al.* (1994).

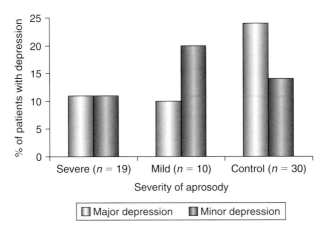

Figure 38.1 Frequency of depression among patients with aprosody for emotional comprehension. Although there were fewer depressions among the mild and severe aprosody groups, these were not significantly different than controls suggesting that comprehension prosody did not inhibit the recognition of depression in the majority of these patients. Data from Starkstein *et al.* (1994).

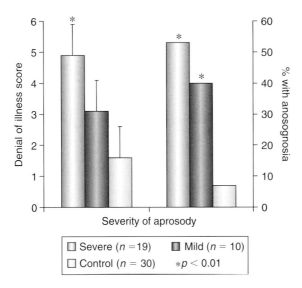

Figure 38.2 The association of aprosody with denial of illness and unawareness of deficits (anosognosia). Patients with the most severe comprehension aprosody were the most unaware of their motor impairments. Data from Starkstein *et al.* (1994).

Patients with severe aprosody were found to have significantly higher scores on the denial of illness scale ($p = 0.0001$) and on the anosognosia scale ($p < 0.01$) compared to patients with mild or no aprosody (Fig. 38.2). Patients with mild or severe aprosody also showed significantly more frequent extinction on double simultaneous

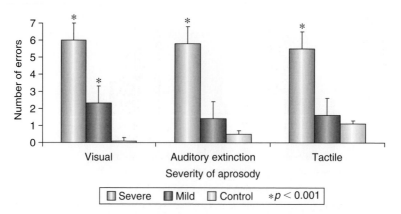

Figure 38.3 Extinction of stimulus perception during double simultaneous stimulation. Patients with severe aprosody demonstrated severe extinction on all three sensory modalities. They did not, however, show visual neglect on drawing tasks. Data from Starkstein *et al.* (1994).

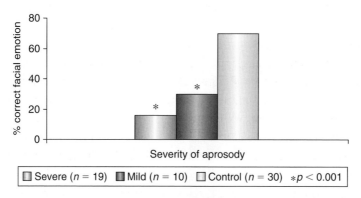

Figure 38.4 The percent of correct identifications of facial emotion in patients with aprosody. Patients with mild or severe aprosody for auditory comprehension of emotional intonation were also unable to correctly identify facial expression of emotion. Data from Starkstein *et al.* (1994).

stimulation on tactile ($p = 0.005$), visual ($p = 0.0001$), and auditory ($p = 0.0001$) modalities (Fig. 38.3). There were, however, no significant differences between the control and aprosody groups in their scores of motor impersistence, hemi-spatial neglect on drawing, or personal neglect, although patients with mild or severe aprosody, showed significantly greater impairments in recognition of facial emotion compared to patients without prosody ($p = 0.0002$) (Fig. 38.4).

A step-wise regression analysis was conducted to examine the independent associations of each of these neuropsychological variables with aprosody. This analysis examined the independent effects of denial of illness scores, the number of errors on recognition of facial emotion, and Ham-D scores. Both denial of illness score

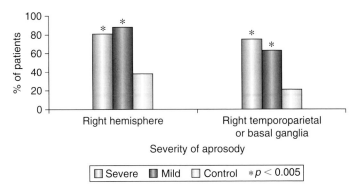

Figure 38.5 Lesion location in patients with aprosody and controls. Patients with mild or severe aprosody had a significantly higher frequency of right hemisphere lesions predominantly in the temporoparietal cortex or basal ganglia compared to stroke patients without aprosody. Data from Starkstein *et al.* (1994).

and the recognition of facial emotion score were significant and independent correlates of aprosody (r for denial $= 0.3$, r for facial emotion $= 0.4$; $p < 0.01$). There was, however, no significant correlation with Ham-D score.

We also examined the relationship between aprosody and the error rate when there was a conflict between the semantic content of the sentence and its emotional intonation. There was a significant group effect, with aprosodic patients showing significantly more deficits when there was incongruence compared to when there was congruence. There were no significant between-group differences in recognition of emotion in congruous sentences. This finding indicates that patients with aprosody improve their ability to recognize emotional intonation when the content of the sentence is consistent with the emotional intonation but deteriorate in their performance when there is a conflict between the emotional intonation and the semantic content of the sentence. There was no difference in performance whether happy or sad sentences were utilized.

The effect of lesion location was also examined. Patients with mild or severe aprosody had a significantly higher frequency of right hemisphere lesions ($p < 0.05$) (Fig. 38.5). We also examined whether patients with right temporoparietal or basal ganglia lesions had a significantly higher frequency of prosody than those without. This was based on the reported lesion correlates found in previous studies (Cancelliere and Kertesz 1990). Of patients with severe aprosody, 75% had a temporoparietal or basal ganglia lesion while 63% of those with mild prosody, and 21% of those with no aprosody had this lesion location (Fig. 38.5).

Patients with mild or severe aprosody also had a significantly larger frontal horn to brain size ratio on the side contralateral to the brain lesion (no aprosody 1.3 ± 0.6, mild aprosody 2.2 ± 0.9, and severe aprosody 1.9 ± 0.7; $p < 0.05$), and a significantly larger third ventricular to brain size ratio than the group without aprosody (no aprosody 0.6 ± 0.4, mild aprosody 1.0 ± 0.6, severe aprosody 1.0 ± 0.5, $p < 0.05$). These findings suggest that patients who developed aprosody had a mild degree of subcortical atrophy which probably occurred prior to the stroke. This finding is similar to findings in studies of a variety of other psychopathologies following stroke, including depression (Chapter 17), mania (Chapter 25), schizophreniform psychosis (Chapter 34), and anosognosia (Chapter 35).

After determining that a number of lesion characteristics are significantly associated with aprosody, we carried out a three-way analysis of variance (ANOVA) looking for potential interactions between lesion side (left versus right), type of emotion being tested (sad versus happy), and congruity of semantic and emotional intonation (congruous versus incongruous). There were significant effects of the side of lesion, congruity, and a significant interaction between the two. These findings demonstrated that patients with right hemisphere lesions had significantly more impairment than patients with left hemisphere lesions in comprehension of emotion when emotional tone and semantic content were incongruous. This effect was even more marked when patients with right temporoparietal or right basal ganglia lesions were compared to patients with lesions in similar areas of the left hemisphere. There were, however, no significant interactions or effects of the type of emotion (i.e., sad, happy, angry), which indicates that the impairments shown by patients with right hemisphere lesions in the recognition of emotional prosody involve both positive and negative emotions.

This was the first study to have examined the relationship between aprosody and depression. We found first that comprehension of emotional prosody was a frequent phenomenon in patients with acute stroke, occurring in 45% of the sample. Comprehensional emotional aprosody was associated with extinction on double simultaneous stimulation, anosognosia, and deficits in comprehension of facial emotions. It was also associated with lesions of the right hemisphere involving temporoparietal cortex and basal ganglia and a mild degree of frontal, subcortical, and diencephalic atrophy. Depression (major or minor) was present in 22% of patients with severe aprosody, 30% of patients with mild aprosody, and 38% of those without aprosody; however, these differences were not statistically significant. Thus, there was no evidence that the existence of aprosody interfered with the patient's ability to recognize their own inner emotional state.

It should be noted in this study that we only examined comprehension aprosody and not expressive aprosody. It is possible that findings in studies of patients with comprehension aprosody may be different than those in studies of expressive or motor prosody. The most accurate way to determine the existence of expressive aprosody is to measure the fundamental frequency and harmonics of the vocal tones to produce intonation contours (Ross *et al.* 1988), methodology which requires experience and the appropriate equipment. In patients with acute stroke, abnormal verbal productions may be due to dysrhythmia, hypophonia, or physical weakness, which may be difficult to differentiate from true aprosody. Thus, the assessment of depression and its relationship with expressive aprosody requires further investigation.

One of the significant findings from this study was the association between aprosody and right temporoparietal and basal ganglia lesions. This finding was consistent with previous case reports that also showed this clinical–pathological correlation (Heilman *et al.* 1975; Ross 1981; Ross *et al.* 1988; Heilman and Valenstein 1993).

This study also replicated the findings of Bowers *et al.* (1987) who showed that right hemisphere lesions are associated with aprosody of incongruent as compared to congruent sentences. They reported that patients with right hemisphere lesions performed significantly worse in the emotional prosody comprehension task when the semantic content conflicted with the emotional prosody. In our study, patients with right hemisphere, particularly right temporoparietal and basal ganglia lesions, had more deficits in recognizing incongruous than congruous sentences compared to patients with comparable lesions of the left hemisphere. Kotz *et al.* (2003), however, examined 12 normal subjects, mean age 24, using functional magnetic resonance imaging (MRI). Positive and negative intonations in speech elicited bilateral fronto-temporal and basal ganglia activation. These findings suggested that emotional prosody may not be exclusively mediated by the right hemisphere.

Pardo *et al.* (1990) demonstrated the importance of the cingulate gyrus in tasks which require subjects to ignore one stimulus in favor of another. In the Stroop test used by Pardo, there was a conflict between the color of the printed word and the meaning of the word. For example, the patient was asked to name the color of the blue print on a word saying red. This task appears to be comparable to the congruous incongruous sentence prosody identification and the result suggests that connections from the anterior cingulate gyrus to the basal ganglia or remote hypometabolic effects in the cingulate gyrus from a basal ganglia lesion could mediate this phenomenon.

Another significant finding of this study (Starkstein *et al.* 1994) was that aprosody was shown to be associated with a variety of neuropsychological disturbances including impairment in recognition of facial emotion, extinction on double simultaneous stimulation, and the presence of anosognosia. Blonder *et al.* (1991) previously demonstrated that patients with right hemisphere lesions ($n = 10$) had more impairments in their ability to discriminate both emotional prosody and facial emotions compared with patients with left hemisphere lesions. They hypothesized that the right hemisphere was involved in perceiving the non-verbal expression of emotion from both facial and prosodic stimuli. Our findings confirmed the results of Blonder *et al.* (1991) and are consistent with this hypothesis. We also found, however, that recognition of facial emotion and recognition of emotion in verbal comprehension were not necessarily tied to each other. Of our 32 patients with deficits in comprehension of facial emotion, 9 (28%) showed no evidence of aprosody. Furthermore, 6 of 29 patients (21%) with comprehensional aprosody showed no deficits in the comprehension of facial emotion. Thus, the perception of facial and language-mediated emotional stimuli may involve independent pathways, or there may be some anatomical regions in which these facial emotion and language emotion recognition tasks are mediated separately. This is another interesting finding which deserves further investigation.

We also found that comprehension of emotional intonation in language was significantly associated with extinction on double simultaneous stimulation. This finding implies that these processes involve similar brain regions but it does not suggest that emotional aprosody is simply a reflection of some general neglect. Other measures of visual neglect did not show significant associations with aprosody.

There have been no treatment trials of aprosody, but a case by Raymer *et al.* (Raymer *et al.* 2001) reported that a man treated in a crossover design with the dopamine agonist, bromocriptine (20 mg), for non-fluent aphasia and emotional aprosodia showed improvement in the fluency of speech, but no change in emotional prosody. Thus, treatment trials are needed for this disorder.

In conclusion, this study found a high frequency of impairment in recognition of facial emotional content, and emotional intonation of sentences among a consecutive series of patients with acute stroke lesions. We replicated the findings of previous investigators, that is, that the comprehension of prosody was associated with right temporoparietal and right basal ganglia lesions. We also found associations between comprehension of emotional prosody and the presence of subcortical brain atrophy, anosognosia, impaired recognition of facial emotion, and extinction on double simultaneous stimulation. Finally, although it appears to be logical that patients unable to comprehend emotional intonation may not be able to recognize their own inner emotional state, we found no evidence to support this hypothesis. The frequency of depression among patients with aprosody was not significantly lower than that of depressive disorder among patients without aprosody. This suggests that there is an important distinction between the recognition of emotional content in external stimuli and the recognition of one's own emotional subjective feelings.

REFERENCES

Blonder, L. H., Bowers, D., and Heilman, K. M. The role of the right hemisphere in emotional communication. *Brain* (1991) 114:1115–1127.

Bowers, D., Coslett, H. B., Bauer, R. M., *et al.* Comprehension of emotional prosody following unilateral hemispheric lesions: processing defect versus distraction defect. *Neuropsychologia* (1987) 25:317–328.

Cancelliere, A. E. B., and Kertesz, A. Lesion localization in acquire deficits of emotional expression and comprehension. *Brain Cogn* (1990) 13:133–147.

De Renzi, E., and Ferrai, C. The reporter's test: a sensitive test to detect expressive disturbances in aphasics. *Cortex* (1978) 14(2):279–293.

Ekman, P., Friesen, W. V., and Ellsworth, T. *Emotion in the Human Face*. Pergamon, New York, 1972.

Heilman, K. M., Scholes, R., and Watson, R. T. Auditory affective agnosia: disturbed comprehension of affective speech. *J Neurol Neurosurg Psychiatr* (1975) 38:69–72.

Heilman, K. M., and Valenstein, E. *Clinical Neuropsychology*. Oxford University Press, Oxford, England, 1993.

Kotz, S. A., Meyer, M., Alter, K., *et al.* On the lateralization of emotional prosody: an event-related functional MR investigation. *Brain Lang* (2003) 86:366–376.

Monrad-Krohn, G. The prosodic quality of speech and its disorders. *Acta Psychol Scand* (1947) 22:225–265.

Pardo, J. V., Pardo, P. J., Janer, K. W., *et al.* The anterior cingulate cortex mediates processing selection in the Stroop attentional conflict paradigm. *Proc Natl Acad Sci USA* (1990) 87:255–259.

Raymer, A. M., Bandy, D., Adair, J. C., *et al.* Effects of bromocriptine in a patient with crossed nonfluent aphasia: a case report. *Arch Phys Med Rehabil* (2001) 82(1):139–144.

Ross, E. D. The aprosodias: functional–anatomic organization of the affective components of language in the right hemisphere. *Arch Neurol* (1981) 38:561–570.

Ross, E. D., and Rush, A. J. Diagnosis and neuroanatomical correlates of depression brain damaged patients. *Arch Gen Psychiatr* (1981) 38:1344–1354.

Ross, E. D., Edmonson, J. A., Seibert, G. B., *et al.* Acoustic analysis of affect prosody during right-side Wada test: a within-subjects verification of the right hemisphere's role in language. *Brain Lang* (1988) 3:128–145.

Starkstein, S. E., Fedoroff, J. P., Price, T. R., *et al.* Neuropsychological and neuroradiological correlates of emotional prosody comprehension. *Neurology* (1994) 44:515–522.

39

Irritability and aggression

Background

Irritability and aggression are common disorders associated with neuropsychiatric conditions, such as stroke, dementia, traumatic brain injury, and Huntington's disease (Burns *et al.* 1990; Paradiso *et al.* 1996; Chemerinski *et al.* 1998; Kim *et al.* 1999). These symptoms create a major stress for the families of patients with stroke (Brooks *et al.* 1986; Williams 1994) and lead to a poorer quality of life for the patient (Angeleri *et al.* 1993). Aggressive behavior is a common reason for referral to geriatric services or admission to a nursing home or hospital (Margo *et al.* 1980; Clarke *et al.* 1981). Aggressive behavior in institutions poses a major management problem and a significant stress on nursing staff (Winger *et al.* 1987).

As with many behaviors, there are multiple etiologies and numerous factors which contribute to the expression of this behavioral disturbance. Environmental precipitants and risk factors for violent behavior associated with neurological disease include social factors such as prior exposure to violence, psychological factors such as loss of job or social position, psychopathological factors, such as the presence of depression, delusions, or hallucinations, and medication effects such as disinhibition associated with benzodiazepines or other medications. In addition to these environmental and psychological factors, violent behavior is also more common in males, those who are younger age, and those of low intelligence (Hodgins 1992). In patients with epilepsy, the location of seizure focus and type of seizure have been reported to play an important role in the occurrence of violent behavior (Falconer 1973; Stevens and Hermann 1981; Herzberg and Fenwick 1988).

Clinical correlates of aggression following stroke

We studied irritability and aggression among our group of 301 patients with acute stroke. As part of the present state examination (PSE), patients were asked if they had displayed irritability with aggressive or violent behavior since the stroke. There were a total of 18 patients who reported episodes of irritability accompanied by angry quarreling, shouting, hitting people, or breaking things. In order to account for demographic variables which may have played a role in the frequency of these violent outbursts, each of the 18 patients reporting violent outbursts were matched to two patients who were, within 5 years of the index patient's age, within 2 years of the index patient's years of education and were the same gender, race, and Hollingshead socioeconomic class. The matching procedure was carried out using the next consecutive patient who met the criteria without knowledge of other clinical variables (Paradiso *et al.* 1996). These patients were also compared with our overall group of 351 patients with acute stroke.

The background characteristics of the self-reported violence group and controls are shown in Table 39.1. Patients with irritability and violent outbursts were significantly younger than patients from the overall acute stroke population ($p = 0.008$). There were no other significant differences between the overall stroke population and the violent group in any background characteristics. It is noteworthy that patients with self-reported violence were not more likely to have abused

Table 39.1. Background characteristics

	Aggression group ($n = 18$)	Control group ($n = 36$)	Overall group ($n = 309$)
Age (mean ± SD in years)	50.9 ± 13.2*	50.9 ± 11.9	58.9 ± 13.4
Race (% African–American)	66	66	66
Gender (% female)	55	53	43
Education (mean number of years ± SD)	9.7 ± 3.0	9.7 ± 3.2	9.4 ± 3.9
Socioeconomic status (% Hollingshead IV, V)	83	80	74
Martial status (% married)	44	42	43
Family psychiatric history (% positive)	17	14	13
Personal psychiatric history (% positive)	22	17	11
Alcohol abuse (% positive)	0	14	13
Time since stroke (mean ± SD days)	14.4 ± 11.3	12.7 ± 8.8	11.1 ± 9.3
History of CVA (% positive)	23.0	26.9	19.8

CVA: cerebrovascular accident.

Reprinted with permission, from Paradiso *et al.* (1996).

*Compared to overall group $p = 0.008$.

alcohol or to have significantly less education. Since medication is a common cause of behavioral change in patients with acute medical illness, patients with violent outbursts and control patients were compared for their use of a variety of medications including benzodiazepines. There were no significant differences in the frequency of antihypertensives, beta blockers, digitalis, diuretics, antiarrhythmics, anticoagulants, corticosteroids, psychoactive drugs, or antiepileptics between the violent and the control patients except that the violent patients were taking more non-steroidal anti-inflammatory drugs (NSAIDs) (i.e., 7 of 18) than controls (i.e., 6 of 36) ($p = 0.03$). No patient was being withdrawn from benzodiazepines or other medications associated with withdrawal symptoms.

Comparison between patients and controls on the basis of neurological findings revealed no significant between-group differences. In the violent group, 78% of patients had motor deficits compared to 67% of the control group. Among violent patients, 35% had sensory deficits compared to 23% in the control group. None of the violent group had visual field deficits compared to 17% of the control group, 14% of the violent group had aphasia compared to 2% of the controls, and 12% of the violent group had cerebellar or brain stem findings compared to 14% of controls. One patient in the violent group and one patient in the non-violent group had clouding of consciousness with impairment of attention and orientation, which indicates that delirium probably did not play a significant role in the irritability and violent behavior.

Depression and impairment scores are shown in Fig. 39.1. Patients with irritability and violence had significantly higher Hamilton depression (Ham-D) scores than the non-violent controls. Consistent with this finding, patients with violent behavior had a diagnosis of major depression in 7 of the 18 cases as compared to only 6 cases of major depression out of the 36 patients in the control group. The number of patients with minor depression was 5 in the violent group and 13 in the control group. Although there was an increased frequency of major depression in the violent group, this difference did not reach statistical difference. There was, however, a significantly greater number of patients in the violent group with abnormal mini-mental state examination (MMSE) scores (i.e., under 24) (66%) compared to the control group (22%) ($p = 0.001$). After covaring for MMSE score, the groups were compared for their Johns Hopkins functioning inventory (JHFI) score and their social functioning. The patients who demonstrated violent outbursts had significantly *less* impairment in activities of daily living than controls (Fig. 39.1). There were no significant differences in social functioning between patients with violent outbursts and those without.

Computed tomography (CT) scans, demonstrating focal brain lesions which were consistent with the neurological examination were available in 31 patients (10 violent patients and 21 controls). In another 5 violent patients and 13 control patients, the

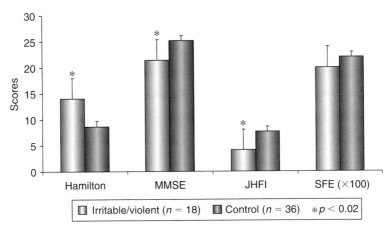

Figure 39.1 Depression severity and impairment scores for acute stroke patients with and without self-reported irritability and violence. Patients reporting angry outbursts had significantly more depressive symptoms as well as greater cognitive impairment (MMSE) but less physical (activities of daily living) impairment (JHFI) and no difference in social functioning examination (SFE) than age-, gender-, and education-matched controls without violent behavior (data from Paradiso *et al.* 1996).

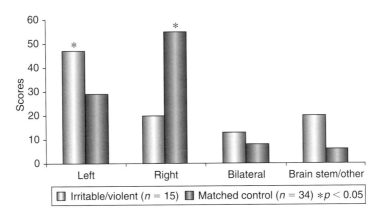

Figure 39.2 Lesion location using either CT imaging or clinical localization in 49 patients with and without self-reported irritable/violent outbursts. Patients with angry outbursts were significantly more likely to have had left hemisphere lesions and less likely to have had right hemisphere lesions compared with controls (data from Paradiso *et al.* 1996).

laterality of lesion was assessed by clinical symptomatology although the imaging scan was negative. Thus, there were only three violent patients and two control patients for whom assessment of lesion was not possible. The frequencies of various lesion locations for the violent and non-violent groups are shown in Fig. 39.2. Irritable, violent patients had a significantly higher frequency of left hemisphere lesions compared with controls ($p = 0.05$). Thus, violent behavior was associated

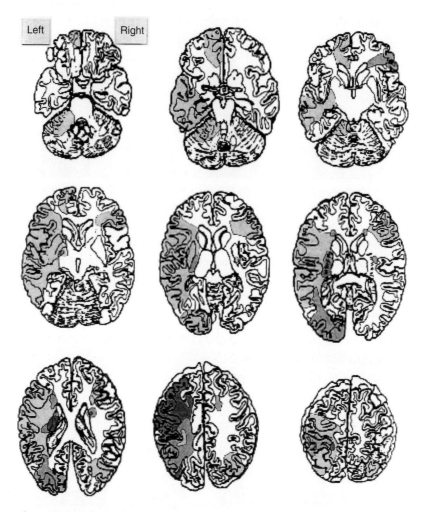

Figure 39.3 Schematic templates showing lesion locations of patients with episodes of angry, violent behavior. Compared to patients who were matched for age, gender, and education, violent patients had a greater frequency of left hemisphere lesions which were closer to the frontal pole (reprinted from Paradiso *et al.* 1996 with permission).

with left anterior lesions. Lesion volume measurements and measurements of the distance of the lesion from the frontal pole were available for 27 subjects (6 violent patients and 21 control patients). A mono-analysis of covariance (MANCOVA) examining the effects of anterior lesion border, posterior lesion border, and lesion volume on the existence of violent outbursts demonstrated a significant effect of anterior lesion location ($p = 0.03$). Lesion volume was not significantly associated with violent behavior even after controlling for proximity of the lesion to the frontal pole.

In the angry outburst group, 66% had cortical lesions, 11% had subcortical lesions, and 22% had both. This was not significantly different from the control group, in which 66% had cortical lesions, 33% had subcortical lesions, and 6% had both (Fig. 39.3 shows schematic drawings of lesion location in the violent group). In order to examine these factors in a larger sample of patients, the CT scan findings in the violent patients were compared to those for the overall group of acute stroke patients. Fisher's exact p-value $= 0.1148$ for 59 cortical and 63 subcortical versus 6 cortical and 1 subcortical.

The χ^2 p-value below ($p = 0.055$) is correct, but we should probably use the Fisher's exact ($p = 0.1148$) because of small NS.

Since left hemisphere lesions close to the frontal pole have been associated with poststroke depression (see Chapter 10), we examined whether the clinical correlates of violent behavior (i.e., cognitive impairment and left frontal lesions) could be explained by the presence of major depression. A two-way analysis of variance (ANOVA) of distance of the lesion from the frontal pole (Factor 1, presence or absence of violent behavior; Factor 2, presence or absence of major depression) showed a significant main effect of violence but no interaction ($p = 0.04$) (Fig. 39.4). *Post hoc* analysis showed that patients with major depression and violent outbursts had significantly more anterior lesions than patients with major depression without violent outbursts ($p = 0.002$).

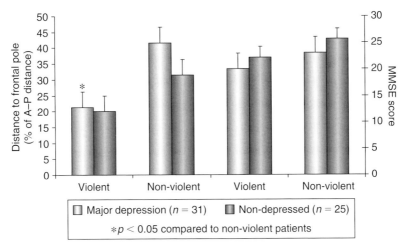

Figure 39.4 Mean ($\pm$SEM) distance of lesion from the frontal pole and mean ($\pm$SE) mini-mental state examination (MMSE) scores for patients with and without violent behavior following stroke) patients were matched for age, gender, and education). Patients were also grouped according to whether they had major depression. A two-way ANOVA (factors: presence or absence of violence and presence or absence of major depression) found that violent patients had the most anterior lesions and the greatest impairment in cognitive function (data from Paradiso *et al.* 1996). A–P: anterior–posterior.

A second two-way ANOVA of MMSE scores was conducted to examine the factors of the presence or absence of major depression and their effect on cognitive impairment. This analysis showed that there is a significant effect of violence ($p = 0.02$), a trend effect for depression ($p = 0.07$) but no interaction between the two (Fig. 39.4). We also examined the effect of cognitive impairment on violence by excluding patients with major depression. Patients who were violent were significantly more cognitively impaired as measured by their MMSE scores than non-violent patients ($p = 0.04$). These findings suggest that the association of violent behavior with anterior lesions and cognitive impairment is not explained by major depression rather they appear to be independent contributors to violent behavior.

We have recently conducted a second study of irritability and aggression using an entirely different group of patients but the same definition of irritability and aggression; that is, answering positively on the PSE to questions about irritability and aggressive behavior (Chan *et al.* in preparation). These reports had to be confirmed by a family member or by rater observation. The items of the PSE included verbal aggression, physical aggression against objects such as throwing things and physical aggression against people. An aggression subscore was calculated by adding the total score of these PSE items with a maximum score of 8. The background characteristics of the aggressive patients compared with non-aggressive control patients with stroke are shown in Table 39.2. In contrast to the first study, the patients were examined almost 2 months following stroke. The increased percent of patients with aggressive behavior probably reflects the greater time since stroke and increased aggressive behavior emerging between weeks 1 and 9 following stroke. The level of aggression was relatively mild with only two patients showing physical aggression against others or objects and the rest reporting only verbal aggression (i.e., shows anger by shouting or quarreling). There were no significant differences between the aggressive and non-aggressive group except for an increased number of patients with a diagnosis of major depression (47.8% versus 17.4%, $p = 0.005$) or generalized anxiety disorder (34.8% versus 7.4%, $p = 0.001$) (Chan *et al.* in preparation).

There were no differences between the aggressive and non-aggressive patients in the type of stroke, side of lesion, neurological deficit, or degree of brain atrophy. Lesion volume, however, was significantly larger in the aggressive patients (Fig. 39.5) and the anterior edge of the lesion was significantly closer to the frontal pole among aggressive compared with non-aggressive patients (Fig. 39.5) ($p = 0.0053$). In addition to the more anterior lesion location among aggressive patients, aggressive patients had significantly higher depression rating scores on the Ham-D than non-aggressive patients (13.2 ± 6.5 SD versus 7.9 ± 5.3 SD, $p = 0.0002$) (Fig. 39.5). Aggressive patients were also significantly more anxious as measured by the Hamilton anxiety (Ham-A) scale (11.3 ± 4.9 SD versus 7.8 ± 4.6 SD, $p = 0.0022$). Cognitive

Table 39.2. Stroke characteristics, neurological findings and radiological findings for aggressive and non-aggressive patients

	Aggressive	Non-aggressive	Significance
Characteristic of stroke	($n = 23$)	($n = 69$)	
Stroke type			
Infarction (%)	91.3	87.0	NS
Hemorrhage (%)	8.7	13.0	NS
Location			
Left hemisphere (%)	34.8	34.8	NS
Right hemisphere (%)	56.5	59.4	NS
Brain stem/other (%)	8.7	5.8	NS
Neurological deficit	($n = 22$)	($n = 60$)	
Motor deficit (%)	81.8	68.3	NS
Sensory deficit (%)	27.3	31.7	NS
Visual field deficit (%)	31.8	25.0	NS
Aphasia (%)	9.1	16.7	NS
Linear brain measurements	($n = 16$)	($n = 51$)	
(mean $\pm$ SD)			
Lateral ventricle/brain ratio	0.1095 ± 0.0437	0.1253 ± 0.0437	NS
Third ventricle/brain ratio	0.0067 ± 0.0034	0.0069 ± 0.0032	NS
Bifrontal ratio	0.3263 ± 0.0865	0.3344 ± 0.0588	NS
Bicaudate ratio	0.1547 ± 0.0577	0.1643 ± 0.0508	NS
Stroke lesion measurements	($n = 10$)	($n = 36$)	
(mean $\pm$ SD)			
Lesion volume (% of total brain volume)	8.77 ± 10.55	4.14 ± 5.84	NS
Anterior location (% of AP diameter of brain)	17.47 ± 8.82	35.43 ± 18.66	$p = 0.0053$

AP: anterior–posterior.

impairment as measured by the MMSE was also significantly more impaired in the aggressive patients than the non-aggressive patients ($p = 0.015$).

The factors which were significantly different between the aggressive and non-aggresssive patients (i.e., HAM-D, HAM-A, MMSE, total PSE score, lesion volume, and proximity of the lesion to the frontal pole) were included in a logistic regression model. Following a stepwise regression, two factors, HAM-A and proximity of the lesion to the frontal pole were independent factors distinguishing the aggressive from the non-aggressive patients. This model had a positive predictive value of 80.4% ($p = 0.0001$).

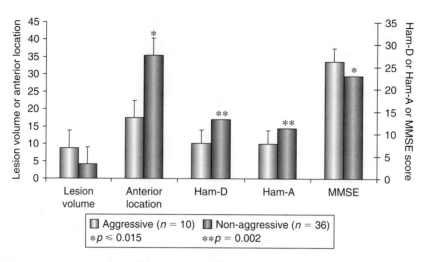

Figure 39.5 Lesion and impairment variables associated with aggressive behavior following stroke. Aggressive patients had more anterior hemisphere lesions, greater depressive, and anxiety symptoms but less cognitive impairment compared with the non-aggressive control patients.

Treatment of poststroke aggression

In addition to confirming many of the findings from our first study of aggression in patients with stroke, in our second study, the patients were participating in our treatment study of poststroke depression (see Chapter 23). Response to antidepressant medication was therefore evaluated in the 23 initially aggressive patients who entered this 12-week treatment trial. Among the active treatment patients, six were treated with fluoxetine titrated from 10 mg/day up to 40 mg/day. Four were treated with nortriptyline titrated from 25 to 100 mg/day and 13 received placebo. Patients given active antidepressant medication during the 12-week treatment trial were not significantly different from the placebo patients in background characteristics, psychometric measures of severity of depression or anxiety or the prevalence of major depression or generalized anxiety disorder prior to treatment. The active treated patients had aggression scores of 2.0 ± 0.87 SD at baseline and 0.2 ± 0.45 SD at 3 months while patients on placebo had scores of 2.0 ± 1.0 SD initially and 0.08 ± 0.28 SD at baseline in 3 months. Intention to treat analysis utilizing the last observation carried forward did not show a significant group by time interaction between the treated and placebo groups. Efficacy analysis comparing only study completers ($n = 13$ placebo, $n = 7$ active treatment) also failed to show a significant effect of treatment.

Since aggression was associated with major depression, we conducted a secondary analysis to determine if response of depression to treatment would be associated with improved aggression. Repeated measures ANOVA of aggressive patients

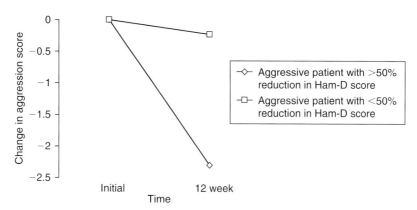

Figure 39.6 Change in aggression score as derived from the PSE at the beginning and end of a 12-week double-blind treatment trial comparing nortriptyline, fluoxetine, and placebo. Active versus placebo analysis did not show a significant time by treatment interaction. Patients who responded to treatment of depression, however, showed a significantly greater decline in aggression scores than patients who did not respond to treatment of depression ($F = 5.79$, df = 1, 18, $p = 0.02$).

who completed the study and had a greater than 50% decline in their Ham-D scores ($n = 7$) compared to aggressive patients who failed to respond to treatment and had less than a 50% decline in Ham-D score ($n = 13$) demonstrated a significant time by treatment interaction (Fig. 39.6) ($p = 0.021$). The number of patients with no aggression after treatment was significantly greater in the responder compared with the non-responder group. These findings suggest that aggression itself does not respond to antidepressant treatment but does suggest that aggression associated with depression can be improved by successful treatment of depression. There were no statistically significant differences between the depression responders and the depression non-responders in background characteristics or severity of impairment but the aggressive group with 50% reduction in Ham-D scores had higher baseline Ham-D scores than non-responders (17.3 ± 5.1 versus 10.4 ± 6.1). The groups, however, were not significantly different in the frequency of major depression (i.e., five versus seven).

Mechanism of aggression

Other investigators have also examined treatment response of aggression in patients with brain damage, particularly traumatic brain injury (Silver and Yudofsky 1994). There are also some controlled trials of treatment of aggression in patients without brain disease. Treatment medications have included antipsychotics, anticonvulsants, such as carbamazepine (Gleason and Schneider 1990), lithium (Haas and Cope

1985), antidepressants (Jackson *et al.* 1985), anti-anxiety agents such as buspirone (Gualtieri 1991; Stanislav *et al.* 1994), valproate (Mazure *et al.* 1992), and beta blockers (Yudofsky *et al.* 1987). Controlled treatment trials have demonstrated the utility of both propranolol and pindolol in the control of violent behavior (Greendyke and Kanter 1986; Yudofsky *et al.* 1987; Mattes 1988). In patients with traumatic brain injury, propranolol was started at a dose of 20 mg and gradually increased until a dose of 12 mg/kg of body weight was achieved (Yudofsky *et al.* 1987). In patients with stroke, low doses of propranolol (i.e., 10 mg) should be used with cautious increases because of the frequent occurrence of cardiovascular disease (Yudofsky *et al.* 1990).

Numerous other investigators have also examined aggression in patients with brain injury. Cohen-Mansfield (1986), for example, found that agitated patients received more medication and tended to have more falls than non-agitated patients. One might also wonder whether poststroke aggression could be a mani-festation of catastrophic reactions. Gainotti (1972) reported that depressive–catastrophic reactions were characterized by shouting, swearing, and refusal. They were also more frequent in patients with left as compared with right hemisphere injury. It seems possible that some of the aggression reported by patients with stroke could have been part of a catastrophic reaction. However, we found that aggression was associated with cognitive impairment, anxiety symptoms, and left anterior lesions which was not the same as our finding that catastrophic reactions were associated with major depression, basal ganglia lesions, and greater activities of daily living (ADL) impairment (see Chapter 36).

Our studies found that irritability and aggression were common (i.e., 25%) among patients within 2 months following stroke but the symptoms were gener-ally mild, consisting predominantly of verbal aggression (i.e., shouting and quar-reling). Irritability and aggression in both studies were associated with higher level of total psychopathology and greater cognitive impairment and closer proximity of the lesion to the frontal pole. Thus, our findings from the first study conducted in a predominantly African–American lower socioeconomic class population were replicated in a different study population that was mainly Caucasian with fewer patients from lower socioeconomic classes. This study also found that although aggression *per se* did not respond to antidepressants, improvement of depression led to a significantly greater reduction in aggression compared to patients who remained depressed.

In both studies, aggressive patients had more frontal lesions compared to the non-aggressive patients. Frontal lobe lesions may have resulted in personality change including disinhibition which led to aggression or alternatively an exacer-bation of a preexisting aggressive personality trait (Burns *et al.* 1990). In addition, both studies found that aggressive behavior was associated with a greater number of depressive symptoms as well as diagnoses of major depression. Since irritability is one of the symptoms of depression, this association was not surprising (American Psychiatric Association 1994). Depression and aggression might share some of the same underlying neurophysiological mechanisms. For example, both depression and aggression have been associated with low cerebrospinal fluid levels of 5-hydroxyindoleacetic acid [5-HIAA], a metabolite of serotonin (Van Praag *et al.* 1986; Bryer *et al.* 1992). Thus, depletion of the neurotransmitter serotonin perhaps caused by stroke lesions, might lead to several behavioral consequences including both depression and aggression.

In both studies aggression was associated with cognitive impairment as measured by the MMSE. Studies among patients with non-stroke related dementia have also found a similar association of aggression with cognitive impairment (Ryden 1988; Cohen-Mansfield *et al.* 1990). This association may be due to a loss of inhibition of aggressive impulses resulting from impaired executive function and judgment. Other hypotheses have also been proposed such as frustration due to impaired ability to communicate, inappropriate response to stimuli such as pain or noise and or misinterpretation of the caretaker (Ryden 1988; Cohen-Mansfield *et al.* 1990).

The association of anxiety with aggression was also to be expected based on the symptomatology of anxiety disorder. In a study of aggression in the elderly, aggressive behavior was attributed to the presence of an anxiety disorder in 31% of patients (Leger *et al.* 2000) suggesting that anxiety is a common association or may even be a cause of aggression in some elderly patients.

Frontal lobe lesions, particularly orbitofrontal lesions, are associated with disinhibited behavior (Fuster 1980). Thus, the association in the present study between violence and a more anterior injury suggests that disinhibited behavior may have contributed to the irritable, angry behavior.

A case history may help to illustrate the nature of these angry outbursts.

CASE STUDY

Mr. M. suffered a stroke during his sleep at age 46 years. After arising from bed to use the bathroom, he was found lying on the floor with a right hemiparesis and aphasia. Although it was initially uncertain whether he would survive the stroke, within 3 days he was able to follow a few simple commands, but could produce only one word. Brain imaging demonstrated an ischemic infarction of the left frontal lobe in the distribution of the left middle cerebral artery. By 6–8 months after the stroke, he was able to do simple reading and could walk with a cane and leg brace. He had previously been an attorney for a private law firm and a judge.

There was no prior history of irritable or violent behavior. The patient had been married for 20 years and had children who were teenagers.

Approximately 6–8 months after the stroke, the patient was trying to fix an appliance in the house. When his wife asked him what he was doing, he suddenly and violently struck her in the neck with a swing of his non-paretic arm. This behavior continued off and on with the patient becoming angry and shouting at his wife over minor issues that would never have caused anger or violence in the past. The patient would periodically grab his wife's arm and would, on some occasions, attempt to strike her. The patient was referred for evaluation and treatment of these violent outbursts.

On mental status examination, the patient denied feelings of depression but stated that he recognized he sometimes lost his temper and was more prone to violent behavior than he used to be. There were no other significant findings on mental status examination. The patient's cognitive functions as measured by the MMSE were intact.

The patient's violent outbursts continued episodically for 3 years. He was tried on courses of doxepin and nortriptyline without improvement in his behavior and the trials had to be discontinued because of complaints of sedation. The patient's wife reported a gradual improvement in this behavior although it did not subside completely.

In summary, we have conducted two systematic studies of patients with aggressive and irritable behavior following stroke. The first study conducted within 2 weeks following stroke, and the second conducted approximately 6 weeks following stroke, found that greater cognitive impairment, greater frequency of depressive symptoms, a higher frequency of major depression, and generalized anxiety disorder as well as lesions that are closer to the frontal pole were significantly associated with self-reported aggressive and irritable behavior. Future research is needed to determine the most effective ways of controlling these aggressive and irritable outbursts in patients without associated depressive disorder. Control of anxiety symptoms or cognitive rehabilitation may be effective means of reducing the aggressive behavior associated with stroke.

REFERENCES

American Psychiatric Association. *Diagnostic and Statistical Manual of Mental Disorders – DSM-IV*. American Psychiatric Press, Inc., Washington DC, 1994.

Angeleri, F., Angeleri, V. A., Foschi, N., *et al*. The influence of depression, social activity, and family stress on functional outcome after stroke. *Stroke* (1993) 24(20):1478–1483.

Brooks, N., Campsie, L., and Symington, C. The five year outcome of severe blunt head injury: a relative's view. *J Neurol Neurosurg Psychiatr* (1986) 49:764–770.

Bryer, J. B., Starkstein, S. E., Votypka, V., *et al.* Reduction of CSF monoamine metabolites in post-stroke depression. *J Neuropsychiatr Clin Neurosci* (1992) 55:377–382.

Burns, A., Folstein, S., Brandt, J., *et al.* Clinical assessment of irritability, aggression, and apathy in Huntington and Alzheimer disease. *J Nerv Ment Dis* (1990) 178(1):20–26.

Chan, K. L., Moser, D. J., Arndt, S., *et al.* Aggressive behavior in patients with stroke: initial findings and response in double blind treatment trial (in preparation).

Chemerinski, E., Petracca, G., Teson, A., *et al.* Prevalence and correlates of aggressive behavior in Alzheimer's disease. *J Neuropsychiatr Clin Neurosci* (1998) 10(4):421–425.

Clarke, M. G., Williams, A. J., and Jones, P. A. A psychogeriatric survey of old people's homes. *Br Med J (Clin Res Ed)* (1981) 283(6302):1307–1310.

Cohen-Mansfield, J. Agitated behaviors in the elderly. II. Preliminary results in the cognitively deteriorated. *J Am Geriatr Soc* (1986) 34(10):722–727.

Cohen-Mansfield, J., Marx, M., and Rosenthal, A. Dementia and agitation in nursing home residents: how are they related? *Psychol Aging* (1990) 5:3–8.

Falconer, M. A. Reversibility by temporal-lobe resection of the behavioral abnormalities of temporal-lobe epilepsy. *New Engl J Med* (1973) 289(9):451–455.

Fuster, J. M. *The Prefrontal Cortex: Anatomy, Physiology and Neuropsychology of the Frontal Lobe.* Raven Press, New York, 1980.

Gainotti, G. Emotional behavior and hemispheric side of the brain. *Cortex* (1972) 8:41–55.

Gleason, R. P., and Schneider, L. S. Carbamazepine treatment of agitation in Alzheimer's outpatients refractory to neuroleptics. *J Clin Psychiatr* (1990) 51:115–118.

Greendyke, R. M., and Kanter, D. R. Therapeutic effects of pindolol on behavioral disturbances associated with organic brain disease: a double-blind study. *J Clin Psychiatr* (1986) 47: 423–426.

Gualtieri, C. T. Buspirone: neuropsychiatric effects. *J Head Trauma Rehabil* (1991) 6:90–92.

Haas, J. F., and Cope, N. Neuropharmacologic management of behavior sequelae in head injury: a case report. *Arch Phys Med Rehabil* (1985) 66:472–474.

Herzberg, J. L., and Fenwick, P. B. The aetiology of aggression in temporal-lobe epilepsy. *Br J Psychiatr* (1988) 153:50–55.

Hodgins, S. Mental disorder, intellectual deficiency, and crime. Evidence from a birth cohort. *Arch Gen Psychiatr* (1992) 49:476–483.

Jackson, R. D., Corrigan, J. D., and Arnett, J. Amitriptyline for agitation in head injury. *Arch Phys Med Rehabil* (1985) 66:180–181.

Kim, S. H., Manes, F., Kosier, T., *et al.* Irritability following traumatic brain injury. *J Nerv Ment Dis* (1999) 187(6):327–335.

Leger, J. M., Moulias, R., Vellas, B., *et al.* Causes and consequences of elderly's agitated and aggressive behavior. *Encephale* (2000) 26(1):32–43.

Margo, J. L., Robinson, J. R., and Corea, S. Referrals to a psychiatric service from old people's homes. *Br J Psychiatr* (1980) 136:396–401.

Mattes, J. A. Carbamazepine vs. propranolol for rage outbursts. *Psychopharmacol Bull* (1988) 24(1):179–182.

Mazure, C. M., Druss, B. G., and Cellar, J. S. Valproate treatment of older psychotic patients with organic mental syndromes and behavioral dyscontrol. *J Am Geriatr Soc* (1992) 40(9):914–916.

Paradiso, S., Robinson, R. G., and Arndt, S. Self-reported aggressive behavior in patients with stroke. *J Nerv Mental Dis* (1996) 184(12):746–753.

Ryden, M. B. Aggressive behavior in persons with dementia who live in the community. *Alzheimer Dis Assoc Disord* (1988) 2(4):342–355.

Silver, J. M., and Yudofsky, S. C. Aggressive disorders. In J. M. Silver, S. C. Yudofsky, and R. E. Hales, eds., *Neuropsychiatry of Traumatic Brain Injury*. American Psychiatric Press, Inc., Washington DC, 1994.

Stanislav, S. W., Fabre, T., Crismon, M. L., *et al.* Buspirone's efficacy in organic-induced aggression. *J Clin Psychopharmacol* (1994) 14:126–130.

Stevens, J. R., and Hermann, B. P. Temporal lobe epilepsy, psychopathology, and violence: the state of the evidence. *Neurology* (1981) 31(9):1127–1132.

Van Praag, H. M., Plutchik, R., and Conte, H. The serotonin hypothesis of (auto)aggression. Critical appraisal of the evidence. *Ann NY Acad Sci* (1986) 487:150–167.

Williams, A. What bothers caregivers of stroke victims? *J Neurosci Nurs* (1994) 26(3):155–161.

Winger, J., Schirm, V., and Stewart, D. Aggressive behavior in long-term care. *J Psychosoc Nurs Ment Health Serv* (1987) 25(4):28–33.

Yudofsky, S. C., Silver, J. M., and Schneider, S. E. Pharmacological treatment of aggression. *Psychiatric Ann* (1987) 17:397–497.

Yudofsky, S. C., Silver, J. M., and Hales, R. E. Pharmacologic management of aggression in the elderly. *J Clin Psychiatr* (1990) 51(Suppl):22–28; discussion 29–32.

40

Pathological laughing and crying

The association of brain injury with uncontrollable episodes of crying, or less frequently laughing, has been recognized as a consequence of brain injury since the 19th century (Wilson 1923; Davison and Kelman 1939). In 1877, Lépine described pseudobulbar palsy as a cranial nerve palsy (i.e., inability to swallow, move the tongue, articulate, forcefully close the eyes) induced by supranuclear lesions (i.e., lesions of the corticobulbar or corticopontine pathway) resulting from bilateral strokes. A frequent accompaniment of pseudobulbar palsy was uncontrollable crying or laughing which was referred to as pseudobulbar affect. Patients would present with an incongruity between the loss of voluntary facial movement and the unimpaired reflexive facial movements associated with spontaneous laughing or crying. Most cases of uncontrollable crying and laughing, however, were not associated with bilateral upper motor neuron or supra tentorial motor pathway lesions. Therefore, most clinicians abandoned the term, pseudobulbar affect, in favor of the more general term, pathological laughing and crying (Davison and Kelman 1939).

Pathological laughing and crying is a phenomenon characterized by outbursts of emotion which are out of proportion to the underlying feelings of happiness and sadness (Wilson 1923). The clinical manifestations of pathological emotions may range from facial expressions of happiness or sadness to loud and uncontrolled outbursts of laughing or weeping. These uncontrolled outbursts of pseudo-emotion are almost uniformly embarrassing to patients. Fears of developing uncontrollable emotional display can lead to social phobia and withdrawal. This phenomenon has been referred to by a variety of names including pathological emotions, emotional lability, emotional incontinence, and emotionalism as well as pseudobulbar affect (Lawson and Macleod 1969; Wolf *et al.* 1979; Ross and Stewart 1987; Hanger 1993). This condition has also been associated with a variety of neurological disorders including stroke, multiple sclerosis, traumatic brain injury, amyotrophic lateral sclerosis, central pontine, myelinolysis and anoxia (Langworth and Hesser 1940).

Poeck (1985) proposed that a diagnosis of pathological laughing and crying should be based on the existence of four characteristics:

1. Response triggered by non-specific stimuli.
2. Lack of relationship between affective change and the observed expression.
3. Absence of a corresponding change in mood during or lasting beyond the actual laughing and crying.
4. No voluntary control of facial expression.

These criteria describe classic pseudobulbar affect and do not describe the majority of cases with pathological emotion.

House *et al.* (1989) suggested that the diagnosis be based on an increased tearfulness with episodes of crying or laughing that were sudden or unheralded and not at all under normal social control. Kim and Choi-Kwon (2000) suggested that both the patient and relatives must agree that pathological laughter or crying occurred on at least two occasions and that the laughter or crying was either excessive or inappropriate to the situation in which it occurred. Assessment of the severity of pathological crying and laughing was first accomplished by developing the pathological laughing and crying scale (PLACS) (Robinson *et al.* 1993) (Table 40.1). Burns *et al.* (1999) proposed the assessment of severity of pathological emotions be based on the House criteria including the following questions scored "1" for yes and "0" for no:

1. Have you been more tearful in the last 2 weeks than you were before your stroke?
2. Have you actually cried more in the last 2 weeks?
3. Does the weepiness come suddenly at times when you were not expecting it?
4. If you feel tears coming on can you control yourself to stop them?
5. Have you been unable to stop yourself crying in front of other people?
6. Is that a new experience for you?

Table 40.1. Pathological laughter and crying scale

Part I. Patient interview

1. Have you recently experienced sudden episodes of laughter?

    _____Rate the frequency of the episodes during the past 2 weeks.

    0. Rarely or not at all
    1. Occasionally
    2. Quite often
    3. Frequently

2. Have you recently experienced sudden episodes of crying?

    _____Rate the frequency of the episodes during the past 2 weeks.

    0. Rarely or not at all
    1. Occasionally
    2. Quite often
    3. Frequently

Table 40.1. (*Continued*)

If you have experienced sudden **episodes of laughter,** *please answer the following questions (3–10) otherwise skip to question 11.*

3.   Have these episodes occurred without any cause in your surroundings?

_____Rate the frequency with which the episodes have occurred without external stimuli in the past 2 weeks.

   0.   Rarely or not at all

   1.   Occasionally

   2.   Quite often

   3.   Frequently

4.   Have these episodes lasted for a long period of time?

_____Rate the average duration of the episodes during the past 2 weeks.

   0.   Very brief

   1.   Few seconds

   2.   Moderate ($<30\,$s)

   3.   Prolonged ($>30\,$s)

5.   Have these episodes been uncontrollable by you?

_____Rate your inability to control the episodes during the past 2 weeks.

   0.   Rarely or not at all

   1.   Occasionally

   2.   Quite often

   3.   Frequently

6.   Have these episodes occurred as a result of feelings of happiness?

_____Rate the frequency with which the episodes have occurred as a result of happiness in the past 2 weeks.

   0.   Frequently

   1.   Quite often

   2.   Occasionally

   3.   Rarely or not at all

7.   Have these episodes occurred without feelings of happiness?

_____Rate the frequency with which the episodes have been disproportionate to the emotional state in past 2 weeks.

   0.   Rarely or not at all

   1.   Occasionally

   2.   Quite often

   3.   Frequently

8.   Have these episodes of laughter occurred with feelings of sadness?

_____Rate the frequency of association between the episode and the paradoxical emotion in the past 2 weeks. The sadness must precede or accompany the episode and not be a reaction to it.

   0.   Rarely or not at all

   1.   Occasionally

   2.   Quite often

   3.   Frequently

Table 40.1. (*Continued*)

9. Have these episodes occurred with any emotions other than happiness or sadness, such as nervousness, anger, fear, etc.?

_____Rate the frequency of association between the episodes and emotions in the past 2 weeks. The emotions must precede or accompany the laughing episode and not be a reaction to it.

    0.   Rarely or not at all

    1.   Occasionally

    2.   Quite often

    3.   Frequently

10. Have these episodes caused you any distress or social embarrassment?

_____Rate the degree of distress or embarrassment caused by the episodes in the past 2 weeks.

    0.   Rarely or not at all

    1.   Occasionally

    2.   Quite often

    3.   Frequently

If you have experienced sudden **episodes of crying** *please answer the following questions (11–18).*

11. Have these episodes occurred without any cause in your surroundings?

_____Rate the frequency with which the episodes have occurred without an external stimuli in the past 2 weeks.

    0.   Rarely or not at all

    1.   Occasionally

    2.   Quite often

    3.   Frequently

12. Have these episodes lasted for a long period of time?

_____Rate the average duration of the episodes during the past 2 weeks.

    0.   Very brief

    1.   Few periods

    2.   Moderate ($<30\,$s)

    3.   Prolonged ($>30\,$s)

13. Have these episodes been uncontrollable by you?

_____Rate your inability to control the episodes during the past 2 weeks.

    0.   Rarely or not at all

    1.   Occasionally

    2.   Quite often

    3.   Frequently

14. Have these episodes occurred without feelings of sadness?

_____Rate the frequency with which the episodes have occurred as a result of sadness in the past 2 weeks. The sadness must proceed or accompany the crying and not be a reaction to it.

    0.   Frequently

    1.   Quite often

    2.   Occasionally

    3.   Rarely or not at all

Table 40.1. (*Continued*)

---

15.   Have these episodes occurred in excess of feelings of sadness?

  _____Rate the frequency with which the episodes have been disproportionate to the emotional state in the past 2 weeks.

  0.   Rarely or not at all

  1.   Occasionally

  2.   Quite often

  3.   Frequently

16.   Have these episodes of crying occurred with feelings of happiness?

  _____Rate the frequency of association between the episode and the paradoxical emotion in the past 2 weeks. The happiness must precede or accompany the crying.

  0.   Rarely or not at all

  1.   Occasionally

  2.   Quite often

  3.   Frequently

17.   Have these episodes occurred with any emotions other than sadness or happiness, such as nervousness, anger, fear, etc.?

  _____Rate the frequency of association between the episodes and emotions in the past 2 weeks. The emotions must precede or accompany the crying episode and not be a reaction to it.

  0.   Rarely or not at all

  1.   Occasionally

  2.   Quite often

  3.   Frequently

18.   Have these episodes caused you any distress or social embarrassment?

  _____Rate the degree of distress or embarrassment caused by the episodes in the past 2 weeks.

  0.   Rarely or not at all

  1.   Occasionally

  2.   Quite often

  3.   Frequently

Ratings are based on clinical assessment. Initial probe questions are given for each item. However, further questions may be used for clarification. Write the number in the spaces provided which most accurately reflects clinical symptoms.

Brown *et al.* (1998) proposed a grading scale modified from Lawson and Macleod (1969) in which 9 grades of severity of pathological emotions were identified as follows:

1. Grade 0: No emotional response throughout.
2. Grade 1: Facial distress provoked by a conversation related to the emotionalism directly.
3. Grade 2: Facial distress provoked by a motive conversation.
4. Grade 3: Facial distress provoked by a neutral topic.

5. Grade 4: Facial distress provoked by an initial introduction.
6. Grade 5: Crying provoked by conversation related to the emotionalism specifically.
7. Grade 6: Crying provoked by a motive conversation.
8. Grade 7: Crying provoked by neutral conversation.
9. Grade 8: Crying provoked by an initial introduction (e.g., hello).

In our initial study of the PLACS (Table 40.1), 82 patients were administered the scale. This is an interviewer-rated instrument that quantifies aspects of laughter and crying, including the relationship of the episodes to external events, their duration, the degree of voluntary control, the appropriateness to underlying emotions, and the magnitude of resultant distress. The scale was administered to patients and relatives or friends who had been in close contact with the patient for the preceding 2 weeks. For each of the items, the examiner made a judgment about the severity of the symptom using a four-point scale (0 – rarely or not at all, to 3 – frequently). Scores for all items were totaled to obtain an overall score. Eight items relate to pathological laughter and eight to pathological crying.

To determine the validity of the PLACS score, diagnoses of emotions were made by examiners blind to the patient's scale scores using their clinical judgment. Clinical ratings of severity using a scale from 1 to 5 were compared to the independently derived PLACS scores. The mean PLACS scores of 17 patients who had a clinical diagnosis of emotional lability made by a psychiatrist who was blind to the patient's PLACS scores was 16.2 ± 3.1 for the pathological emotions group versus 2.7 ± 4.8 for 50 stroke patients without pathological emotions ($p < 0.001$). Using a cutoff score of 13 or greater (arbitrarily selected because it seemed to distinguish two bimodally separated groups), we found that the sensitivity of the PLACS for clinically diagnosed emotional lability was 88% ($n = 67$), specificity was 96%, and the positive predictive value was 83%. The Pearson correlation coefficient between the PLACS scores obtained from patient interviews and PLACS scores obtained from relatives' reports of patient's behavior and feelings was 0.86 ($n = 28$) indicating that there was good agreement between what the relatives were observing and what the patients were reporting using this scale. Furthermore, there were no significant correlations between the PLACS score, and the Hamilton depression scores ($r = 0.09$), the mini-mental state examination (MMSE) scores ($r = 0.01$), or Johns Hopkins functioning inventory (JHFI) scores ($r = 0.05$), indicating that the PLACS was measuring something other than depression or impairment. Finally, a subgroup of 15 patients was randomly selected and administered the PLACS independently by two psychiatrists to assess inter-rater reliability of the instrument. The interclass correlation coefficient for assessments made by two psychiatrists, who separately administered the PLACS to 15 patients, was 0.93 ($p < 0.01$). The Pearson correlation coefficient for test–retest reliability of this instrument when administered by the same rater at 2-week intervals was 0.85 ($n = 21, p < 0.01$).

Studies of the prevalence of pathological emotions have mainly come from studies of patients with stroke. Table 40.2 lists all of the studies which have examined the prevalence and clinical correlates of pathological laughing and crying following stroke.

Table 40.2. Pathological emotions following stroke

Study	n	Setting	Findings	Clinical correlates
Murai et al. (2003)	15	Acute		SPECT, lower serotonin transporter in path cry group
Piamarta et al. (2004)*	33	Acute	Prevalence 48.5% path cry, 57.6% depression	
Langhorne et al. (2000)*	311	Acute and rehabilitation	12% emotionalism	Emotionalism correlated depression
Calvert et al. (1998)*	448	Acute	21.5% (101) had emotionalism, of 101 with emotionalism, 38% had mood disorder versus 18% without emotionalism	Irritability and ideas of reference associated with emotionalism
MacHale et al. (1998)	55	Acute	Single lesion, 18% of depressed had emotionalism	
Allman et al. (1992)	30	Rehabilitation	All had emotionalism, no subtypes found	
Tang et al. (2004)*	127	Acute	17.9% had emotionalism	Logistic regression: history of depression and cortical infarct associated with emotionalism
Kim (2002)	25	Outpatient		Lesions <2 cm, lenticulocapsular stroke, 52% associated with globus pallidus (dorsal) lesion
Choi-Kwon and Kim (2002)	70	Acute	34% had emotionalism 3-month poststroke, resolved by 2 years	

Table 40.2 (*Continued*)

Study	*n*	Setting	Findings	Clinical correlates
Kim and Choi-Kwon (2000)	148	Outpatient	34% emotionalism (18% MDD)	Frontal lenticulocapsular lesion associated with emotionalism
House *et al.* (1989)*	128	Acute	15% emotionalism at 1 month, 11% emotionalism at 1 year	
Andersen (1995)*	211	Acute	14% acute, 11% at 1 year (19% overall)	
Morris *et al.* (1993)*	66	Acute	18% emotionalism	
Robinson *et al.* (1993)*	67	Acute	25% emotionalism	
Burvill *et al.* (1995)	42 with MDD at 4 months	Community	7% (of 42) with emotionalism at 12 months	

Overall estimate of prevalence of emotionalism is 14.9%.

MDD: major depressive disorder.

*Studies that contributed to overall estimate of prevalence of emotionalism.

Although pathological crying is the most common manifestation, some individuals have episodes of laughing without episodes of crying and some have both laughing and crying episodes. Some patients will gradually change from having predominantly crying episodes to having laughing episodes over the first year following stroke.

The largest studies to examine pathological emotions were conducted by Calvert *et al.* (1998) in which 448 patients who were within 1 month of stroke, living independently before the stroke and had no severe language or cognitive impairment were examined for pathological emotions based on the House criteria for emotionalism (House *et al.* 1989). A total of 101 (22.5%) participants reported emotionalism since the stroke. Of these, 83 reported symptoms of crying only, 16 reported symptoms of laughter and crying, and only 2 patients reported symptoms of laughter only. House *et al.* (1989) reported in a community-based study of 128 first ever stroke patients that the frequency of pathological emotions was 15% at 1 month and 11% at 1 year. Overall, during the first year 21% of the patients experienced this condition. Andersen (1995) reported that 14% of patients in a community-based study of 211 first ever stroke patients developing pathological crying and 11% demonstrated this symptom at 1 year. During the overall 1-year evaluation, a total of 19% of patients experienced this condition. Morris *et al.*

(1993) reported that pathological emotions were found in 12 of 66 patients (18%) admitted to a stroke rehabilitation hospital following a first ever stroke.

Langhorne *et al.* (2000) examined 311 patients admitted to hospital with acute stroke. Patients were recruited within 7 days following stroke onset and were examined during the acute hospitalization based on the criteria of House *et al.* (1989). A total of 37 patients (12%) were diagnosed with emotionalism. The prevalence rate after hospital discharge, however, was not evaluated. Based on all of the studies that examined pathological emotions following stroke (Table 41.2), the pooled data estimate of the prevalence of pathological emotions was 14.9%. The prevalence rates, however, ranged from 48.5% among 33 patients with first ever stroke and single supratentorial lesions (Piamarta *et al.* 2004) to 7% in a community study of 211 patients assessed 1 year following stroke (Burvill *et al.* 1995).

There have been a number of interesting clinical–pathological correlations which have been reported in studies of pathological emotions. Poeck (1985) reviewed the pathology reports of 30 patients with pathological crying. He concluded that a lesion in the supranuclear motor pathways was a sufficient, but not a necessary, condition for this disorder. Interruption of these descending motor pathways, frequently bilaterally, may produce denervation of the bulbar motor nuclei producing bulbar palsy and also producing, through some undetermined mechanism in the base of the brain stem, interruption of the motor pathways that control laughing and crying (Lieberman and Benson 1977).

House *et al.* (1989) reported that left anterior lesions were associated with increased emotionalism (i.e., pathological crying) in their community-based study of first ever stroke. Emotionalism was more common among patients with lesions of the left frontal and left temporal lobes compared with other lesion locations. Morris *et al.* (1993) found no association between emotional lability and the occurrence of either right or left hemisphere infarctions. However, patients with frontal or temporal lesions in either hemisphere were found to have a significantly greater frequency of emotional lability than patients with lesions in any other brain region (35% versus 11%) (odds ratio (OR): 4.4; 95% confidence interval (CI): 1.1–19.9). Adjusting for potential confounding demographic factors (i.e., age, gender, marital status, social class) and clinical variables (i.e., stroke type, impairment in activities of daily living, cognitive impairment, depression diagnosis), a logistic regression showed an association between pathological emotions and frontal or temporal lesions.

In addition to the association with frontal and temporal lesions, Morris *et al.* (1993) found that patients with pathological laughing and crying had lesions whose anterior border was closer to the frontal pole of the brain compared to patients without this condition (i.e., the anterior border was $19 \pm 7\%$ of the anterior–posterior distance in patients with pathological emotions while in patients without emotional lability it was $35 \pm 16\%$ of the anterior–posterior distance, $p = 0.02$).

Andersen *et al.* (1993) reported on the association between lesion size and the location and severity of pathological crying in 12 selected stroke patients with pathological emotions. Patients were divided into three groups. The group with the most frequent episodes of crying had bilateral, relatively large pontine lesions without hemispheric infarction. The intermediate group had bilateral relatively large anterior hemispheric lesions involving the basal ganglia or periventricular structures. The least affected group had mainly unilateral large subcortical lesions. Andersen *et al.* (1993) concluded that poststroke pathological crying may be the consequence of a partial destruction of serotonergic raphe nuclei in the brain stem or their ascending projections to the hemispheres. This hypothesis that serotonergic pathways are involved in pathological laughing and crying was also based on the finding that the selective serotonin reuptake inhibitors (SSRIs) citalopram or fluoxetine rapidly and effectively alleviated this condition (Seliger *et al.* 1992; Andersen *et al.* 1993).

Kim and Choi-Kwon (2000) in a study of 25 outpatients found that the lenticulo-capsular lesions were associated with pathological emotions. Tang *et al.* (2004) examined 127 patients with acute stroke and found that both depression and cortical infarctions were independent correlates of pathological emotions based on a multivariate regression analysis. The study by Calvert *et al.* (1998) found that among the 101 patients with pathological emotions, this emotionalism was associated with the existence of depression (38% of those with pathological emotions had depressive disorder compared to 18% depression among patients without pathological emotions). Based on logistic regression, pathological emotions were also independently associated with ideas of reference and irritability. Finally, MacHale *et al.* (1998) found that pathological emotions occurred in 18% of 145 patients at 6 months following stroke and was associated with the existence of depression (i.e., 62% of the pathological emotionalism patients were depressed while only 11% of the non-emotionalism patients were) ($p < 0.001$). Pathological emotions were also associated with right anterior lesions (OR: 5.3; 95% CI: 1.2–22.9; $p = 0.03$).

Currently, there are four double-blind placebo-controlled treatment trials assessing the treatment of pathological emotions. A summary of the treatment studies of pathological emotions is shown in Table 40.3. The first treatment trials were reported by Andersen *et al.* (1993) and Robinson *et al.* (1993).

The background characteristics of 28 patients included in our double-blind-randomized study of nortriptyline in the treatment of pathological laughing and crying are shown in Table 40.4 (Robinson *et al.* 1993). The patients were predominantly Caucasian, in their later 50s and approximately 8–12 months had passed since their stroke. These patients were recruited separately from our other stroke studies and so represent a different group of patients than those previously described in our longitudinal studies. There were no statistically significant differences between the nortriptyline-treated and placebo groups in terms of age, gender, race,

Table 40.3. Treatment of pathological emotions following stroke

Study	n	Weeks of treatment	Rx type	Methodology	Results
Robinson et al. (1993)*	28	6 weeks	Nortriptyline versus placebo	Double blind	Nortriptyline > placebo at weeks 4 and 6
Brown et al. (1998)*	19	10 days	Fluoxetine versus placebo	Double blind	Diminished tearfulness, fluoxetine > placebo
Burns et al. (1999)*	28	8 weeks	Sertraline versus placebo	Double blind	50% reduction in emotionalism, sertraline > placebo
Andersen et al. (1993)*	13	9 weeks	Citalopram versus placebo	Double-blind crossover	Citalopram > placebo, all citalopram versus two placebo patients had decreased crying
Sloan et al. (1992)	6 (5 stroke)	1 week	Fluoxetine open label		All improved
Ramasubbu and Patten (2003)	1	4 weeks	Lamotrigine		Recovered
Derex et al. (1997)	1	8 weeks	Paroxetine		Recovered
Mukand et al. (1996)	2	Unknown	Sertraline		Both recovered

*Using the four double-blind studies: 48 of 50 (96.0%) treated patients improved versus 14 of 51 (27.5%) placebo patients, Fisher's exact test $p \leq 0.0001$.

Table 40.4. Characteristics of patients in a study of pathological laughing and crying

Characteristic	Nortriptyline (n = 14)	Placebo (n = 14)
Age (mean ± SD in years)	57.8 ± 10.1	58.5 ± 11.8
Gender (n, female)	6	10
Race (n, white)	7	12
Married (n)	7	10
Socioeconomic class IV or V (n)	7	4
Right handed (n)	10	14
Time since stroke (months ± SD)	8.1 ± 9.9	15.7 ± 13.5

socioeconomic status, marital status, previous cerebrovascular accident, handedness, or time since stroke.

The active and placebo treatment groups were also not significantly different in any
of their neurological or computed tomographic (CT) scan findings. Of the 26 patients
in whom neurological findings were available, 10 patients had a single right hemisphere lesion and 8 had bilateral or multiple lesions. There were no significant differences, however, in the frequency of right, left, bilateral, cortical, or subcortical lesion
location or lesion volume (mean volume for the nortriptyline group was 9.1 ± 6.4%
(SD) of brain volume and for the placebo group mean was 8.0 ± 7.8% (SD)).

Prior to the onset of treatment, there were no significant differences between the
active and placebo treatment groups in terms of scores on the MMSE, the JHFI
(activities of daily living), or the social ties checklist. The placebo group, however,
had significantly higher mean pretreatment Hamilton depression scores than the
nortriptyline treatment group (nortriptyline treatment group mean 12.1 ± 7.3,
placebo group mean was 18.6 ± 5.2, $p < 0.02$). Based on Diagnostic and Statistical
Manual, 3rd ed., revised (DSM-III-R) criteria for major depression, 8 of the 14
patients treated with nortriptyline and 11 of the 14 patients treated with placebo
had major depression. The active- and placebo-treated groups both had significantly improved in Hamilton depression scores, but, of the two, the improvement
shown by the nortriptyline-treated group was significantly greater ($p < 0.001$).

The PLACS score over the 6 weeks of treatment were evaluated using a repeated-
measures analysis of variance (ANOVA) (Fig. 40.1). There was a significant

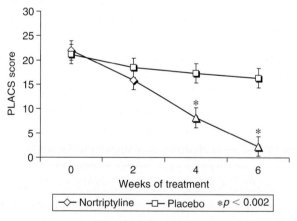

Figure 40.1 Comparison of PLACS scores over 6 weeks of double-blind treatment with nortriptyline or
placebo using parametric analysis (repeated-measures ANOVA). There was a significant
treatment (i.e., nortriptyline versus placebo) by time interaction ($p = 0.0001$). The active
treatment was superior to placebo at both 4 and 6 weeks of treatment. Using non-
parametric analog of repeated measures, there was again a significant treatment-by-time
interaction ($p < .001$) and significantly greater improvement in the active-treated group at
4 and 6 weeks (reprinted from Robinson *et al.* 1993 with permission).

group-by-time interaction ($p = 0.001$) (i.e., the group treated with nortriptyline improved more quickly than the placebo group) (Fig. 40.1). Planned comparisons revealed that the two groups were not significantly different in their PLACS scores at the beginning of the study and at 2 weeks, but the nortriptyline group was significantly more improved (i.e., lower PLACS scores) than the placebo group at weeks 4 ($p = 0.005$) and 6 ($p = 0.001$) (Fig. 40.1).

Since the nortriptyline-treated group had significantly lower Hamilton depression scores than the placebo group prior to the onset of treatment, we matched eight pairs of patients in the two groups according to their Hamilton depression scores (± 4 points). Although the pretreatment Hamilton depression scores were not significantly different (15.9 ± 4.2 for the nortriptyline group versus 16.5 ± 5.3 for the placebo group), the nortriptyline group showed a significantly greater improvement in terms of their PLACS scores than the placebo group ($p = 0.002$), and repeated-measures ANOVA revealed a significant time by group interaction ($p = 0.001$) (i.e., the nortriptyline-treated group showed a significantly faster improvement than the placebo group).

We also investigated the effect of lesion location on the response to treatment. Patients with single right hemisphere lesions ($n = 4$ in the nortriptyline group, $n = 6$ in the placebo group) were compared to patients with bilateral lesions ($n = 4$ in the nortriptyline-treated group, $n = 3$ in the placebo group). Two-way repeated-measures ANOVA revealed that the effect of nortriptyline treatment was significant ($p = 0.001$), while that of lesion location was not (i.e., the right hemisphere and bilateral groups improved to the same degree with nortriptyline).

We also examined the effect of time since stroke on the response to treatment. Since the nortriptyline-treated patients were evaluated an average of 8.1 months after their stroke and placebo patients an average of 15.7 months after their stroke, we wanted to be sure that the placebo patients were not a more treatment-resistant, chronic group than the nortriptyline patients. We matched eight pairs of patients for time since stroke (i.e., the exact number of months for patients up to 12 months poststroke, within ± 3 months up to 24 months and within ± 6 months for more than 24 months). The mean time since stroke for the nortriptyline-treated group was 10.9 ± 11.2 months and 11.3 ± 10.3 months for the placebo group. Repeated-measures ANOVA revealed a significant treatment-by-time interaction ($p = 0.001$) (i.e., patients given nortriptyline treatment improved significantly faster than placebo-treated patients). Finally, in order to ensure that parametric and non-parametric analysis did not give different results, we analyzed the data using non-parametric statistical procedures (Conover and Iman 1981) which demonstrated a significant time-by-treatment interaction ($p = 0.0001$) (i.e., the patients treated with nortriptyline improved at a significantly faster rate than patients treated with placebo). *Post hoc* analysis demonstrated that the nortriptyline-treated group had significantly lower PLACS scores at 4- and 6-week

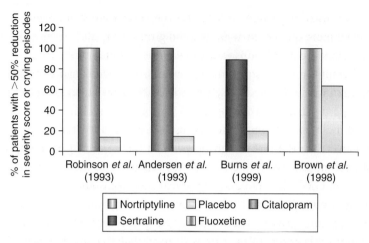

Figure 40.2 Comparison of double-blind treatment studies using nortriptyline, citalopram, sertraline, or fluoxetine in patients with pathological crying. The mean, pooled data response rates were 96% for active medication and 27.5% for placebo. These findings suggest that all of the medications are effective in the treatment of poststroke pathological crying.

post-treatment while there was no significant affect at weeks 0 and 2. These findings are identical to those using a parametric statistical analysis.

Although the number of patients with pathological laughing was small ($n = 2$), one patient who was given nortriptyline responded by PLACS scores falling from 27 before treatment to 0 at week 6 while the PLACS score of another patient given placebo did not change significantly (i.e., 32 at week 0, 31 at week 2, 31 at week 4, and 27 at week 6). Thus, this preliminary evidence suggests that nortriptyline may be as effective in the treatment of pathological laughing as it is in the treatment of pathological crying.

Andersen et al. (1993) evaluated 16 patients who were given 1 week of baseline measurement of the frequency of episodes of crying or laughing, 3 weeks of citalopram (20 mg less than age 65, 10 mg 65 or older), 1 week of washout, 1 week of baseline, and 3 weeks of crossover treatment. All 13 completers had a reduction in the number of crying episodes by at least 50% while 2 patients responded to placebo (Fig. 40.2); 8 patients responded within 24 h, 3 patients within 3 days, and 4 patients responded after 1 week. Brown et al. (1998) in a study of 9 patients treated with fluoxetine (20 mg) or placebo over 10 days found that by day 3 there was greater than 50% reduction in the number of crying episodes in 8 of 9 fluoxetine-treated patients compared to 2 of 10 placebo-treated patients. The most recent double-blind treatment trial was reported by Burns et al. (1999) who found that 14 patients treated with sertraline (50 mg) for 8 weeks improved significantly more than a comparable group of 14 patients given placebo treatment. Episodes of tearfulness were significantly decreased in 93% of the sertraline-treated patients after 2 weeks of an 8-week treatment trial compared with 50% of the placebo-treated patients. After 8 weeks of treatment, patients had a 2-week placebo washout and a final evaluation. The 10-week evaluation found only 5 patients (36%) treated with sertraline and 9 patients (64%) treated with placebo had an improved lability scale. Thus, within 2 weeks of withdrawal of antidepressant treatment, the patients had relapsed to no significant effect of prior treatment. The response rates across all the double-blind treatment trials are displayed in Fig. 40.2.

Perhaps the most fundamental question about the finding of an improvement in emotional lability associated with antidepressant treatment is its relationship to depression. Could the decrease in the frequency of crying in response to antidepressant treatment be ascribed to an improvement in patients' mood symptoms? The significant improvement in Hamilton depression scores among patients in our treatment study and the Andersen treatment study is consistent with this hypothesis. Ross and Stewart (1987) suggested that in some patients, the combination of depression and a right hemisphere lesion involving neocortical control of limbic-associated motor behaviors was necessary to produce pathological laughing and crying. These authors also suggested that pathological affect in these patients was indicative of the presence of depression. The majority of patients in our treatment study met criteria for major depression (19 out of 36 patients). Changes in PLACS scores among patients with depression ($n = 8$ nortriptyline treatment, $n = 11$ placebo treatment) were compared to patients without depression ($n = 6$ nortriptyline treatment, $n = 3$ placebo treatment). Two-way repeated-measures ANOVA of the scores of depressed versus non-depressed groups revealed a significant effect of active treatment versus placebo over time, but no effect of depression (i.e., depressed and non-depressed patients responded equally). In fact, there was a trend ($p = 0.06$) for the non-depressed patients to improve more on the PLACS scale than the depressed patients. Furthermore, as indicated previously, when patients were matched for Hamilton depression scores (± 4 points), the significant effect of active treatment was still demonstrable ($p = 0.002$).

Although the mechanism of pathological laughing and crying remains unknown, Andersen et al. (1993) hypothesized that pathological crying may be the consequence of partial destruction of serotonergic raphe nuclei in the brain stem or to the ascending serotonergic projections in the hemispheres. The only study to directly examine a potential mechanism for pathological crying was reported by Murai et al. (2003). Six stroke patients with pathological crying were compared with 9 comparable stroke patients without pathological crying for serotonin transporter densities in the midbrain–pons and thalamus–hypothalamus. The patients were not significantly different in age, gender distribution, time since stroke (i.e., 6.2 ± 2.4 days pathological crying group, 8.7 ± 5.9 days non-pathological crying group) as well as lesion location and neurological findings. Using 2β-carbomethoxy-3β-(4-indophenyl) tropane ($[^{123}I]\beta$-CIT) with high affinity for serotonin transporter receptors and single photo-emission computed tomography (SPECT) imaging, binding ratios (i.e., ipsilateral to contralateral radioactivity counts) of the pathological crying group were found to be significantly lower in the midbrain and pons (1.26 ± 0.51 versus 1.93 ± 0.59, $p = 0.025$) compared to the non-pathological crying group. This study is consistent with the hypothesis that serotonergic neurotransmission is more severely impaired in patients who develop pathological crying compared to patients without pathological crying following stroke. Obviously, further research is needed to identify the mechanisms as well as the reason for such rapid response to SSRI medications in the treatment of pathological emotions.

In summary, pathological laughing and crying is a frequent problem in patients with stroke occurring in approximately 15% of patients during the acute post-stroke period and approximately 20% of patients during the first year following stroke. This is a socially debilitating disorder than may occur as frequently as 100 times a day and last from a few seconds to several minutes. It is associated with the existence of depression in a significant number of cases but is a comorbid condition that is independent of depression. The clinical pathological correlates of pathological emotions have included unilateral lesions of the basal ganglia, frontal or temporal cortex as well as lesions of the brain stem or periventricular structures. The most frequent clinical correlate of pathological emotions is depression. Four double-blind treatment trials have demonstrated that nortriptyline, fluoxetine, citalopram, and sertraline have all been effective in treating this clinically important condition. Combining the four double-blind treatment trials, a greater than 50% reduction in the number of crying episodes at the end of the treatment trial occurred in 96% of patients receiving active antidepressant therapy compared with 27.5% of patients receiving placebo (Fisher exact <0.0011). The onset of the effect of fluoxetine, sertraline, and citalopram may occur within 24 h. The doses used for treatment of this condition are similar to those used for antidepressant treatment. The cause of pathological emotions is unknown but the existing evidence suggests that disruption of the serotonergic pathways perhaps to the limbic areas of cortex or the descending bulbar motor pathways may play a central role. Further research is needed to determine the mechanism of this disorder as well as the effect of pathological emotions on long-term outcome from stroke, both in patients receiving treatment and those without treatment.

REFERENCES

Allman, P., Hope, T. and Fairburn, C. G. Crying following stroke. A report on 30 cases. *Gen Hosp Psychiatr* (1992) 14(5):315–321.

Andersen, G. Treatment of uncontrolled crying after stroke. *Drug Aging* (1995) 6:105–111.

Andersen, G., Vestergaard, K., and Riis, J. Citalopram for post-stroke pathological crying. *Lancet* (1993) 342(8875):837–839.

Brown, K. W., Sloan, R. L., and Pentland, B. Fluoxetine as a treatment for post-stroke emotionalism. *Acta Psychiatr Scand* (1998) 98(6):455–458.

Burns, A., Russell, E., Stratton-Powell, H., *et al.* Sertraline in stroke-associated lability of mood. *Int J Geriatr Psychiatr* (1999) 14(8):681–685.

Burvill, P. W., Johnson, G. A., Jamrozik, K. D., *et al.* Prevalence of depression after stroke: the Perth Community Stroke Study. *Br J Psychiatr* (1995) 166:320–327.

Calvert, T., Knapp, P., and House, A. Psychological associations with emotionalism after stroke. *J Neurol Neurosurg Psychiatr* (1998) 65(6):928–929.

Choi-Kwon, S., and Kim, J. S. Poststroke emotional incontinence and decreased sexual activity. *Cerebrovasc Dis* (2002) 13(1):31–37.

Conover, W. J., and Iman, R. L. Rank transformations as a bridge between parametric and non-parametric statistics. *Am Stat* (1981) 35:124–129.

Davison, C., and Kelman, H. Pathological laughing and crying. *Arch Neurol Psychiatr* (1939) 1442:595–643.

Derex, L., Ostrowsky, K., Nighoghossian, N., *et al.* Severe pathological crying after left anterior choroidal artery infarct. Reversibility with paroxetine treatment. *Stroke* (1997) 28(7):1464–1466.

Hanger, H. C. Emotionalism after stroke (letter). *Lancet* (1993) 342:1235–1236.

House, A., Dennis, M., Molyneau, A., *et al.* Emotionalism after stroke. *Br Med J* (1989) 198:991–994.

Kim, J. S. Post-stroke emotional incontinence after small lenticulocapsular stroke: correlation with lesion location. *J Neurol* (2002) 249(7):805–810.

Kim, J. S., and Choi-Kwon, S. Poststroke depression and emotional incontinence: correlation with lesion location. *Neurology* (2000) 54(9):1805–1810.

Langhorne, P., Stott, D. J., Robertson, L., *et al.* Medical complications after stroke: a multicenter study. *Stroke* (2000) 31(6):1223–1229.

Langworth, O., and Hesser, F. Syndrome of pseudobulbar palsy. *Arch Intern Med* (1940) 65:106–121.

Lawson, J. R., and Macleod, R. D. M. The use of imipramine ("Tofranil") and other psychotropic drugs in organic emotionalism. *Br J Psychiatr* (1969) 115:281–285.

Lépine, R. Note sur la paralysie glosso-labiée cérébrale à forme pseudo-bulbaire. *Revue Mensuelle de Médecine et de Chirurgie* (1877) 1:909–922.

Lieberman, A., and Benson, D. F. Control of emotional expression in pseudobulbar palsy. *Arch Neurol* (1977) 34:717–719.

MacHale, S. M., O'Rourke, S. J., Wardlaw, J. M., *et al.* Depression and its relation to lesion location after stroke. *J Neurol Neurosurg Psychiatr* (1998) 64:371–374.

Morris, P. U., Robinson, R. G., and Raphael, B. Emotional lability following stroke. *Aust NZ J Psychiatr* (1993) 27:601–605.

Mukand, J., Kaplan, M., Senno, R. G., *et al.* Pathological crying and laughing: treatment with sertraline. *Arch Phys Med Rehabil* (1996) 77(12):1309–1311.

Murai, T., Barthel, H., Berrouschot, J., Sorger, D., von Cramon, D. Y., *et al.* Neuroimaging of serotonin transporters in post-stroke pathological crying. *Psychiatr Res Neuroimag* (2003) 123:207–211.

Piamarta, F., Iurlaro, S., Isella, V., *et al.* Unconventional affective symptoms and executive functions after stroke in the elderly. *Arch Gerontol Geriatr Suppl* (2004) (9):315–323.

Poeck, K. Pathological laughter and crying. In J. A. M. Fredricks, ed., *Handbook of Clinical Neurology*, Vol. 1(45): *Clinical Neuropsychology*. Elsevier Science, Amsterdam, 1985, 219–225.

Ramasubbu, R., and Patten, S. B. Effect of depression on stroke morbidity and mortality. *Can J Psychiatr* (2003) 48(4):250–257.

Robinson, R. G., Starr, L. B., Kubos, K. L., *et al.* A two year longitudinal study of post-stroke mood disorders: findings during the initial evaluation. *Stroke* (1983) 14:736–744.

Robinson, R. G., Parikh, R. M., Lipsey, J. R., *et al.* Pathological laughing and crying following stroke: validation of measurement scale and double-blind treatment study. *Am J Psychiatr* (1993) 150:286–293.

Ross, E. D., and Stewart, R. S. Pathological display of affect in patients with depression and right frontal brain damage. *J Nerv Ment Dis* (1987) 175:165–172.

Seliger, G. M., Hornstein, A., Flax, J., *et al.* Fluoxetine improves emotional incontinence. *Brain Injury* (1992) 6(3):267–270.

Sloan, R. L., Brown, K. W., and Pentland, B. Fluoxetine as a treatment for emotional lability after brain injury. *Brain Injury* (1992) 6(4):315–319.

Tang, W. K., Chan, S. S., Chiu, H. F., *et al.* Emotional incontinence in Chinese stroke patients – diagnosis, frequency, and clinical and radiological correlates. *J Neurol* (2004) 251(7):865–869.

Wilson, S. A. K. Some problems in neurology. II. Pathological laughing and crying. *J Neurol Psychopathol* (1923) 4:299–333.

Wolf, J. K., Santana, H. B., and Thorpy, M. Treatment of "emotional incontinence" with levodopa. *Neurology* (1979) 29:1435–1436.

41

Summary and future directions

In this second edition of *The Clinical Neuropsychiatry of Stroke*, I have attempted to review and summarize the world's literature on the many types of disorders which are a consequence of stroke. The only major group of mental disorders which was not discussed in detail is the cognitive disorders. Although much of our work has been devoted to examining the effect of depression, anxiety, mania, and other post-stroke disorders on cognitive function, we have not systematically studied the neuropsychological impairments of specific lesion site or the syndrome of vascular dementia. In the absence of psychopathology, brain lesions themselves, of course, produce cognitive impairment. There are many texts of neuropsychology [e.g., Gazzaniga's *Cognitive neuroscience* (2002); Lezak's *Neuropsychological Assessment* (2004); Heilman's *Clinical Neuropsychology* (2003)] which discuss cognitive impairment in relationship to vascular infarction.

In addition to the wide variety of neuropsychiatric disorders which occur following stroke, perhaps the most striking aspect of our findings and the findings of other investigators is the high prevalence rate for many of these disorders. Table 41.1 provides a summary of all of the disorders discussed in this book including their prevalence, clinical symptoms, and associated neuropathology. As one reads down the column of prevalence of each of these disorders, it is obvious that the total is greater than 100%. Thus, these neuropsychiatric disorders of stroke are not occurring as a single disorder but are, in many patients, comorbid disorders. Although the identification of each of these disorders requires experience and background in clinical neuropsychiatry, family members and caregivers are often extremely important to clinicians when they report changes in patients' behaviors or mental state. Poststroke patients need to be asked at regular intervals during the first several years following the stroke whether they feel depressed, anxious, apathetic, irritable, or euphoric. If their emotional state has changed, a clinical assessment to examine for other accompanying symptoms such as loss of interest or pleasure in usual activities, difficulty sleeping, etc. should be obtained. The Diagnostic and Statistical Manual of Mental Disorder, IV Text Revised (DSM-IV-TR) diagnostic criteria for

Table 41.1. Clinical syndromes associated with cerebrovascular disease

Syndrome	Prevalence	Clinical symptoms	Associated lesion location
Major depression	22%	Depressed mood, diurnal mood variation, loss of energy, anxiety, restlessness, worry, weight loss, decreased appetite, early morning awakening, delayed sleep onset, social withdrawal, and irritability	Left frontal lobe, left basal ganglia
Minor depression	20%	Depressed mood, anxiety, restlessness, worry, diurnal mood variation, hopelessness, loss of energy, delayed sleep onset, early morning awakening, social withdrawal, weight loss, and decreased appetite	Right or left posterior parietal and occipital regions
Mania	Unknown, rare	Elevated mood, increased energy, increased appetite, decreased sleep, feeling of well being, pressured speech, flight of ideas, grandiose thoughts	Right basotemporal or right orbitofrontal or right subcortical
Bipolar mood disorder	Unknown, rare	Symptoms of major depression alternating with mania	Right basal ganglia or right thalamic lesions
Anxiety disorder	18%	Symptoms of major depression, intense worry and anxious foreboding in addition to depression, associated light-headedness or palpitations and muscle tension or restlessness, and difficulty concentrating or falling asleep	Left cortical lesions, usually dorsal lateral frontal lobe
Psychotic disorder	Unknown, rare	Hallucinations or delusional beliefs	Right temporoparietal–occipital junction

Apathy			
Without depression	11%	Loss of drive, motivation, interest, low energy	
With depression	11%	uncommon	Posterior internal capsule
Pathological laughing and crying	15%	Frequent, usually brief laughing and/or crying; crying not caused by sadness or out of proportion to it; and social withdrawal secondary to emotional outbursts	Frequently bilateral hemispheric Can occur with almost any location
Anosognosia	24%	Denial of impairment related to motor function, sensory perception, visual perception or other modality with an apparent lack of concern	Right hemisphere and enlarged ventricles
Catastrophic reaction	19%	Anxiety reaction, tears, aggressive behavior, swearing, displacement, refusal, renouncement, and compensatory boasting	Left anterior-subcortical
Aprosodias			
Motor	Unknown	Poor expression of emotional prosody and gesturing, good prosodic comprehension and gesturing, and denial of feelings of depression	Right hemisphere posterior inferior frontal lobe and basal ganglia
Sensory	32%	Good expression of emotional prosody and gesturing, poor prosodic comprehension and gesturing, and difficulty empathizing with others	Right hemisphere posterior inferior parietal lobe and posterior superior temporal lobe

depression, mania, or anxiety disorder due to stroke may be used to diagnose the presence of these disorders. Suspicion of an emotional disorder remains the first step in the appropriate management of patients who are within the first 2 years following stroke.

In addition to the identification of neuropsychiatric disorders in the patient with stroke, there are now several controlled treatment trials which have established standards for the care of these patients. For many years, investigators had demonstrated that clinicians caring for patients with stroke failed to recognize and therefore to treat these neuropsychiatric disorders (Feibel and Springer 1982; Schubert *et al.* 1992). Chapter 22 has described in some detail the controlled trials demonstrating the effectiveness of antidepressants in the treatment of poststroke depression. Chapter 33 described the first study which demonstrated the potential treatment of anxiety disorder, at least in the presence of comorbid depressive disorder, in alleviating anxiety symptoms. In addition, Chapter 40 detailed the several controlled studies which have demonstrated the effectiveness of antidepressants in the treatment of pathological laughing and crying. Although there are numerous disorders (e.g., mania, apathy, catastrophic reactions, etc.) in which control trials have not been conducted. Clinical management including treatments such as stimulants, antipsychotic medications, and antianxiety medications are all potential avenues for improving the symptoms that these patients suffer. Although many of the research questions relevant to each of the topics covered in this book have been cited in the specific chapter dealing with that disorder, ultimately effective treatments based on double-blind controlled randomized trials is the most pressing need to alleviate the suffering and consequences of these conditions in the poststroke population.

Although the development of effective treatment is the major research need in poststroke neuropsychiatric disorders, rational treatment will only be possible when the mechanisms of these disorders can be identified. Whether these emotional behavioral disorders result from imbalance of the biogenic amine neurotransmitters or whether they result from the effect of proinflammatory cytokines released by stroke or whether they result from a psychological response to impairment, development of treatments targeted at the etiological abnormality require that the cause and mechanism of these disorders be identified. Both pharmacological and psychological treatments may be helpful to these patients if specific abnormalities can be identified.

In most specialties of medicine, we have been unable to achieve truly rational therapy. It is perhaps only in the realm of infectious diseases where our treatments can be described as rational and targeted to the etiological agent. Nevertheless, our ultimate goal should be to find the etiology and mechanism of these disorders so that rational treatments may replace empirical treatments and lead to the most effective and fullest response.

The following case study demonstrates both the progress that is made in caring for patients with poststroke depression as well as the many unresolved issues of treatment.

CASE STUDY

Mr. N., a 59-year-old white, married male, had suffered a large right hemisphere thromboembolic stroke in the distribution of the middle cerebral artery 2 years prior to his initial neuropsychiatric evaluation. At the time of the initial evaluation, the patient had a chief complaint of severe depression and anxiety of 3-month duration.

The patient had retired following his stroke after 35 years as the director of security for a large company. The patient's father was 80 years old and had arthritis but no other major medical conditions. His mother had been hospitalized for depression just prior to the patient's birth. She died, 20 years before the patient's index stroke, of heart failure after several strokes in the few months prior to her death. The only other family history of stroke was a brother who had diabetes and several strokes.

The patient had been married for 34 years and had four children. None of the children had a psychiatric disorder and all were doing well. The patient denied any marital conflict, but felt that he was "driving his wife crazy" because of his irritability and depression.

The patient's past medical history included a mitrolotomy approximately 20 years before his stroke secondary to mitral stenosis following rheumatic heart disease.

One year following the patient's stroke he developed seizure disorder. The patient was treated with phenytoin and phenobarbital and had no further seizures. The patient was also taking warfarin and digoxin for prevention of cardiac thrombosis or embolism and congestive cardiac damage secondary to mitral stenosis and rheumatic heart disease.

Following the stroke the patient was hospitalized for physical rehabilitation for 2 months. During this period, he reported having a depression but recovered from this and was in good spirits for approximately 18 months when he began to have increasing anxiety and depression about having another seizure and fear of dying. He was brought for neuropsychiatric evaluation because of continued feelings of hopelessness and depression.

On mental status examination, the patient stated that he felt he was no longer able to manage his finances. He had lost interest in his usual activities and had a constant fear of dying. The patient also complained of physical symptoms, such as mucous in his throat which made it difficult to swallow and caused respiratory distress. The patient also complained of light-headedness, sweating, and cramps in his stomach associated with anxiety. The patient also had difficulty making decisions and trouble falling asleep as well as frequent awakening during the night and terminal insomnia. He also noted a decrease in his appetite with an 8 lb (3.6 kg) weight loss during the past month.

Because of his hemiparesis, the patient was sitting in a wheelchair, and he smoked cigarettes continually through the interview. His leg was constantly bouncing and he had a noticeable tremor of his right hand. The patient stated that he felt extremely depressed and was feeling hopeless about the future. He stated that he wanted to return to work and felt he was a failure because he was unable to do so. He had lost interest in all of his previous activities and did not go out of the house. His son had just bought a new car and wanted to take the patient for a ride but the patient refused to leave his home. He left home only to see his doctors.

On cognitive examination, the patient was not oriented to the year nor did he know the date of the month or the place where the interview was being conducted. The patient's recall was intact, and he was able to serially subtract 7s beginning with 100 but was unable to write a sentence and was unable to draw the intersecting pentagons on the mini-mental state examination.

The patient was started on amitriptyline and his dose was increased to 75 mg daily. Exactly 2 weeks after reaching a dose of 100 mg amitriptyline, the patient's depression remitted. He no longer had feelings of anxiety, depression, thoughts of death, feelings of hopelessness, or sleep disturbance. The patient, however, complained of sedation and marked constipation. He was switched to 75 mg nortriptyline and was able to tolerate this mediation.

The patient was not seen after that for 18 months. When seen again, he reported that he had been doing well during the interim although he continued to be unable to walk. The patient, for the first time, was able to take care of many of his complex daily activities, such as settling his father's estate, and managing his financial investments. He stated that he had no sleep or appetite disturbance and had gained approximately 10 lbs (4.5 kg) during the past year. The patient then stated that he would like to taper off his 75 mg nortriptyline, which was scheduled to occur over a 3-month period.

Three months later the patient returned and stated that when his nortriptyline dose got to 25 mg he began to experience increasing anxiety, irritability, depression, sleep difficulty, low energy, and felt that he was unable to cope with the daily stresses. His dose was increased back to 75 mg and within 3 weeks he reported that his mood was stable, that he was sleeping well, and his appetite was good. Three months later, after the patient's daughter had married, he reported that he planned to get an electric wheelchair so that he could get around more easily. He stated that he had had no periods of depression and was sleeping well. The patient reported no change in interests although his energy seemed low. The patient requested a taper of his 75 mg nortriptyline again and over a 3-month period the nortriptyline was stopped. After that time, the patient had no further episodes of depression and was able to carry out his daily activities and to go out regularly with his wife. Four years later he suffered another large stroke and died.

This patient demonstrates the problems of knowing the proper maintenance dose of antidepressants for patients who have suffered poststroke depression, how long treatment should be maintained in order to prevent relapse of depression and perhaps more importantly, how best to prevent the occurrence of poststroke depression. Some patients may develop depression over at least 2 years following stroke and the longest prevention trials have only been conducted for 1 year. Questions such as whether all patients should be placed on antidepressant medication to prevent the development of depression or to enhance recovery or to decrease mortality rate are questions which are vital to the care of patients with stroke. Which medications are most effective in prevention versus treatment of poststroke depression is another issue needing investigation. The prevention of relapse in patients who have developed depression and treatment methodologies for treatment resistant depressions are areas which have not even begun to be systematically investigated.

I am heartened by the marked increase in the number of investigations of neuropsychiatric disorders following stroke which have emerged between the publication of the first edition of this text and the present edition. This worldwide interest raises the hope that many of these areas needing further research will be investigated and that further research will lead to an expanded version of the third edition of this text. I am hopeful that significant advances will be made in our understanding of the mechanism and treatment of these neuropsychiatric disorders. Great progress have been made within the past 7 years and the next 7 years should bring even greater advances in our knowledge of this disorder which afflicts more than 600,000 patients per year in the US and continues to be the third leading cause of death in the elderly.

REFERENCES

Feibel, J. H., and Springer, C. J. Depression and failure to resume social activities after stroke. *Arch Phys Med Rehabil* (1982) 63:276–278.

Gazzaniga, M. S., Ivry, R. B., and Mangun, G. R. *Cognitive neuroscience: the biology of the mind.* New York: Norton, 2002.

Heilman, K. M. *Clinical Neuropsychology.* Oxford University Press, Oxford, New York, 2003.

Lezak, M. D. *Neuropsychological Assessment.* Oxford University Press, Oxford, New York, 2004.

Schubert, D. S. P., Taylor, C., Lee, S., *et al.* Detection of depression in the stroke patient. *Psychosomatics* (1992) 33:1–5.

Index